The Prefrontal Cort

The Prefrontal Cortex

Executive and Cognitive Functions

Edited by

A.C. ROBERTS
Department of Anatomy, University of Cambridge

T.W. ROBBINS
Department of Experimental Psychology, University of Cambridge

and

L. WEISKRANTZ
Department of Experimental Psychology, University of Oxford

*Originating from contributions
to a Discussion Meeting
of the Royal Society of London*

Oxford · New York · Tokyo

OXFORD UNIVERSITY PRESS

1998

Oxford University Press, Great Clarendon Street, Oxford OX2 6DP
Oxford New York
Athens Auckland Bangkok Bogota Bombay Buenos Aires Calcutta
Cape Town Chennai Dar es Salaam Delhi Florence Hong Kong Istanbul
Karachi Kuala Lumpur Madrid Melbourne Mexico City Mumbai
Nairobi Paris São Paolo Singapore Taipei Tokyo Toronto Warsaw
and associated companies in
Berlin Ibadan

Oxford is a trade mark of Oxford University Press

Published in the United States
by Oxford University Press, Inc., New York

A catalogue record for this book is available from the British Library

Library of Congress Cataloging in Publication Data
The prefrontal cortex: executive and cognitive functions/edited by
A. C. Roberts, T. W. Robbins, and L. Weiskrantz.
"Originating from contributions to a discussion meeting of the
Royal Society of London."
Also published in Philosophical transactions of the Royal Society
of London. Series B, Biological sciences, v. 351, 1996, under title:
Executive and cognitive function of the prefrontal cortex.
Includes bibliographical references and index.
1. Prefrontal cortex–Congresses.   I. Roberts, A. C. (Angela C.)
II. Robbins, Trevor W.   III. Weiskrantz, Lawrence.   IV. Royal
Society (Great Britain).   Discussion Meeting.   V. Executive and
cognitive functions of the prefrontal cortex.
[DNLM: 1. Prefrontal Cortex–physiology–congresses.
WL 307 P923 1998]
QP383. 17.P74   1998
612.8'25–dc21
DNLM/DLC
for Library of Congress   97–51746   CIP

ISBN 0 19 852442 0 (Hbk)
0 19 852441 2 (Pbk)

Typeset by Puretech India Ltd,
Printed in Great Britain by Biddles Ltd., Guildford, Surrey

Contents

Contributors

Alan Baddeley Department of Psychology, University of Bristol, 8 Woodland Road, Bristol BS8 1TN, UK.

Karen Faith Berman Clinical Brain Disorders Branch, National Institute of Mental Health, Neuroscience Center at St Elizabeths, 2700 Martin Luther King Jr Ave SE, Washington, DC 20032, USA.

Todd S. Braver Department of Psychology, Carnegie Mellon University, Pittsburgh, PA 15213, USA.

Paul Burgess Institute of Cognitive Neuroscience, c/o Department of Psychology, University College London, Gower Street, London WC1N 3BT, UK.

Jonathon D. Cohen Department of Psychology, Carnegie Mellon University, Pittsburgh, PA 15213, USA, and Department of Psychiatry, University of Pittsburgh, Pittsburgh, PA 15213, USA.

Antonio R. Damasio Department of Neurology, University of Iowa Hospitals and Clinics, Iowa City, Iowa 52242, USA.

Sergio Della Sala Department of Psychology, University of Aberdeen, King's College, Old Aberdeen AB9 2UB, UK.

Adele Diamond Department of Brain and Cognitive Sciences, Massachusetts Institute of Technology, Building E10–044, Cambridge, MA 02139, USA. Current address: Department of Behavioral Sciences, Kennedy Shriver Center, 200.

Chris Frith Wellcome Department of Cognitive Neurology, Institute of Neurology, Queen Square, London WC1N 3BG, UK.

P. S. Goldman-Rakic Section of Neurobiology, Yale University School of Medicine, 333 Cedar Street, New Haven, CT 06520–8001, USA.

Randall C. O'Reilly Department of Psychology, Carnegie Mellon University, Pittsburgh, PA 15213, USA.

D. N. Pandya Department of Anatomy and Neurobiology, Boston University School of Medicine, 80 East Concord Street, Boston, MA 02118, USA.

R. E. Passingham Department of Experimental Psychology, University of Oxford, South Parks Road, Oxford OX1 3UD, UK.

Michael Petrides Montreal Neurological Institute, 3801 University Street, McGill University, Quebec, Canada H3A 2BA.

T. W. Robbins Department of Experimental Psychology, University of Cambridge, Downing Street, Cambridge CB2 3EB, UK.

A. C. Roberts Department of Anatomy, University of Cambridge, Downing Street, Cambridge CB2 3DY, UK.

Edmund T. Rolls Department of Experimental Psychology, University of Oxford, South Parks Road, Oxford OX1 3UD, UK.

Tim Shallice Institute of Cognitive Neuroscience, c/o Department of Psychology, University College London, Gower Street, London WC1N 3BT, UK.

Daniel R. Weinberger Clinical Brain Disorders Branch, National Institute of Mental Health, Neuroscience Center at St Elizabeths, 2700 Martin Luther King Jr Ave SE, Washington, DC 20032, USA.

L. Weiskrantz Department of Experimental Psychology, University of Oxford, South Parks Road, Oxford OX1 3UD, UK.

E. H. Yeterian Department of Psychology, Colby College, 5557 Mayflower Hill, Waterville, ME 04901-8855, USA.

1

Introduction

A. C. Roberts

One of the major debates in studies of the prefrontal cortex has been whether this cortical region should be considered unitary or heterogeneous in function. In the past, progress in addressing this issue was hampered by an inadequacy in our understanding of the complex cognitive and emotional processes that may be subserved by this region of the brain. Whilst poor judgement, planning, and decision making were recognizable characteristics of damage to the prefrontal cortex, the component psychological processes that contributed to these complex cognitive capacities were poorly understood, making it difficult to characterize the precise role of the prefrontal cortex in the expression of these functions. Moreover, the commonly used but ill-defined terms of 'executive processing' and 'higher-order cognitive processing', used to describe the overall function of the prefrontal cortex, only added to the confusion.

From the early ablation studies in monkeys, two cognitive processes emerged that appeared to be dependent upon an intact prefrontal cortex: 'short-term memory', as measured primarily by performance on the delayed response paradigm and 'behavioural inhibition', as measured by performance on discrimination reversal and go–no go paradigms. Deficits in these processes became associated with damage to the dorsal and ventral regions of the prefrontal cortex, respectively (Mishkin 1964; Iversen & Mishkin 1970; Fuster 1980). However, on closer examination, the anatomical differentiation of these two processes within the prefrontal cortex was far from clear. For example, Diamond & Goldman-Rakic (1989) identified disinhibitory components to the impaired performance of monkeys with lesions of the dorsolateral prefrontal cortex on the spatial delayed response task. Conversely, lesions of the inferior prefrontal convexity, commonly associated with perseverative responding on a visual discrimination reversal task (Iversen & Mishkin 1970), subsequently were shown to impair an object version of the delayed response task (Kowalska *et al.* 1991). Thus, from ablation studies in monkeys it was proving difficult to identify a set of general principles that could account for all the experimental findings and which would thereby characterize the overall functional organization within the primate prefrontal cortex.

In parallel with the studies in monkeys, functional differences between the dorsal and ventral surfaces of the prefrontal cortex also emerged from investigations in humans although, in contrast to monkeys, the distinction was between cognitive and social/emotional aspects of behaviour rather than between short-term memory and behavioural inhibition. However, while deficits in cognitive tasks following dorsolateral prefrontal lesions in humans were easily captured in the laboratory in a large range of tests, including tests of planning, such as the Tower of London (Shallice 1982), and tests of cognitive flexibility such as the Wisconsin Card Sort Test (WCST) (Milner 1963; 1982), it proved harder to capture the deficits in patients with ventral frontal damage in the laboratory even though these patients had profound social and emotional abnormalities and were severely disrupted in their everyday activities. This highlights one of the discrepancies between studies of prefrontal function in monkeys and humans since in monkeys, unlike humans, it has been relatively easy to obtain deficits in performance of standard laboratory tests following damage to ventral regions of prefrontal cortex (see above). Another discrepancy between monkey and human studies has been that cognitive inflexibility (or behavioural disinhibition) is associated with damage to dorsolateral regions of prefrontal cortex in humans, as shown, for example, by impaired performance on the WCST (Milner 1963), while perseverative deficits in monkeys are associated primarily with damage to ventral regions of the prefrontal cortex (Mishkin 1964; Iversen & Mishkin 1970).

Such inconsistencies both within species as well as between species, regarding the functional organization of the prefrontal cortex, along with a paucity in our knowledge of the complex psychological processes subserved by this region, have begun to be addressed over the last few years, with new theoretical, as well as technical, advances. It was these issues that were the focus of the Discussion Meeting held at the Royal Society. One obvious advance has been in our understanding of the anatomical organization of the prefrontal cortex, particularly with respect to the non-human primate brain, a topic that is taken up by the paper of Pandya & Yeterian (Chapter 5). A far greater number of regions within the prefrontal cortex are recognized today than as little as ten years ago, based largely upon studies of cyto- and myeloarchitecture (Preuss & Goldman-Rakic 1991; Carmichael & Price 1994; Petrides & Pandya 1994) and patterns of connectivity (Carmichael & Price 1995a,b) within the frontal lobes of the Macaque. Since the majority of ablation studies in monkeys have been based upon the subdivisions proposed by Walker (1940), it is evident that in many of these studies the lesions inadvertently extended across a number of different subdivisions of prefrontal cortex. Therefore, with hindsight, this may have contributed to the difficulty in identifying functional distinctions between the various regions of prefrontal cortex in the monkey. In addition, discrepancies between functional studies in monkeys and humans may, in part, have been due to an inadequate understanding of the comparable regions of prefrontal cortex in monkey and man. However, this too has been addressed recently by a comparative study of the neural architecture of the prefrontal cortex in humans and monkeys by Petrides & Pandya (1994) which will provide us with a far better framework for relating experimental studies in monkeys and humans.

The ability to extrapolate findings in monkeys to humans has also been improved by another major advance in prefrontal research, namely the use of comparable tests of cognition in human and non-human primates, an approach that was illustrated in many of the papers presented at this Proceedings including those of Petrides and Robbins (Chapters 8 and 9). Such an approach, the merits of which were first realized in the study of human memory and vision (Weiskrantz 1977), is now being used in all fields of cognitive brain research as it increases considerably the likelihood that the same cognitive function is being studied in both species (Roberts 1996). Notably, it has been used successfully to advance our understanding of the neural basis of memory (Squire *et al.* 1988; Gaffan 1991; Gaffan *et al.* 1991) and visuospatial attention (Petersen *et al.* 1987; Posner *et al.* 1988) and to identify the neural and neurochemical basis of a variety of neurodegenerative disorders such as Parkinson's disease and Alzheimer's disease (Flicker *et al.* 1984; Morris *et al.* 1987; Freedman & Oscar-Berman 1989), and neuropsychiatric disorders such as schizophrenia (Frith & Done 1983; Ridley *et al.* 1988). With respect to the study of the prefrontal cortex, Milner & Petrides have taken various frontal lobe tests classically used in monkeys and adapted them for use in humans, including their self-ordered pointing task (Petrides & Milner 1982) (which was adopted from the internal and external generated sequencing tasks used to study frontal lobe function in monkeys by Brody & Pribram (1978)) and the visual conditional associative learning tasks (Petrides 1985). Similarly, Freedman & Oscar-Berman (1986) and Verin *et al.* (1993) have tested patients on the spatial delayed response and alternation tasks as well as visual discrimination tasks. Whilst originally, these tests were considered to be too 'easy' for humans and therefore unlikely to be sensitive to frontal lobe damage in humans, this has been shown not to be the case. Patients with frontal lobe damage can be impaired on these delayed response tasks and the saccade-response version of the spatial delayed response task, described by Goldman-Rakic (1995), is now used successfully in functional neuro-imaging studies (Jonides *et al.* 1993). In addition, a recent study by Rolls *et al.* (1994) has reported deficits on reversal of a go–no go task in patients with damage restricted to the orbitofrontal cortex. Not only is this latter finding consistent with the original studies in monkeys, demonstrating reversal deficits following damage to the orbitofrontal cortex, but it demonstrates, in addition, that it is possible to find impairments following orbitofrontal damage in humans using standard laboratory tests.

Moving in the opposite direction, Roberts *et al.* (1988) have adapted a clinical test of frontal lobe function, for use in monkeys, namely the Wisconsin Card Sort Test. Using this paradigm it has been shown that the deficits in frontal patients shifting an attentional set from one perceptual dimension to another, such as shifting from colour to shape, as required in the WCST, are probably the result of damage to a different region of prefrontal cortex to the perseverative deficits seen in monkeys on the visual discrimination reversal task which requires monkeys to shift responding from one specific visual stimulus to another (Dias *et al.* 1996). These findings not only raise the possibility that 'response inhibition' may be a general process carried out by a number of different regions of prefrontal cortex, but also that different regions of prefrontal cortex are involved in different aspects of cognitive processing even within the same modality. In this example, the attentional processing of visual patterns is carried out in an area distinct from that involved in the 'affective' processing of visual patterns.

Of course, this organization must be integrated with another level of organization within the prefrontal cortex based upon sensory-specific domains that has been proposed by Wilson *et al.* (1993) from their electrophysiological recording studies. This leads us onto a third major advance in the field of prefrontal research which has been in our understanding of the relationship between neuronal activity within the prefrontal cortex and ongoing behaviour. In humans this has been at the 'macro-level' of analysis, studying event-related potentials over the scalp, in intact as well as frontal lesioned patients. This work has identified, for example, the importance of the prefrontal cortex in 'inhibition' and 'novelty detection' (Knight 1991). In monkeys, such analysis can be performed at the cellular level and has been used successfully to study the role of the prefrontal cortex in mnemonic (Goldman-Rakic 1995) and associative (Thorpe *et al.* 1983) processes, issues that will be considered in detail in the papers by Rolls and Goldman-Rakic (Chapters 6 and 7). Together, this approach is providing insight into the neuronal operations that are performed by the prefrontal cortex, an important step towards an understanding of the component cognitive mechanisms that contribute to higher-order executive processing.

A fourth major advance has come with the use of functional neuroimaging which is providing further insight into the functional organization of the prefrontal cortex in humans. For example, a recent study by Courtney *et al.* (1996) has highlighted a dissociation between object and spatial working memory within ventrolateral and dorsolateral prefrontal cortex, respectively, in agreement with the findings of Wilson *et al.* (1993) in monkeys. This finding supports the hypothesis that one level of organization within the prefrontal cortex is based upon sensory-specific processing. Yet another level of organization to have been identified with functional neuroimaging is hierarchical in nature and will be discussed in the paper of Petrides (Chapter 8) with respect to a two-stage model of working memory (Petrides 1994). In addition, this technique is also providing us with insight not only into the functional interactions between the prefrontal cortex and the rest of the brain including the basal ganglia (Goldberg *et al.* 1990), the processing modules of posterior cortex (Frith *et al.* 1991), and the non-specific arousal systems of the reticular formation (Daniel *et al.* 1991; Grasby *et al.* 1992; Dolan *et al.* 1995), but also between different regions, and thus potentially different processing modules, within the prefrontal cortex itself. Many of these are highlighted in the papers by Passingham, Weinberger, and Frith (Chapters 10, 12 and 13). Of course, functional neuroimaging, using the 2-deoxyglucose method, can also be used to visualize the interactions of the prefrontal cortex with other brain areas in monkeys and has been used successfully by Friedman & Goldman-Rakic (1994) to identify those areas, in addition to the dorsolateral prefrontal cortex, that are involved in performance of the spatial delayed response task, including the parietal cortex.

Finally, major conceptual advances in human neuropsychology and cognitive psychology, drawing upon artificial intelligence and connectionism, have contributed greatly to our understanding of executive functioning. These have brought to the fore the issues that have to be addressed when referring to 'executive' function and whether it is helpful or not to think of this as a 'unitary' system or as a 'multiple processing' system. Aspects such as these were discussed in the papers of Baddeley & Della Sala and Shallice & Burgess (Chapters 2 and 3). Shallice & Burgess (1991) in attempting to fractionate 'executive' functioning into a number of distinct component processes have developed a concept of 'markers' which act to interrupt ongoing behaviour and trigger new plans of action, if appropriate. They have suggested that this 'marker' process may be particularly impaired in patients with orbitofrontal damage and may explain the profound organizational deficits apparent in the daily activities of such patients. This concept of markers has also been introduced, independently, by Damasio in his 'somatic marker hypothesis' which focuses on the role of emotional processing in the orbitofrontal cortex in the control of complex decision-making (Damasio *et al.* 1991). Whether these different, but perhaps related, concepts of 'markers' can be integrated into an overall model of prefrontal function remains to be determined. Interestingly, Damasio proposes that possible neural substrates of his somatic markers may include the non-specific arousal pathways that innervate the prefrontal cortex, including the monoaminergic and cholinergic systems. Few studies have investigated the role of these systems specifically with respect to the modulation of prefrontal function and even fewer have assessed their possible differential contribution to prefrontal function (Brozowski *et al.* 1979; Sawaguchi *et al.* 1990; Sawaguchi & Goldman-Rakic 1991; Roberts *et al.* 1992, 1994). However, the role of one of these, dopamine, was considered at the cellular level in the paper by Goldman-Rakic (Chapter 7) and at the behavioural level in the papers of Robbins and Diamond (Chapters 9 and 11), the latter drawing upon evidence from her studies on PKU deficiency in children. The role of dopamine was taken up again in the final paper by Cohen *et al.* (Chapter 14) which, drawing upon neurobiological as well as psychological evidence, illustrated the use of computational models in making explicit the mechanisms within prefrontal cortex that may underlie executive processing.

Acknowledgements

Supported by the Wellcome Trust.

References

Brody, B. A. & Pribram, K. H. 1978 The role of frontal and parietal cortex in cognitive processing. Tests of spatial and sequence functions. *Brain* **101**, 607–33.

Brozowski, T. J., Brown, R. M., Rosvold, H. E. & Goldman, P. S. 1979 Cognitive deficit caused by regional depletion of dopamine in prefrontal cortex of rhesus monkey. *Science* **205**, 929–32.

Carmichael, S. T. & Price, J. L. 1994 Architectonic subdivision of the orbital and medial prefrontal cotex in the macaque monkey. *J. Comp. Neurol.* **346**, 403–34.

Carmichael, S. T. & Price, J. L. 1995*a* Limbic connections of the orbital and medial prefrontal cortex in macaque monkeys. *J. Comp. Neurol.* **363**, 615–41.

Carmichael, S. T. & Price, J. L. 1995*b* Sensory and premotor connections of the orbital and medial prefrontal cortex of macaque monkeys. *J. Comp. Neurol.* **363**, 642–64.

Courtney, S. M., Ungerleider, L. G., Keil, K. & Haxby, J. V. 1996 Object and spatial visual working memory activate separate neural systems in human cortex. *Cerebral Cortex* **6**, 39–49.

Damasio, A. R., Tranel, D. & Damasio, H. 1991 Somatic markers and the guidance of behaviour: theory and preliminary testing. In *Frontal lobe function and dysfunction* (ed. H. S. Levin, H. M. Eisenberg & A. L. Benton), pp. 217–229. New York: Oxford University Press.

Daniel, D. G., Weinberger, D. R., Jones, D. W., Zigun, J. R., Coppola, R., Handel, S., Bigelow, L. B., Goldberg T. E., Berman, K. F. & Kleinman, J. E. 1991 The effect of amphetamine on regional cerebral blood flow during cognitive activation in schizophrenia. *J. Neuroscience* **11**, 1907–17.

Diamond, A. & Goldman-Rakic, P. S. 1989 Comparison of human infants and rhesus monkeys on Piaget's AB task: evidence for dependence on dorsolateral prefrontal cortex. *Exp. Brain Res.* **74**, 24–40.

Dias, R., Robbins, T. W. & Roberts, A. C. 1996 Dissociation in prefrontal cortex of affective and attentional shifts. *Nature* **380**, 69–72.

Dolan, R. J., Fletcher, P., Frith, C. D., Friston, K. J., Frakowiac, R. S. J. & Grasby, P. M. 1995 Dopaminergic modulation of impaired cognitive activation in the anterior cingulate cortex in schizophrenia. *Nature* **378**, 180–83.

Flicker, C., Bartus, R. T., Crook, T. & Ferris, S. F. 1984 Effects of aging and dementia upon recent visuospatial memory. *Neurobiol. Aging* **5**, 275–83.

Freedman, M. & Oscar-Berman, M. 1986 Bilateral frontal lobe disease and selective delayed response deficits in humans. *Behavioural Neuroscience* **100**, 337–42.

Freedman, M. & Oscar-Berman, M. 1989 Selective delayed response deficits in Parkinson's and Alzheimer's disease. *Arch. Neurol.* **44**, 394–98.

Friedman, H. R. & Goldman-Rakic, P. S. 1994 Coactivation of prefrontal cortex and inferior parietal cortex in working memory tasks revealed by 2DG functional mapping in the rhesus monkey. *J. Neuroscience* **14**, 2775–88.

Frith, C. D. & Done, J. 1983 Stereotyped responding by schizophrenic patients on a two-choice guessing task. *Psychol. Med.* **13**, 779–86.

Frith, C. D., Friston, K. J., Liddle, P. F. & Frackowiak, R. S. J. (1991) Willed action and the prefrontal cortex in man: a study with PET. *Proceedings of the Royal Society of London, Serires B* **244**, 241–6.

Fuster, J. M. 1980 *The prefrontal cortex*. New York: Raven Press.

Gaffan, D. 1991 Spatial organisation of episodic memory. *Hippocampus* **1**, 262–64.

Gaffan, E. A., Gaffan, D. & Hodges, J. R. 1991 Amnesia following damage to the left fornix and to other sites. *Brain* **114**, 1297–313.

Goldberg, T. E., Berman, K. F., Moore, E. & Weinberger, D. R. 1990 rCBF and cognition in Huntington's disease and schizophrenia: a comparison of patients matched for performance on a prefrontal-type task. *Arch. Neurol.* **47**, 418–22.

Goldman-Rakic, P. S. 1987 Circuitry of primate prefrontal cortex and regulation of behaviour by representational memory. In *Handbook of physiology, the nervous system, higher functions of the brain* (ed. F. Plum), sect. I, vol. V, pp. 373–417. Bethesda, MD: American Physiological Society.

Goldman-Rakic, P. S. 1995 Cellular basis of working memory. *Neuron* **14**, 477–85.

Grasby, P. M., Friston, K. J., Bench, C. J., Frith, C. D., Paulescu, E., Cowen, P. J., Liddle, P. F., Frakowiac, R. S. J. & Dolan, R. 1992 The effect of apomorphine and buspirone on regional cerebral blood flow-measuring neuromodulatory effects of psychotropic drugs in man. *Eur. J. Neurosci.* **4**, 1203–12.

Iversen, S. D. & Mishkin, M. 1970 Perseverative interference in monkeys following selective lesions of the inferior prefrontal convexity. *Exp. Brain. Res.* **11**, 376–86.

Jones, B. & Mishkin, M. 1972 Limbic lesions and the problem of stimulus–reinforcement associations. *Exp. Neurol.* **36**, 362–77.

Jonides, J., Smith, E. E., Koeppe, E. A., Minoshima, S. & Mintun, M. A. 1993 Spatial working memory in humans as revealed by PET. *Nature* **363**, 623–25.

Knight, R. T. 1991 Evoked potential studies of attention capacity in human frontal lobe lesions. In *Frontal lobe function and dysfunction* (ed. H. S. Levin, H. M. Eisenberg & A. L. Benton), pp. 139–56. New York: Oxford University Press.

Kowalska, D. M., Bachevalier, J. & Mishkin, M. 1991 The role of the inferior prefrontal convexity in performance of the delayed nonmatching-to-sample. *Neuropsychologia* **29**, 583–600.

Milner, B. 1963 Effects of different brain lesions on card sorting. *Arch. Neurol.* **9**, 100–10.

Milner, B. 1982 Some cognitive effects of frontal lobe lesions in man. *Phil. Trans. R. Soc. Lond.* **286**, 211–26.

Mishkin, M. 1964 Perseveration of central sets after frontal lesions in man. In *The frontal granular cortex and behavior* (ed. J. M. Warren & K. Akert), pp. 219–94. New York: McGraw-Hill.

Morris, R. G., Evenden J. L., Sahakian, B. J. & Robbins T. W. 1987 Computer-aided assessment of dementia: comparative studies of neuropsychological deficits in Alzheimer-type dementia and Parkinson's disease. In *Cognitive neurochemistry* (ed. S. M. Stahl, S. D. Iversen & E. C. Goodman) pp. 21–36. Oxford: Oxford University Press.

Passingham, R. 1975 Delayed matching after selective prefrontal lesions in monkeys (Macaca mulatta). *Brain Res.* **92**, 89–102.

Petersen, S. E., Robinson, D. L. and Morris, J. D. 1987 Contributions of the pulvinar to visual spatial attention. *Neuropsychologia* **25**, 97–105.

Petrides, M. 1985 Deficits on conditional associative learning tasks after frontal- and temporal-lobe lesions in man. *Neuropsychologia* **23**, 601–14.

Petrides, M. 1994 Frontal lobes and working memory: evidence from investigations of the effects of cortical excisions in nonhuman primates. In *Handbook of neuropsychology*, vol. 9 (ed. F. Boller & J. Grafman), pp. 59–82. Amsterdam: Elsevier.

Petrides, M. & Milner, B. 1982 Deficits on subject-ordered tasks after frontal- and temporal-lobe lesions in man. *Neuropsychologia* **20**, 249–62.

Petrides, M. & Pandya, D. N. 1994 Comparative architectonic analysis of the human and the macaque frontal cortex. In *Handbook of neuropsychology*, vol. 9 (ed. F. Boller & J. Grafman), pp. 17–58. Amsterdam: Elsevier.

Posner, M. I., Petersen, S. E., Fox, P. T. & Raichle, M. E. 1988 Localisation of cognitive operation in the human brain. *Science* **240**, 1627–31.

Preuss, T. M. & Goldman-Rakic, P. S. 1991 Myelo- and cytoarchitecture of the granular frontal cortex and surrounding *Galago* and the anthropoid primate *Macaca*. *J. Comp. Neurol.* **310**, 429–74.

Ridley, R. M., Baker, H. F., Frith, C. D., Dowdy, J. & Crow, T. J. 1988 Stereotyped responding on a two-choice guessing task by marmosets and humans treated with amphetamine. *Psychopharmacology* **95**, 560–64.

Roberts, A. C. 1996 Comparison of cognitive function in human and non-human primates. *Cognitive Brain Research* **3**, 319–27.

Roberts, A. C., Robbins, T. W. & Everitt, B. J. 1988 The effects of intradimensional and extradimensional shifts on visual discrimination learning in humans and non-human primates. *Q. J. Exp. Psychol.* **40**, 321–41.

Roberts, A. C., Robbins, T. W., Everitt, B. J., & Muir, J. L. 1992 A specific form of cognitive rigidity following excitotoxic lesions of the basal forebrain in the marmoset. *Neuroscience* **47**, 251–64.

Roberts, A. C., De Salvia, M. A., Wilkinson, L. S., Collins, P., Muir, J. L., Everitt, B. J. & Robbins, T. W. 1994 6-Hydroxydopamine lesions of the prefrontal cortex in monkeys enhance performance on an analog of the Wisconsin Card Sort Test: possible interactions with subcortical dopamine. *J. Neuroscience* **14**, 2531–44.

Rolls, E. T., Hornak, J., Wade, D. & McGrath, J. 1994 Emotion-related learning in patients with social and emotional changes associated with frontal lobe damage. *J. Neurol. Neurosurg. Psychiat.* **57**, 1518–24.

Sawaguchi, T. & Goldman-Rakic, P. S. 1991 D1 dopamine receptors in prefrontal cortex: involvement in working memory. *Science* **251**, 947–50.

Sawaguchi, T., Matsumura, M. & Kubota, K. 1990 Catecholaminergic effects on neuronal activity related to a delayed response task in monkey prefrontal cortex. *J. Neurophysiol.* **63**, 1385–95.

Shallice, T. 1982 Specific impairments of planning. *Phil. Trans. R. Soc. Lond. B* **298**, 199–209.

Shallice, T. & Burgess, P. W. 1991 Deficits in strategy application following frontal lobe damage in man. *Brain* **114**, 727–41.

Squire, L. R., Zola-Morgan, S. and Chen, K. 1988 Human amnesia and animal models of amnesia: performance of amnesic patients on tests designed for the monkey. *Behav. Neuroscience* **102**, 210–21.

Thorpe, S. J., Rolls, E. T. & Maddison, S. 1983 The orbitofrontal cortex: neuronal activity in the behaving monkey. *Exp. Brain Res.* **49**, 93–115.

Verin, M., Partiot, A., Pillon, B., Malapani, C., Agid, Y. & Dubois, B. 1993 Delayed response tasks and prefrontal lesions in man—evidence for self-generated patterns of behaviour with poor environmental modulation. *Neuropsychologia* **31**, 1379–96.

Walker, A. E. 1940 A cytoarchitectural study of the prefrontal area of the macaque monkey. *J. Comp. Neurol.* **73**, 59–86.

Weiskrantz, L. 1977 Trying to bridge some neuropsychological gaps between monkey and man. *Br. J. Psychol.* **68**, 431–45.

Wilson, F. A., O'Scalaidhe, S. P. & Goldman-Rakic, P. S. 1993 Dissociation of object and spatial processing domains in primate prefrontal cortex. *Science* **260**, 1955–58.

2

Working memory and executive control

Alan Baddeley and Sergio Della Sala

2.1 Introduction

The so-called 'frontal syndrome' is one of the most dramatic and readily recognizable neuropsychological behaviour patterns involving 'disturbed attention, increased distractibility, a difficulty in grasping the whole of a complicated state of affairs . . . well able to work along routine lines . . . (but) . . . cannot learn to master new types of task' (Rylander 1939, p. 20). While this pattern is classically associated with frontal lobe damage however, by no means all patients with damage to the frontal lobes show such behaviour, and where deficits do occur, the pattern of deficits will typically vary from one patient to another.

The classic neuropsychological approach has been to attempt to use lesion data, mapping the location of the lesion onto the nature of the deficit (Milner 1964; Reitan & Wolfson 1994). While this has certainly had some success, the approach is limited by the lack of any obvious coherent pattern in the tasks impaired by frontal damage, which range from concept formation and verbal fluency through the capacity for making cognitive approximations to judgements of recency and the performance of various complex learning tasks (Stuss & Benson 1986). Attempts to look for meaningful clusters of tasks within this array using factor analytic techniques have in general proved disappointing: the various tasks tend to correlate modestly but significantly, without falling into any very clear pattern (Della Sala *et al.* 1996*a*). Furthermore, none of the classic 'frontal' tests seem to capture the frequent gross behavioural derangements that typify patients with frontal lobe damage (Harlow 1868). Indeed dissociations between such tests and behaviour have frequently been reported (Eslinger & Damasio 1985; Shallice & Burgess 1991; Brazzelli *et al.* 1994).

We suggest that these difficulties stem in part, at least, from the failure of cognitive psychology to provide an adequate characterization of the executive processes that form one of the principal functions of the frontal lobes, and we describe below the early stages of one attempt to remedy this.

2.2 Separating anatomy from function

We would suggest first of all that the very use of the term 'frontal syndrome' compounds the problem by stressing anatomical location rather than function and potentially interferes with its solution. It is both common and useful for neuropsychological syndromes to be defined functionally rather than anatomically. We talk about aphasia, dyslexia, dysgraphia, agnosia and amnesia, accepting that in many cases the exact anatomical underpinning of these disorders represents an important but separate question from their functional analysis. We would suggest that this is highly appropriate. There is no good evidence to suggest within the amnesic syndrome for example, that patients who are amnesic following hippocampal damage are necessarily functionally different from those whose damage is based on the mammillary bodies or indeed from temporal lobe damage, despite many attempts to argue for such differences. It is also the case that examples of 'frontal' behaviour may occur in the absence of frontal localization. Examples include generalized infections such as syphilis, where behaviour shown by Nietzsche was distinctly 'frontal' (Kaufmann 1974), or in metabolic diseases such as porphyria which led to the 'madness' of King George III (Bennett 1995).

The approach to be described developed from an attempt to understand working memory, the system necessary for holding and manipulating information while performing a wide range of tasks including learning, reasoning and comprehending (Baddeley & Hitch 1974). Our studies of the functioning of normal subjects prompted us to propose a sub-component of working memory, the central executive, that was responsible for attentional control of working memory. In attempting to conceptualize it in more detail we were strongly influenced by Shallice's (1982) paper in which a model of the control of action is proposed and related to the functioning of the frontal lobes and the breakdown of behavioural control in the frontal syndrome (Baddeley 1986). For a number of reasons however, we were anxious to dissociate the functional from the anatomical aspects of the executive concept.

While the work described by Shallice strongly suggested that bilateral frontal damage might disrupt executive processes, we did not wish to preclude the possibility that other parts of the brain might be involved. Indeed, given that executive processes involve communication between subsystems located elsewhere in the brain, it seemed entirely possible that they could be disrupted before or after the involvement of frontal systems. Given that the frontal lobes occupy a large proportion of the cortex, it seemed entirely possible that they are concerned with functions other than executive processing, with the result that frontal lobe damage need not necessarily lead to executive deficits.

A further constraint was entirely practical. We often did not have precise and accurate anatomical information about many of the patients we studied. One can of course continue to use the 'frontal' label, as indeed is often the case in the neuropsychological literature for patients who show a clear pattern of executive deficit, but to do so assumes the very relationship between anatomy and function that we are trying to test. For that reason we introduced the term dysexecutive syndrome as a functional description of a pattern of behaviour that explicitly leaves open its anatomical underpinning (Baddeley 1986; Baddeley & Wilson 1988). Note that this terminological distinction does not deny the importance of a more traditional anatomically-based approach, in which attempts are made to investigate the function of specific anatomical structures. It does however suggest the need for a parallel approach that emphasizes a functional analysis, which can then as a separate step be related to brain structure. Both the structure and function of the executive system is known to be highly complex: attempting to solve both simultaneously may result in a problem with too many unknowns.

2.3 Analysing the dysexecutive syndrome

Having made this decision to separate the functional from the anatomical, we were left with a major problem, namely that the central executive was by far the least understood component of working memory. The problem was highlighted by an attempt to analyse the cognitive dysfunction associated with Alzheimer's disease. An initial study of patients suffering from dementia of the Alzheimer Type (DAT) suggested that in addition to the clear deficit in episodic long-term memory, there appeared to be an impairment in working memory that was most readily attributable to the central executive (Spinnler *et al.* 1988). How should one investigate it? It was tempting to opt for using the classic frontal lobe measures, but to do so would mean that our argument for separating the functional from the anatomical was merely cosmetic. We therefore decided to use the Baddeley–Hitch working memory model to postulate functions that would certainly be required if the model were to operate along the lines implied. We began with a very obvious prediction that is suggested by the representation of the model in figure 2.1, where the central executive is seen as coordinating the operation of two subsidiary slave systems, the phonological loop which deals with speech based information, and the sketchpad which handles visuospatial information. We argued that a defective executive should have difficulty in

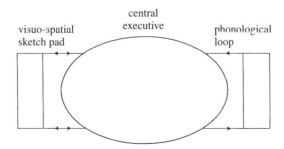

Fig. 2.1   The Baddeley & Hitch (1974) model of working memory.

coordinating the simultaneous operation of these two systems, with the result that dual-task performance should be particularly susceptible to the effect of DAT.

Our first study combined verbal processing with a visuospatial task in which subjects attempted to keep a stylus in contact with a moving spot of light; by varying the speed of movement the task could be adjusted so that equivalent levels of accuracy were achieved by our DAT patients and by age-matched and young control subjects. In one study, subjects combined tracking with a digit span task in which they were required to repeat back sequences of numbers, with the length of sequence set so that the error rate was constant across the three groups. When the two tasks were combined, the young and elderly controls performed in a similar manner, suggesting that age *per se* does not markedly influence the capacity to combine tasks, given that level of difficulty is appropriately adjusted. In contrast, DAT patients showed a marked decrease in performance levels on both the digit span and the concurrent tracking, when required to combine them (Baddeley *et al.* 1986).

A subsequent longitudinal study required DAT patients and controls to perform the tracking and digit span tasks singly and in combination on successive occasions separated by six months (Baddeley *et al.* 1991). As figure 2.2 shows, the capacity to perform either of the tasks singly showed little or no deterioration, while combined performance showed a steady decline over the three successive tests.

While we were pleased with the results obtained, we were concerned about the generality and the logistic practicality of the procedure used. The tracking task in particular was problematic since it requires a light pen that is not a standard piece of most people's laboratory equipment, together with a program

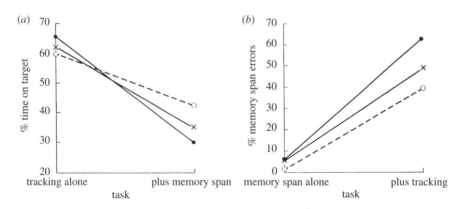

Fig. 2.2 Longitudinal decline in the capacity of DAT patients to combine tasks. (*a*) Effects of memory span on tracking; (*b*) effects of tracking on memory span errors. Patients were tested at six-monthly intervals (open circles denote test 1; crosses denote test 2; closed circles denote test 3); performance on the individual tasks when performed alone was maintained, but both tracking and serial digit recall decline over time, when concurrent performance was required. (Data from Baddeley *et al.* 1991).

which we found did not readily transfer even to other computers that were nominally identical. We therefore began the search for a paper and pencil alternative to tracking. After a surprisingly long and frustrating search, we eventually developed a task in which the subject is required to place a cross in a chain of boxes arrayed on a response sheet. Having practised the task, subjects are required to fill as many boxes as possible in two minutes. The digit span task then involves selecting a length at which the subject recalls the sequence virtually perfectly, followed by a two minute test run in which tasks are performed simultaneously (Della Sala et al. 1995).

The test was validated using a sample of 12 DAT patients and 12 control subjects. Of 13 subjects originally tested within the presumed AD group, all but one showed a decrement in span when combined with tracking that was greater than that obtained in any of the control subjects. The atypical subject subsequently proved not to have a progressive neurological disease and was excluded. Tracking performance showed a similar but less clear cut tendency for patients to show a greater dual task decrement than controls, although this did not reach significance (Della Sala et al. 1995).

The same task was used by Greene et al. (1995) in a study comparing minimally and mildly impaired DAT patients with age-matched control subjects. Again, there was a clear tendency for the combined task to be particularly susceptible to the disease, whether in the minimally or mildly impaired group, but in contrast to the Italian subjects in the Della Sala et al. study, these patients showed their principal decrement on the tracking task. The reason for the discrepancy is not clear, but could stem from the rather higher proportion of memory tasks within the Greene et al. study, which may have suggested to the patients that memory performance was more important than tracking. It is worth noting that had the differences in strategy occurred between different patients within the two studies rather than between studies, it is possible that neither of them would have demonstrated a statistically significant difference between the two groups on any single one of the component tasks, thus highlighting the need for a score that combines both of the concurrent tasks. Unfortunately, deriving such a score is likely to depend crucially on the particular assumptions underlying the method of combination. Ideally, such a score should be based on a more detailed analysis of the processes underlying performance at different levels of difficulty, together with an understanding of the process involved in combining them. This is likely to demand a substantial research effort, and in the meantime the following formula has been proposed:

$$mu = \left[1 - \frac{P_m + P_t}{2}\right] \times 100$$

where mu is the combined dual task score, P_m is the proportional loss in span performance between single (P_s) and dual task (P_d) conditions, $((P_s - P_d)/P_s)$ while P_t is the equivalent proportional tracking decrement (Baddeley et al. 1996). When this formula was applied to the validating study, there was a clear separation between performance of DAT patients and control subjects.

One potential theoretical objection to the claim that dual task performance is particularly vulnerable to DAT stems from the suggestion that the results are a simple reflection of level of task difficulty. Baddeley *et al.* (1991) attempted to test this hypothesis by manipulating difficulty within a categorization task by increasing the number of sorting alternatives. While performance deteriorated with the progress of the disease, there was no evidence that the deterioration was particularly marked for the harder conditions, as would be predicted by an interpretation of our earlier results in terms of level of difficulty. A further problem with an interpretation in terms of level of difficulty is the danger of circularity; unless there is some independent measure of difficulty level, then any differential impairment in AD patients can be attributed *post hoc* to hypothetical differences in underlying difficulty. The strength of the working memory model is that it attempts to specify sources of difficulty in a principled way. However, there clearly remains a need to understand the underlying process in more detail, and to contrast the effects of increasing the level of difficulty of a single task with that of requiring task combination.

Another basic question regarding the dual task technique concerns its generality of application. If it reflects a basis executive function, then one might expect dual task performance decrements to occur more widely than simply in DAT patients. Evidence is beginning to accumulate that this is indeed the case, with a study by Dalrymple-Alford (1994) showing significant though smaller dual task decrement in Parkinson's disease, while Hartman *et al.* (1992) observed a dual task decrement in patients suffering from traumatic brain injury, with a suggestion that the impairment may have been greater for subjects showing impaired performance on tasks typically associated with frontal lobe dysfunction. This study had the further aim of exploring the possible implications of dual task deficit on the process of rehabilitation, demonstrating that concurrent conversation, although not simple encouragement, had a detrimental effect on motor performance in brain damaged patients, while having no such effect on the performance of control subjects. They conclude that, while it may be appropriate for physiotherapists to chat to their patients while treating them, in the case of brain damaged patients this could be counter-productive.

Another potentially important clinical application of the dual task method is described by Alderman (1996), a clinical neuropsychologist operating within a programme attempting to assist brain damaged patients with severe behavioural problems. The programme is based on a token economy system whereby patients are rewarded for behaving in a socially acceptable way. In general, the programme is very effective in helping patients to deal with the antisocial behaviour that would otherwise prevent them participating in a rehabilitation programme. However, a small but important minority of patients failed to benefit from the regime; Alderman set himself the task of attempting to predict who these would be. He chose to test all incoming patients on a range of measures including both classic 'frontal' tests such as verbal fluency and the Wisconsin card sorting test, and also a range of variants of dual task performance. The behaviour of the subjects was subsequently monitored, and patients assigned to separate groups depending on whether they did or did not benefit from the rehabilitation regime. The results of the study are shown in figure 2.3, from which it is clear that whereas single task performance does not differentiate between the groups, subjects who do not thrive within the system tend to perform badly on a tracking task under dual task conditions. The differential decrement occurred whether the concurrent task involved digit span forward, digits backward, conversation or a task requiring judgment of how long specified activities such as travelling from London to Glasgow by train might take. As in the Hartman *et al.* (1992) study, when the secondary task involved only non-specific encouragement, all three groups showed a tendency for the tracking task to improve over the single task baseline. Of the four more traditional frontal lobe tests used (cognitive estimates, verbal fluency, Wisconsin card-sorting and trails A and B), only trails B showed a clear inter-group difference, with the rest showing a small and marginally significant tendency to poorer performance in the non-responding group.

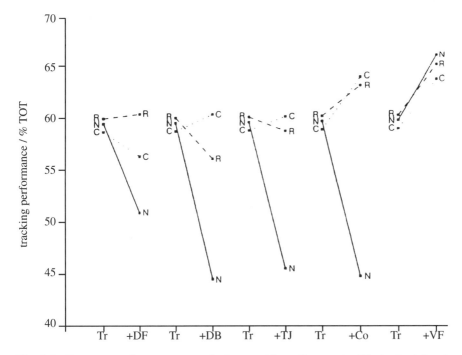

Fig. 2.3 Percentage time on target during tracking of controls (C), brain injured patients who responded to therapy (R) and non-responders (N) when performing alone, and in combination with a range of auditory verbal secondary tasks. Tr denotes tracking only; +DF denotes tracking and digits forward; +DB denotes tracking and digits backwards; +TJ denotes tracking and temporal judgment; +Co denotes tracking and conversation;+VF = tracking and verbal feedback. Data from Alderman (1996).

2.4 Dual task performance and frontal lobe function

Preliminary evidence therefore suggests that the capacity for combining the performance of two tasks may be an executive process of some generality, and potentially of practical as well as theoretical significance. It appears to have a degree of overlap with more traditional measures of frontal lobe function, but with evidence from Alderman's study that it may allow better prediction of certain types of behavioural breakdown. The final study to be described is concerned with investigating the relationship between dual task performance and frontal lobe function and is based on a sample of patients selected on the basis of known frontal lesions (Baddeley *et al.* unpublished results).

A total of twenty-seven patients with radiologically verified lesions of the frontal lobes were assessed using the box crossing task combined with concurrent digit span. All subjects were also assessed on Nelson's shortened form of the Wisconsin Card Sort Test, and on letter fluency, being required to generate as many words as possible beginning with the letters F, P and L, each within a one-minute period. Finally, each patient was independently assessed by two neurologists on the basis of whether they showed behavioural disturbances of a type characteristically associated with the dysexecutive syndrome. One of the raters based the assessment on the patient's notes, while the other used comments by the patient's relatives, together with observed behaviour during testing as a basis for the classification. The estimates agreed for all but three patients who were subsequently discarded from the analysis, leaving two groups of patients, a dysexecutive and non-dysexecutive group both containing twelve subjects. The nature of the behavioural disturbance varied, with a slight preponderance of patients tending to show apathetic behaviour ($N = 7$), with four tending to be disinhibited, and one oscillating between the two. These differences were not subsequently reflected in test performance.

Considering the combined group of 24 subjects with frontal lobe damage, there was a significant tendency for patients to score below the cut-off based on population norms for both the Wisconsin Card Sort Test (20 below cut-off) and on verbal fluency (17). When the two sub-groups were compared however, there was no significant difference in verbal fluency or card sorting performance between the group showing dysexecutive behaviour and those who appeared to behave normally, although there was a non-significant trend for poorer performance in dysexecutive patients.

When performance of the two groups on dual task performance was compared, as figure 2.4 shows, there was a significant tendency for the dysexecutive group to show a decline in performance when the two tasks were combined, an effect that was significant for the memory score ($p < 0.02$), the combined task ($p < 0.02$), but not for the tracking score.

This study therefore reinforces the conclusions drawn from that of Alderman, in suggesting that dual task performance is a potentially useful marker of dysexecutive behaviour. The fact that it is found in half our sample of patients with frontal lobe damage clearly implicates the frontal lobes, while suggesting

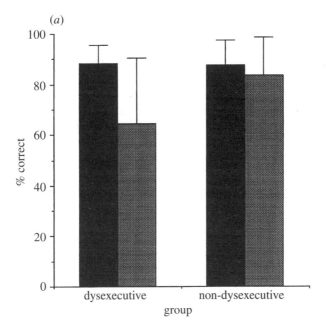

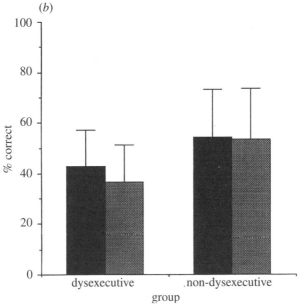

Fig. 2.4 Effect of dual task on (*a*) memory span and (*b*) tracking performance in two groups of frontal lobe patients. Those patients showing dysexecutive behaviour were impaired on dual task performance while patients showing no behavioural disturbance showed no such decrement (data from Baddeley *et al*. 1996*b*). (Solid bars denote single task; hatch bars denote dual task.)

that by no means all patients with frontal lobe damage will show either dual task deficit or the characteristic behavioural disorder. It is interesting to contrast the pattern of dual task performance with those shown by the two more traditional frontal tasks, which appear to be clearly associated with frontal damage, but dissociable from dual task performance. As such, our findings are consistent with the view that both the frontal lobes and executive processes may be fractionable into subsystems, possibly with different anatomical locations, although our own results provide no direct evidence on this last point.

Our finding of a clear association between dual task performance and behavioural disorder was serendipitous, but in combination with Alderman's results are very encouraging. It is perhaps worth noting at this point that Shallice & Burgess (1991) have observed a subgroup of patients with frontal lobe damage who appear to be able to pass virtually all the standard tests, and yet are sufficiently disturbed in their social activities as to make it impossible for them to return to a structured occupation. One of the clearest predictors of this behavioural disturbance is the six elements test, in which subjects are required to perform a task comprising six parallel subtasks which must be performed in a coordinated manner in order to receive a high score. It seems plausible to assume that Shallice & Burgess's richer and more complex six task coordination measure may rely on a similar function to our dual task test.

2.5 Further fractionation of the central executive

We have so far confined our attention principally to one executive capacity, with what we regard as encouraging results. It is, however, clearly the case that any adequate model of the central executive must have a range of other subprocesses if it is to be capable of serving the role of attentional controller, organizer of learning and retrieval planner. We have therefore begun to apply the same logic to the postulation of further potentially separable executive processes (Baddeley 1996). One important function must be that of selective attention, the capacity to focus attention on one stream of information while shutting out irrelevant material. Another is presumably involved in the capacity to switch attention from one source to another, a process that we suggest may underlie the difficulty experienced in attempting to generate random sequences, where subjects become locked into retrieval patterns and tend to produce stereotyped responses under time pressure (Baddeley 1966). A very important executive demand on working memory is provided by the need to access and manipulate information in long-term memory. We suspect that it is this function of the central executive that plays an important role in individual difference measures of working memory span such as that developed by Daneman & Carpenter (1980). The processes of comprehending a complex prose passage also seem likely to make demands on the capacity of the central executive to set up and manipulate models within long-term memory, as recently proposed by Ericsson & Kintsch (1995). It seems unlikely that this list is exhaustive, and since we have very little understanding of most of the processes outlined, we clearly have a good way to go in understanding the functioning of the central executive.

There are obvious dangers in postulating an unlimited number of executive processes. Simply inventing new tasks on *a priori* principles and then nominating them as measures of basic executive processes is clearly not a satisfactory solution to the problem of analysing the central executive. It is necessary, first of all, to postulate only processes that have some chance of operating across a range of different materials and situations, and then to demonstrate this generality. In due course, when adequate measures of a number of supposedly different executive processes have been developed, it will be necessary to carry out larger scale correlational studies using patients who are likely to have a range of executive problems. If we have been successful in isolating a number of separable executive processes, then we would expect a higher correlation across different tasks that are assumed to measure the same process, with clear separation from other clusters of proposed executive processes. This leads on to the question of how the component sub-processes are related; we do not propose a multiplicity of executives, but wish to leave open to empirical investigation the question of whether the organization is hierarchical, with one or more subsystems dominating, or whether a more heterarchical structure is involved.

Another potential source of validating data comes from studying the pattern of executive deficits across different subject populations who might be expected to have differential disruption of the functioning of the central executive. It seems likely that some executive processes for example, will deteriorate with normal aging. Our own data suggest this will not be true of all executive processes since the capacity for dual task performance appears to be preserved, provided the level of difficulty of the relevant tasks is matched across groups, whereas as we have seen, dual task performance appears to be an area of clear deficit in DAT patients.

Finally, a clearly formulated and well structured functional model will provide a much sounder basis for studies concerned with the anatomical localization of executive processes. While lesion studies have been, and will continue to be important, the rapid developments in neuroimaging are particularly promising. Working memory has already proved a fruitful area for PET studies with models initially based on studies within cognitive psychology showing very good correspondence with neuroanatomical distinctions based on functional imaging. The fruitfulness of this approach has already been established in studies of the phonological loop (Paulesu *et al.* 1993) and the visuospatial sketchpad (Jonides *et al.* 1993). Work has now begun to appear on the functional imaging of dual task performance (D'Esposito *et al.* 1995), suggesting, we are happy to note, a frontal lobe involvement. Recent studies of learning suggest the possibility that the executive processes involved in organizing and encoding incoming material may have a left frontal location, whereas those involved in episodic retrieval seem to be mediated by areas in the right frontal cortex (Shallice *et al.* 1994; Tulving *et al.* 1996). Conclusions in this area are still preliminary, but if established, these latter findings may represent a new stage in the application of functional imagery to the analysis of cognitive function. The pattern so far has been one of establishing the viability of the imaging method by demonstrating that it is capable of giving clear and replicable anatomical answers to the location of functions that have typically already been specified and broadly localized on the basis of cognitive and earlier lesion studies. Having established its viability, functional imaging is now in a position to suggest hypotheses which will enrich and may well change our functional models of cognition.

Acknowledgements

This paper draws heavily on collaborative work with a range of colleagues; we are particularly grateful to Robert Logie, Costanza Papagno, Hans Spinnler and Barbara Wilson.

References

Alderman, N. 1996 Central executive deficit and response to operant conditioning methods. *Neuropsychological Rehabilitation* **6**, 161–86.

Baddeley, A. D. 1966 The capacity for generating information by randomisation. *J. Exptl. Psychol.* **18**, 119–29.

Baddeley, A. D. 1986 *Working memory*. Oxford: Clarendon Press.

Baddeley, A. D. 1996 Exploring the central executive. *Q. J. Exptl. Psychol.* **49**A (1), 5–28.

Baddeley, A. D., Bressi, S., Della Sala, S., Logie, R. & Spinnler, H. 1991 The decline of working memory in Alzheimer's disease: a longitudinal study. *Brain* **114**, 2521–42.

Baddeley, A. D., Della Sala, S., Gray, C., Papagno, C. & Spinnler, H. 1996a Testing central executive functioning with a paper and pencil test. In P. Rabbitt (ed.), *Methodology of frontal and executive functions*, pp. 61–80. Hove: Psychology Press.

Baddeley, A. D., Della Sala, S., Papagno, C. & Spinnler, H. 1996b. Dual task performance in dysexecutive and non-dysexecutive patients with a frontal lesion. *Neuropsychology* **11**, 187–94.

Baddeley, A. D. & Hitch, G. 1974 Working memory. In I. G. A. Bower (ed.), *The psychology of learning and motivation*. pp. 47–90. New York: Academic Press.

Baddeley, A. D., Logie, R., Bressi, S., Della Sala, S. & Spinnler, H. 1986 Dementia and working memory. *Q. J. Exptl. Psychol.* **38**A, 603–18.

Baddeley, A. D. & Wilson, B. 1988 Frontal amnesia and the dysexecutive syndrome. *Brain & Cognition* **7**, 212–30.

Bennett, A. 1995 *The madness of King George*. London: Faber and Faber.

Brazzelli, M., Colombo, N., Della Sala, S. & Spinnler, H. 1994 Spared and impaired cognitive abilities after bilateral frontal damage. *Cortex* **30**, 27–51.

D'Esposito, M., Detre, J. A., Alsop, D. C., Shin, R. K., Atlas, S. & Grossman, M. 1995 The neural basis of the central executive system of working memory. *Nature, Lond.* **378**, 279–81.

Dalrymple-Alford, J. C., Kalders, A. S., Jones, R. D. & Watson, R. W. 1994 Central executive deficit in patients with Parkinson's Disease. *Journal of Neurology, Neurosurgery and Psychiatry*, **57**, 360–67.

Daneman, M. & Carpenter, P. A. 1980 Individual differences in working memory and reading. *Journal of Verbal Learning and Verbal Behavior* **19**, 450–66.

Della Sala, S., Baddeley, A. D., Papagno, C. & Spinnler, H. 1995 Dual task paradigm: A means to examine the central executive. In *Structure and functions of the human prefrontal cortex* pp. 161–90. New York: Annals of the New York Academy of Sciences.

Della Sala, S., Gray, C., Spinnler, H. & Trivelli, C. 1998 Frontal lobe functioning in man: The riddle revisited. *Archives of Clinical Neuropsychology*. (In the press).

Ericsson, K. A. & Kintsch, W. 1995 Long-term working memory. *Psychol. Rev.* **102**, 211–45.

Eslinger, P. J. & Damasio, A. R. 1985 Severe disturbance of higher cognition after bilateral frontal lobe labation: Patient E.V.R. *Neurology* **35**, 1731 41.

Greene, J. D. W., Hodges, J. R. & Baddeley, A. D. 1995 Autobiographical memory and executive function in early dementia of Alzheimer type. *Neuropsychologia* **33**, 1647–70.

Harlow, J. M. 1868 Recovery from the passage of an iron bar through the head. *Massachusetts Medical Society Publications* **2**, 327–46.

Hartman, A., Pickering, R. M. & Wilson, B. A. 1992 Is there a central executive deficit after severe head injury? *Clinical Rehabilitation* **6**, 133–40.

Jonides, J., Smith, E. E., Koeppe, R. A., Awh, E., Minoshima, S. & Minturn, M. A. 1993 Spatial working memory in humans as revealed by PET. *Nature, Lond.* **363**, 623–25.

Kaufmann, W. 1974 *Nietzsche: Philosopher, Psychologist, Antichrist*. Princeton, New Jersey: Princeton University Press.

Milner, B. 1964 Some effects of frontal lobectomy in man. In *The frontal granular cortex and behavior* (ed. J. M. Warren and K. Akert) pp. 313–34. New York: McGraw-Hill.

Paulesu, E., Frith, C. D. & Frackowiak, R. S. J. 1993 The neural correlates of the verbal component of working memory. *Nature, Lond.* **362**, 342–45.

Reitan, R. M. & Wolfson, D. 1994 A selective and critical review of neuropsychological deficits and the frontal lobes. *Neuropsychol. Rev.* **4**, 161–98.

Rylander, G. 1939 Personality changes after operation on the frontal lobes, a clinical study of 32 cases. *Acta Psychiatrica Neurologica*, **30** (20), 3–327.

Shallice, T. 1982 Specific impairments of planning. *Phil. Trans. R. Soc. Lond.* B **298**, 199–209.

Shallice, T. & Burgess, P. W. 1991 Deficits in strategy application following frontal lobe damage in men. *Brain* **114**, 727–41.

Shallice, T., Fletcher, P., Frith, C. D., Grasby, P. M., Frackowiak, R. S. J. & Dolan, R. J. 1994 Brain regions associated with acquisition and retrieval of verbal episodic memory. *Nature, Lond.* **368**, 633–35.

Spinnler, H., Della Sala, S., Bandera, R. & Baddeley, A. D. 1988 Dementia, ageing and the structure of human memory. *Cognitive Neuropsychology* **5**, 193–211.

Stuss, D. T. & Benson, D. F. 1986 *The frontal lobes*. New York: Raven Press.

Tulving, E., Markowitsch, H. J., Craik, F. I. M., Habib, R. & Houle, S. 1996 Novelty and familiarity activation in PET studies of memory encoding and retrieval. *Cerebral Cortex* **6**, 71–9.

3

The domain of supervisory processes and the temporal organization of behaviour

Tim Shallice and Paul Burgess

3.1 Introduction

In recent accounts of the cognitive processes carried out by the prefrontal cortex it has been common to characterize them in terms of some key single type of process. The most common characterization has been in terms of working memory (e.g. Kimberg & Farah 1993). However, rival unitary accounts exist. Thus Duncan (1993) argued that 'goal-weighting'—the weighting of candidate goals to control behaviour in the next period of time— underlies general intelligence *g* and is the key process carried out by prefrontal cortex. We have argued for what may seem to be a related position, namely that prefrontal cortex is the seat of one overriding system—the supervisory system (Norman & Shallice 1986; Shallice & Burgess 1991). However, on this approach a 'system' is viewed as such because of how it interacts with other systems outside itself and not because it carries out only a single process.

In this paper we will present three lines of argument that even if it is appropriate to view the supervisory system as a single system, it is not correct to view it as carrying out only a single type of process. Indeed the evidence points to the existence of a variety of processes carried out by different subsystems but operating together to have a globally integrated function.

The processes carried out in human prefrontal cortex are, in causal terms, relatively far from both stimulus input and response output. Therefore they do not map transparently into the stimulus or response parameters of simple tasks. Characterizing these processes therefore is best achieved by a form of converging operations. In addition, one of these operations needs to be a theoretical framework of the types of processes likely to be present.

In the approach we have adopted, like in most of the competing characterizations, the prefrontal cortex is the seat of high-level processes that modulate lower-level ones. On such an approach it is essential that the lower-level modulated processes are adequately characterized. In an earlier version of the present theory (Norman & Shallice 1986; Shallice 1988) the more detailed aspects of the theorizing concerned the modulated system—so-called 'contention scheduling'. Contention scheduling has recently been simulated (Cooper *et al*. 1995). When noise is added in the implementation to produce an analogue of a lesion it gives rise to behaviour analogous to utilization behaviour (Lhermitte 1983; Shallice *et al*. 1989) and the core characteristics of the action disorganization syndrome (Schwartz *et al*. 1993). As these are both existing neurological syndromes this increases the plausibility of the approach.

In this paper we continue to adopt the contention scheduling/supervisory system framework and address the question of how one should proceed in the fractionation of the supervisory system into its basic subcomponents. We begin by broad theoretical considerations and then discuss two types of empirical evidence—neuropsychological dissociations and localization by functional imaging.

3.2 Theoretical considerations

We use the term situation to refer to a particular combination of environmental and internal states, particularly goals. Under the theory, a routine situation is one where thought and action schemas, essentially subroutines which are capable of realizing the relevant goals effectively, are selected through the automatic triggering on-line of well-learned perceptual or cognitive cues. Various types of evidence exist that the prefrontal cortex is, however, critically involved in coping with novel situations in contrast to routine ones—neuropsychological (e.g. Luria & Tsetkova 1964; Shallice & Evans 1978; Walsh 1978; Shallice 1982), electrophysiological (Knight 1984) and from functional imaging (Raichle *et al*. 1994).

While computational theories such as *Soar* (Newell 1990) show that the distinction between 'novel' and 'routine' can be effectively implemented, no existing computational theory of confronting novel situations is psychologically plausible (see Cooper & Shallice 1995 for discussion). The following position is therefore essentially speculative. The first basic premise of this paper is that coping with a novel situation involves a variety of different types of process operating over at least three stages. The second basic premise is that a key element in coping with a novel situation is the construction and implementation of a temporary new schema, which can take the place of the source schema triggered by the situation for routine control of behaviour, and which will in turn be capable of controlling lower-level schemas so as to provide a plausible procedure for achieving the situation goals. This temporary new schema can be an existing one, which is not directly triggered by the situation but more usually is an adaptation of an existing schema or schemas. Its phenomenological equivalent is the strategy the subject is carrying out (see also Robbins, this volume, Chapter 9).

The processes assumed to be involved are:
Stage 1
As will be discussed shortly, a variety of processes can be involved in constructing the temporary new schema.

Stage 2
A process (process 1) is required for implementing the operation of the tempo-rally active schema constructed in stage 1. This will require a working memory. However, this will be far from a general-purpose working memory, but one for the specific purpose of holding the temporally active schema since the schema is not triggered automatically in the situation.

Stage 3
A process (process 2) is needed for monitoring how well the type 2 processes are effected as with both the schemas and the situation being novel, temporary schemas cannot be known to be effective. This process can lead on to the rejection or alteration of the existing temporary schema (process 3).

The processes involved in stage 1 (strategy generation) are more complex. Strategy generation can occur spontaneously or through a process of problem solving. 'Spontaneous' strategy generation refers to the way that a procedure for tackling the situation can come to mind without any explicit attempt to solve a problem, but merely following a sense of dissatisfaction with the preceding method of tackling the situation. To implement it would necessarily be far more complex than say the running of a program (process 1) but in this paper we merely assume it to be a distinct process (process 4).

The second alternative is to use problem solving which frequently occurs in situations which do not explicitly require it (see Burgess & Shallice 1996a). Problem solving involves processing passing through a series of phases which, at the grossest level, are the phase of problem formation or orientation, the phase of the deepening of a solving attempt, then the phase of the assessment of a solution attempt followed by a return to the first phase or of a phase of recapitulation and checking (see De Groot 1966, p. 148). The control of the sequence of phases must require a process for the determination of what we call the processing mode in operation for that particular phase, by analogy with Tulving's (1983) conception of 'retrieval mode' (process 5). The one of these phases which would seem to require a process different to those previously discussed is that of the initial problem formation or orientation and in parti-cular what De Groot (1966) calls the 'evaluative moment', the process which leads to 'goal-setting' and 'quantitative expectancy' about what is to be achieved (process 6). This process is critical in that it provides the criteria for the later assessment of the solution attempt.

A final category of process consists of special purpose processes to assist in appropriate strategy generation. One is the formation and realization of inten-tions (process 7), so that one can prepare a strategy and plan action for a later time. A second is episodic memory retrieval (process 8) which according to Schank (1982) has the function of providing the raw material of related experi-ences for confronting novel situations (Burgess & Shallice 1996d). These pro-cesses all clearly relate to Fuster's (1980) conception of the prefrontal cortex as responsible for the structuring of behaviour over time, (see figure 3.1).

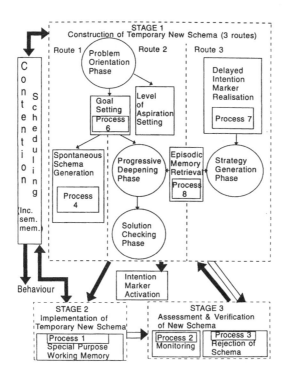

Fig. 3.1 Diagram of the relation between the theoretical constructs discussed. Within the dotted rectangles representing the different stages, temporally distinct phase of supervisory system processing is depicted by a circle. An operation, which corresponds to a change-of-state of one or more control variables, is depicted by a solid rectangle. Solid lines between the stage represent flow of control between the operation of different stages or between the supervisory system and contention scheduling. Unfilled lines represent information transfer used in monitoring operations.

It seems likely that all of these eight processes involve prefrontal structures. However, in the discussion of empirical evidence that follows we will not attempt to separate processes 1 and 4 (to be called process 1/4) or processes 2 and 3 (to be called process 2/3) and we will not be concerned with process 6 (but see Duncan 1986 and Damasio this volume) or process 8 (but see Burgess & Shallice 1996a). This leaves four processes to be considered later.

A key element in this approach is the temporary schema with its pheno- menological correspondence, the subject's strategy. Since the 1960s it has been known in cognitive psychology that to understand the performance of subjects in many tasks it is necessary to know which strategy has been used, which they can typically report. Prefrontal patients often have a striking deficit in this domain, in that they do not use the strategy normal subjects typically generate. For instance, Shallice & McGill (unpublished) carried out an experiment which was an analogue of Corsi's experiments (see Milner 1971) on recency judgments except that Corsi's time dimension was replaced by an importance dimension. Stimuli (words or faces) were presented and at the same time the subject was told 'important' for some of the stimuli. On interspersed test trials subjects were presented with two types of forced choice in a mixed sequence, namely ones based on relative importance and ones based on simple forced-choice recognition. Most normal subjects develop the strategy of paying less attention to stimuli not labelled important at input, to facilitate the first and more difficult of the discriminations. Of the 46 posterior patients, 78% indicated that they developed the strategy compared to only 50% of the 46 patients whose lesions involved the frontal lobes.

In a quite different situation Owen *et al.* (1990) found that frontal patients have a deficit on a spatial working memory task. However, they also showed a significant deficit on a measure which reflected the consistency in the search strategy they employed. The basic deficit in the group appeared to concern their strategies (see Robbins, Chapter 9). Finally we have recently studied the ability of patients to inhibit a prepotent verbal response (Burgess & Shallice 1996*b*). Subjects were given a sentence with its final highly constrained word removed. They were instructed to give a word which had no relation to the sentence frame. Again, normal subjects were typically found to adopt a strategy, in order to avoid the need to inhibit the prepotent response. They used one of two procedures to generate a candidate word prior to the response and then checked it for suitability or rather unsuitability after the sentence frame was presented. Frontal patients used such a strategy significantly less than patients with posterior lesions, although this time the original deficit was still present when the strategy score was used as a covariate. Process 1/4 therefore seems to be impaired by frontal lesions.

In none of these studies does one know to what extent the problem of the prefrontal patients was in strategy generation or in a strategy realization. However, strategy realization would involve the holding of a small programme of internal commands based on previously learned operations (schemas) and if/ then operations using perceptual or cognitive signals (triggers). It would take the form of a temporarily active schema, but being not well learned it would need to be retained in a specific working memory store; this is a plausible candidate function for the working memory stores described in dorsolateral prefrontal cortex (e.g. Goldman-Rakic 1987).

The process of monitoring for errors (process 2) is discussed in section 3.4, and determination of processing mode (process 5) in the next section. The final process to be considered (process 7) intention generation and realization—we held to be the critical component giving rise to the impaired performance of three patients with frontal head injuries in carrying out so-called strategy application disorder tasks (Shallice & Burgess 1991). These are tasks in which it is necessary for the subject to carry out a set of unrelated subtasks without any specific triggering of individual subtasks by relevant instructions as to when they should have been carried out, and to do this while obeying certain simple rules of task execution. When starting the experiment, the subject needs to set up intentions both to carry out the individual tasks and to obey the rules, which requires process 7. These frontal patients spent much longer on individual subtasks seemingly forgetful of the other tasks that needed to be carried out (see also Goldstein *et al.* 1993; Cockburn 1995). Later research has shown that performance on one such task—the six elements task—is the most highly correlated (0.46) of a set of executive tasks with relatives' assessments of the difficulty patients had in realizing plans (Burgess et al. 1996). It has also been shown in a group study that frontal patients are strongly impaired on this task by comparison with normal controls, even though the two groups did not differ on Raven's matrices (Burgess *et al.* unpublished).

We have so far shown that of the four processes to be considered two are impaired by frontal lobe lesions. However, before considering the other two, the issue of the empirical separability of subprocesses will be discussed.

3.3 Low correlations between tasks which load on supervisory functions

Classically within neuropsychology the way to determine whether two processes involve separable systems is to begin by establishing cross-over double dissociations between certain tasks which load heavily on one of the processes and tasks which load heavily on the other. The use of individual case studies is, however, primarily of value when three conditions hold. The range of performance of normal subjects must leave an ample region in which to observe clearly impaired performance. Normal performance must be approximately stationary, and theoretically interesting variations on the basic task must be effectively usable on the individual subject. These three conditions are frequently not all satisfied with tasks that load heavily on 'frontal functions'. For exceptions with respect to single dissociations see the example of the selective inability to modulate strategies in working memory tasks (Robbins *et al.* 1995) and the selective inability to carry out multiple unscheduled tasks (Shallice & Burgess 1991; Goldstein *et al.* 1993).

Group study methodology, however, offers an apparently analogous approach, namely to show low correlations between frontally loaded tasks in a group of patients with frontal lobe lesions. At least three recent studies have reported relatively low correlations in tasks known to be frontally loaded— word fluency and Wisconsin Card Sort Test—patients who perform poorly on them (0.35, 0.25 and 0.37 for fluency-Wisconsin categories and −0.40, −0.13, −0.41 for fluency-Wisconsin perseverative errors (Crockett *et al.* 1986; Shoqeirat *et al.* 1990; Kopelman 1991).

There are a number of problems in drawing inferences to fractionation within the frontal lobes from such evidence. First, word fluency and Wisconsin card sorting use different sorts of material and require different sorts of non-frontal processes in their performance. Thus they load on different non-frontal processes and indeed the patients in these studies would all be expected to have lesions which extend outside the frontal lobes. Moreover on a working memory hypothesis, working memory for different types of material would be expected to involve different regions of the frontal lobe, given that different locations are relevant in animal working memory studies with different material (Goldman-Rakic 1987; Kowalska *et al.* 1991). Second, little is known of the reliability of measures of frontal lobe tests. Finally a characteristic found in many frontal lobe patients is variability of performance over sessions (Stuss *et al.* 1994); a suggested explanation is that this arises from impairments in the setting up stage of temporary schemas for task solution (see Stuss *et al.* 1995), given that by definition the task is not well learned.

Consideration of these factors means that for observations of low correlations across frontal tasks to be theoretically interesting the tasks must at least involve the same type of material. As an example consider the Hayling sentence completion test developed by us (Burgess & Shallice 1996b), which was discussed briefly in the previous section. Subjects are presented with a sentence minus the final word with the completion word being strongly cued by the sentence frame. For instance, 99% of subjects completed the sentence frame 'He mailed the letter without a ...' with the word 'stamp' (Bloom & Fischler 1980). In the first condition (A) the subject merely completed the sentence as quickly as possible. In the second condition (B) the subject had to complete the sentence with any word that made no sense given the sentence frame. In both Hayling A and B frontal patients performed significantly worse than either controls or patients with posterior lesions. Surprisingly there were no effects of hemisphere. Critically the correlation between Hayling A and Hayling B was only 0.19 which reduced to 0.07 when age and Wechsler Adult Intelligence Scale. WAIS IQ were partialled out, both values being not significantly different from zero. Taking into account split-half reliabilities of the test, performance on the two parts doubly dissociate in individual frontal patients (e.g. patient X, A 1 percentile, B 76 percentile; patient Y, A 66 percentile, B 0.1 percentile). Here at least three of the conditions for separability are met, the possible exception being that test–retest reliability has yet to be established.

We see later that the relation between performance on this test and separability of function is more complex than it might seem. However, from the theoretical standpoint the results are straightforward. Hayling A requires the operation only of the contention scheduling system since one must merely allow the prepotent response to occur. However, to produce an inappropriate response in Hayling B some temporary schema or novel strategy needs to come into operation and indeed as discussed in the previous section normal subjects typically develop a particular strategy such as using a heuristic to generate a response prior to the sentence presentation and use of such a heuristic is affected by frontal damage.

If one considers the two types of correct responses—those that fit with one of the two strategies and those that do not—they both correlate negatively with the number of completion errors (−0.66 and −0.45 respectively). However, they do not correlate with each other (−0.10) and their correlations with semantically related responses are very different (−0.65 and −0.16 n.s.). This suggest they arise from different processes. As partialling out the number of strategy-related responses still left an overall effect of lesion site this implies that there is indeed a second separable process in addition to those involved in strategy production and realization which was also frontally based. This second process is presumably related to the monitoring or error correction processes discussed in the previous section. Thus both process 1/4 and process 2/3 are impaired by frontal lesions but appear to be separable.

The Brixton spatial anticipation test (Burgess & Shallice 1996c) gives rise to a similar effect. The Brixton test is a non-verbal analogue of the Wisconsin Card Sort Test except that the rules are more abstract and unlike the Wisconsin no response is prepotently triggered by the stimulus situation. The subject is presented with a card containing a 2×5 display of circles numbered in sequence of which one only is filled, the rest being in outline only. The subject must predict where on the next card the circle would be completed. Nine simple rules exist which are each in operation for three to eight trials, typical examples are moving to the next lowest number and alternating between circle 4 and circle 10. On three different measures frontal patients score significantly worse then either posterior patients or controls. One measure is simply the number of correct responses (measure A) but two measures of error type are also significantly higher in frontal patients. Interestingly neither of these is related to perseveration of previous responses or rules. One is concerned with the number of responses never given by any normal control subject in a position (measure B) and the other is the number of times switching away from a rule that had been attained occurs without any negative reinforcement being given (measure C). All three measures are roughly equally sensitive to the anterior/posterior location of the lesion. Measures A and B correlate 0.6 with each other and with age and IQ. However, measure C correlates with neither of the other measures (A: 0.13; B: 0.13).

This strongly suggests that there are two separable frontal factors involved in performance on the Brixton test too and this is supported by structural equation modelling. Simple explanations of either factor in terms of distractibility are implausible since the frontal group were no worse than the posterior patients on WAIS IQ. We associate the first factor with an inability to produce a new hypothesis which would be equivalent to the strategy generation (process 1/4) factor discussed in the previous section. Guesses then would reflect the situation in which the patient cannot come up with an appropriate strategy. The measure C, by contrast, relates to behaviour observed on the Heaton version of Wisconsin Card Sort Test by Stuss et al. (1983). Within the theoretical framework laid out in the previous section these errors would relate to an error in selecting the appropriate processing mode (process 5) by being in temporary schema-search mode (stage 1) instead of realization of temporary schema mode (stage 2). More critically, however, a dissociation-related methodology supports fractionation of supervisory functions.

3.4 Localization by means of PET

Within neuroscience the standard way of inferring separability of different subsystems is through demonstrating that the corresponding processes have different localizations. However, this criterion like both the previous ones is not conclusive; in this case processing in different regions may be strongly correlated. The previous studies being based on patients with a variety of aetiologies were not very suitable for precise localization. In any case functional imaging is now the most suitable procedure for addressing issues of localization of function in the human brain. Recently Nathaniel-James *et al.* (1996) have given normal volunteers the Hayling sentence completion test in the positron emission tomography (PET) camera. Using reading the last word of the sentence as the control condition they find that Hayling A activates the left frontal operculum (Brodmann's area 45) and right anterior cingulate (Brodmann's area 32). Hayling B activates the very same regions to roughly the same extent.

Initially these results were surprising as Hayling B is much the more difficult of the two parts for frontal patients. However, as Nathaniel-James *et al.* point out the localizations are very similar to those obtained by Warburton *et al.* (1996) for verb retrieval given the corresponding noun. Now this underlines a conceptual problem for localizing the processes involved in many frontal tests such as the Hayling test. Performance on the test of many normal subjects is not qualitatively stationary. As discussed in section 1 of this paper normal subjects frequently develop a strategy after which the on-line processing underlying task performance changes drastically. The typical strategy is to prepare a response before the sentence frame occurs, for instance, by looking round the room for objects, and then to check that the candidate word does not in fact make sense given the sentence frame. Once it is operative the process becomes that of generation from a given set and then checking. The similarity of activation sites with the Warburton *et al.* study becomes more comprehensible. However, this leads to a problem. Many severe frontal patients show no sign of using the strategy and it is more plausible that this is occurring because they failed to develop the strategy rather than because they cannot carry it out. Thus patient performance and normal subject PET performance would reflect different stages of task execution. Of course, the strategy development phase can occur in the normal subject too in the PET camera but it will occur relatively infrequently and possibly only once so it may occur in only one of the four experimental scans. The average PET activation results will be insensitive to it. Analogous problems will occur in attempting to interpret PET analysis of tasks like Wisconsin card sorting where the critical strategy-change process occurs only fairly rarely. Ideally what is required for critical processes to be detected by PET is to use a task where performance remains qualitatively stationary and critical processes occur on presentation of each stimulus. For this reason we will consider memory experiments.

In two recent PET studies (Tulving *et al.* 1994; Shallice *et al.* 1994) memory retrieval led to the activation of the right prefrontal cortex when related studies of memory encoding had led to activation of left prefrontal cortex. In the two studies different hypotheses were advanced for the processes underlying the right frontal activation, both being related to different supervisory system subprocesses discussed earlier. Tulving *et al.* argued that the critical factor was the subject being in retrieval mode (related to the mode-setting concept discussed earlier—process 5). The London group argued that the cause was monitoring and verification of putative responses related to process 2/3.

A recent experiment (Fletcher *et al.* 1996) carried out for a different purpose indirectly provides strong evidence on the choice between the alternatives. The experiment principally investigated the contrast between retrieval of imageable and non-imageable word-pairs from memory. It was concerned with a hypothesis on the functions of the precuneus activated in our previous memory retrieval study. Variation in the semantic distance between stimuli and responses in the word pairs was included as a factor to check that differences in degree of training between the two types of word-pair was not critical. Sets of pairs with six different semantic distances were included—five with semantic relations going from close (5) to distant (1) and then a sixth set of randomly related pairs (0). For both imageable and non-imageable stimuli all pairs were given appropriate amounts of pre-training so that subjects were approximately equally accurate at retrieval for all semantic distances. This involved from 1 to 4 pre-scan presentations for the imageable pairs and from 1 to 8 for the non-imageable pairs.

The results were very striking. For related pairs there was a general decline in activation at retrieval with increasing amount of training (and increase in semantic distance) supporting the position of Raichle *et al.* (1994). However, for the random pairs there was a highly significant reversal (see figure 3.2) particularly in the medial frontal and right prefrontal regions. Retrieval of randomly related pairs led to as high activation in that region as did retrieval of closely related pairs even though the former had been seen on many previous trials. Why should this be? It is difficult to account for this highly nonlinear effect on the retrieval mode explanation. However, random pairs make a much larger demand on verification processes than do related pairs. If a putative response is produced it can be simply determined with which stimulus it could be paired in the related condition but not for the random condition. As the response set can be learned partially independently of the S-R bonds, subjects will have a much more difficult verification process in the random conditions than in the otherwise comparable related conditions since they cannot easily be sure without checking whether the response elicited by the stimulus actually went with that stimulus or another one in the list. This suggests that verification processes are responsible for the activation shown in the right prefrontal cortex. They are the analogue in the memory domain of the monitoring processes in the tasks discussed earlier.

This would mean that one of the processes discussed in section 3.2 is lateralized within the frontal lobes and that a program of localization of the subprocesses discussed in section 3.2 may be practicable.

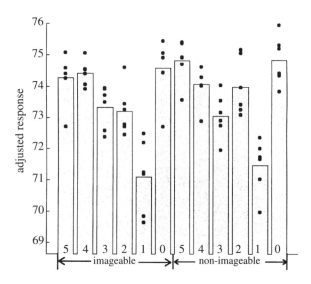

Fig. 3.2   rCBF equivalent values from a medial frontal pixel (coordinates $x, y, z = -2$, 50, 32) showing that the frontal decrease in activity associated with weakening semantic linkage (figure shown at the base of rCBF bars) is relatively linear across the linked pairs (5 to 1) but that this is reversed for the unlinked pairs (0) predominantly in the right frontal region (reproduced from Fletcher *et al.* 1996).

3.5 Conclusion

We have presented three lines of argument for the idea that the prefrontal cortex contains a set of subsystems which implement different processes. Arguments are derived from differences in the computations that are required to realize the processes, from the dissociations that occur between neurological patients who have frontal lobe lesions and from the possible specific localization of a particular process. Clearly this has been a very preliminary discussion. The computational distinctions between the processes the individual hypothesized subsystems are held to carry out have essentially been asserted rather than proved. The group-study dissociation methodology adopted is experimental and only two pairs of dissociations were discussed. Moreover, as only one process was considered from a localization point-of-view, the argument was insufficient to show that processes localize differently. In addition, no systematic attempt was made to show that a consistent pattern occurs from all three types of argument. However, a programme of research to investigate a possible convergence seems practicable.

   Finally, if there are a variety of subsystems carrying out different processes and differently localized within prefrontal cortex, is it useful to characterize them as different parts of a single system? We would argue that it is if they have a common overall function within the overall processing system and if they are characteristically used in a related fashion. Both these criteria seem to apply. The processes hypothesized are ones involved in confronting situations which are not routine when routine processes are assumed to be controlled by contention scheduling. They are therefore the set of processes which modulate contention scheduling from above. Moreover in confronting a typical non-routine situation most of the processes would be involved. It seems appropriate to view them as subsystems of the supervisory system.

Acknowledgement

Work discussed in this paper has been supported by a grant from the Medical Research Council and one from the Wellcome Trust.

References

Bloom, P. A. & Fischler, I. 1980 Completion norms for 329 sentence contexts. *Memory and Cognition* **38**, 631–42.

Burgess, P. W., Alderman, N., Emslie, H., Evans, J., Wilson, B. A. & Shallice, T. 1996 The modified Six Element Test. In *Behavioural assessment of the dysexecutive syndrome* (ed. B. A. Wilson, N. Aldeman, P. W. Burgess, H. Emslie & J. J. Evans). Thames Valley Test Company, Bury St Edmunds: UK.

Burgess, P. W. & Shallice, T. 1996*a* Confabulation and the control of recollection. *Memory* **4**(2), 359–412.

Burgess, P. W. & Shallice, T. 1996*b* Response suppression, initiation and strategy use following frontal lobe lesions. *Neuropsychologia*, **34**, 263–76.

Burgess, P. W. & Shallice, T. 1996*c* Bizarre responses, rule detection and frontal lobe lesions. *Cortex* **32**, 241–60.

Burgess, P. W. & Shallice, T. 1996*d* Autobiographical recollection and prospective remembering. In *Cognitive models of memory* (ed. M. A. Conway). pp. 81–123. London: UCL Press.

Cockburn, J. 1995 Task interruption in prospective memory: A frontal lobe function? *Cortex* **31**, 87–97.

Cooper, R. & Shallice, T. 1995 Soar and the case for unified theories of cognition. *Cognition* **55**, 115–149.

Cooper, R., Shallice, T. & Farringdon, J. 1995 Symbolic and continuous processes in the automatic selection of actions. In *Hybrid problems, hybrid solutions* (ed. J. Hallam). IOS Press: Amsterdam.

Crockett, D., Bilsker, D., Hurwitz, T. & Kozak, J. 1986 Clinical utility of three measures of frontal dysfunction in neuropsychiatric samples. *Int. J. Neurosci.* **30**, 241–48.

De Groot, A.D. 1966 *Thought and choice in chess.* Mouton: The Hague.

Duncan, J. 1986 Disorganisation of behaviour after frontal lobe damage. *Cognitive Neuropsychol.* **3**, 271–90.

Duncan, J. 1993 Selection of goal and input in the control of behaviour. In *Attention: selection, awareness and control* (ed. A. D. Baddeley & L. Weiskrantz). Clarendon Press: Oxford.

Fletcher, P. C., Shallice, T., Frith, C. D., Frackowiak, R. S. J. & Dolan, P. J. 1996 Brain activity during memory retrieval: the influence of imagery and semantic cuing. *Brain*, **119**, 1587–96.

Fuster, J. M. 1980 *The prefrontal cortex: anatomy, physiology and neuropsychology of the frontal lobe*. Raven: New York.

Goldman-Rakic, P. 1987 Circuitry of primate prefrontal cortex and regulation of behaviour by representational knowledge. In *Handbook of physiology* (eg. F. Plum & V. Mountcastle), vol 5, pp. 373–417. American Physiological Society: Bethesda, MD.

Goldstein, L. H., Bernard, S., Fenwick, P. B. C., Burgess, P. W. & McNeil, J. 1993 Unilateral frontal lobectomy can produce strategy application disorder. *J. Neurol., Neurosurg. Psychiat.* **56**, 274–76.

Kimberg, D. Y. & Farah, M. J. 1993 A unified account of cognitive impairments following frontal lobe damage: The role of working memory in complex organized behaviour. *J. Exptl Psychol.* **122**, 411–28.

Knight, R. T. 1984 Decreased response to novel stimuli after prefrontal lesions in man. *EEG Clin. Neurophysiol.* **59**, 9–20.

Kopelman, M. D. 1991 Frontal dysfunction and memory deficits in the alcoholic Korsakoff syndrome and Alzheimer-type dementia. *Brain* **114**, 117–37.

Kowalska, D. M., Bachevalier, J. & Mishkin, M. 1991 The role of inferior prefrontal convexity in performance of delayed matching-to-sample. *Neuropsychologia* **29**, 583–600.

Lhermitte, F. 1983 'Utilisation behaviour' and its relation to lesions of the frontal lobes. *Brain* **106**, 237–55.

Luria, A. R. & Tsetkova, L. D. 1964 The programming of constructive ability in local brain injuries. *Neuropsychologia* **2**, 95–108.

Milner, B. 1971 Interhemispheric differences in the localisation of psychological processes in man. *Br. Med. Bull.* **27**, 272–77.

Nathaniel-James, D. A., Fletcher, P. & Frith, C. D. 1996 The functional anatomy of verbal initiation and suppression during the Hayling Test *Neuropsychologia* **35**, 559–66.

Newell, A. 1990. *Unified theories of cognition*, Cambridge MA: Harvard University Press.

Norman, D. A. & Shallice, T. 1986 Attention to action: willed and automatic control of behaviour. In *Consciousness and self-regulation* (ed. G. E. Schwartz & D. Shapiro), vol 4. Plenum Press: New York.

Owen, A. M., Downes, J., Sahakian, B. J., Polkey, C. E. & Robbins, T. W. 1990 Planning and spatial working memory following frontal lobe lesions in man. *Neuropsychologia* **28**, 1021–34.

Raichle, M. E., Fiez, J. A., Videen, T. I., Macleod, A. M. K. & Fox, P. T. 1994 Practice-related changes in human brain functional anatomy during non-motor learning. *Cerebral Cortex* **4**, 8–26.

Robbins, T. W., Shallice, T., Burgess, P. W., James, M., Rogers, R. D., Warburton, E. & Wise, R. S. 1995 Selective impairments in self-ordered working memory in a patient with an unilateral striatal lesion. *Neurocase* **1**, 217–30.

Schank, R. C. 1982 *Dynamic memory*. Cambridge: Cambridge University Press.

Schwartz, M. F., Mayer, N. H., Fitzpatrick, E. J. & Montgomery, M. W. 1993 Cognitive theory and the study of everyday action disorders after brain damage. *J. Head Trauma Rehabil.* **8**, 59–72.

Shallice, T. 1982 Specific impairments of planning. *Phil. Trans. R. Soc. Lond.* B **298**, 199–209.

Shallice, T. 1988 *From neuropsychology to mental structure*. Cambridge University Press: Cambridge.

Shallice, T. & Burgess, P. W. 1991 Deficits in strategy application following frontal lobe damage in man. *Brain* **114**, 727–41.

Shallice, T., Burgess, P. W., Schon, F. & Baxter, D. W. 1989 The origins of utilisation behaviour. *Brain* **11**, 1587–98.

Shallice, T. & Evans, M. E. 1978 The involvement of the frontal lobes in cognitive estimation. *Cortex* **14**, 294–303.

Shallice, T., Fletcher, P., Frith, C. D., Grasby, P., Frackowiak, R. S. J. & Dolan, R. J. 1994 Brain regions associated with the acquisition and retrieval of verbal episodic memory. *Nature, Lond.* **386**, 633–35.

Shoqeirat, M. A., Mayes, A., MacDonald, C., Meudell, P. & Pickering, A. 1990 Performance on tests sensitive to frontal lobe lesions by patients with organic amnesia: Leng and Parkin revisited. *Br. J. Clin. Psychol.* **29**, 401–08.

Stuss, D. T., Benson, D. F., Kaplan, E. F., Weir, W. S., Naeser, M. A., Liberman, I. & Ferill, D. 1983 The involvement of orbitofrontal cerebrum in cognitive tasks. *Neuropsychologia* **21**, 235–48.

Stuss, D. T., Shallice, T., Alexander, M. P. & Picton, T. W. 1995 A multidisciplinary approach to anterior attentional functions. *Ann. N. Y. Acad. Sci.* **769**, 191–211.

Tulving, E. 1983 *Elements of episodic memory*. Clarendon Press: Oxford.

Tulving, E., Kapur, S., Markowitsch, H. J., Craik, F. I. M., Habib, R. & Houle, S. 1994 Neuroanatomical correlates of retrieval in episodic memory: auditory sentence recognition. *Proc. Nat. Acad. Sci.* **91**, 2012–15.

Walsh, K. W. 1978 *Neuropsychology: a clinical approach*. Edinburgh: Churchill Livingstone.

Warburton, E., Wise, R. J. S., Price, C. J., Weiller, C., Hadar, U., Ramsay, S. & Frackowiak, R. S. J. 1996 Noun and verb retrieval by normal subjects: studies with PET. *Brain*, **119**, 159–79.

4

The somatic marker hypothesis and the possible functions of the prefrontal cortex

Antonio R. Damasio

4.1 Introduction

This text is about a hypothesis, known as the somatic marker hypothesis, which concerns the possible role of some regions of the prefrontal cortex in the processes of reasoning and decision making. The text follows closely, in form and substance, several reviews in which my colleagues and I have presented the hypothesis and its preliminary testing (see Damasio 1994, 1995*a*).

The hypothesis developed as a response to a number of intriguing observations made in neurological patients with focal damage in the frontal lobe. Briefly, patients with damage to the prefrontal region, especially when the damage is centred in ventral and medial aspects of this region, present with severe impairments in personal and social decision making, in spite of otherwise largely preserved intellectual abilities (Damasio 1979, 1994). Before the onset of brain damage the patients may be described as intelligent, creative and successful; but after damage occurs the patients develop a pattern of abnormal decision making which is most notable in personal and social matters. Specifically, patients have difficulty planning their work day; difficulty planning their future over immediate, medium and long ranges and difficulty choosing suitable friends, partners and activities. The plans they organize, the persons they elect to join, or the activities they undertake often lead to financial losses, losses in social standing and losses to family and friends. The choices these patients make are no longer personally advantageous, socially inadequate and are demonstrably different from the choices the patients were known to have made in the premorbid period.

The patients' intellect remains normal, as measured by conventional IQ tests, so does the learning and retention of factual knowledge at both unique and non-unique levels and the learning and retention of skills. The ability to use logic in the solution of problems commonly posed in neuropsychological testing is also normal, so is language. Basic attention and working memory are not affected, nor is the ability to make estimates (as tested in a paradigm developed by Shallice & Evans 1978), to perform normally in the Wisconsin Card Sort Test and to judge recency and frequency of events (see Milner 1963, 1964;

Petrides & Milner 1982; Milner *et al.* 1985). The patients' repertoire of social knowledge is still retained and can be accessed in a laboratory situation (Saver & Damasio 1991). The disturbance shown by this particular class of patients cannot be explained in terms of defects in (a) pertinent knowledge; (b) intellectual ability; (c) language; (d) basic working memory; or (e) basic attention. As if this challenge were not enough, the patients pose yet another. Although their impairment is obvious in everyday life, there has not been, until recently, a laboratory probe to detect it or measure it.

In the text below, I outline the somatic marker hypothesis, which is part of a framework to account for the condition, and describe new laboratory probes designed to detect and measure aspects of the condition. I do not address the condition of patients whose frontal lesions are located in anatomical sectors other than the ventromedial. Some of those patients may also have defects in reasoning or decision making, but those defects are accompanied by impairments in abilities which are preserved in patients with ventromedial lesions. The conditions with which such other patients present may or may not be accountable by the somatic marker hypothesis. The hypothesis should not be seen as a general theory for how prefrontal cortices work as, in all likelihood, this large and parcellated sector of the brain accomplishes several separate albeit cooperative functions.

4.2 The somatic marker hypothesis

The idea for the somatic marker hypothesis came from the realization that, while the ventromedial patients were intact in neuropsychological laboratory tests they did have a compromised ability to express emotion and to experience feelings in situations in which emotions would normally have been expected and would presumably have been present during the premorbid period. In other words, along with normal intellect and abnormal decision making, there were abnormalities in emotion and feeling. In the absence of other cognitive impairments that might effectively account for the salient aspects of the condition, I reasoned that the defect in emotion and feeling, along with its neurobiological underpinnings, would play an important role in the pathological process; and on the basis of the pathological process I then specified a number of structures and operations to be found in the normal condition. Because I see emotion as expressing itself most importantly, though not solely, through changes in the representation of body state, and because I believe that the results of emotion are primarily represented in the brain in the form of transient changes in the activity pattern of somatosensory structures, I designated the emotional changes under the umbrella term 'somatic state.' Note that by somatic I refer to musculoskeletal, visceral, and internal milieu components of the soma rather than just to the musculoskeletal aspect; and note also that a somatic signal or process, although related to structures which represent the body and its states does not need to originate in the body in every instance (see

Damasio 1994, 1995*b* for details). The summary of the proposal's background assumptions and specific structures and operations is presented below.

Background assumptions

In addition to an operative self and consciousness, the basis for neither of which I will discuss, the mechanisms I envision require four main assumptions:

1. that human reasoning and decision making depend on many levels of neurobiological operation, some of which occur in mind (i.e. are conscious, overt cognitive), and some of which do not. Minded (conscious, overt cognitive) operations depend on sensory images which are based on the coordinated activity of early sensory cortices.
2. that all mind operations regardless of the content of images, depend on support processes such as attention and working memory.
3. that reasoning and decision making depend on the availability of knowledge about situations, actors, options for action and outcomes. Such knowledge is stored in 'dispositional' form throughout higher-order cortices and some subcortical nuclei. (By the term dispositional I mean coded, implicit and non-topographically organized; see Damasio 1989*a, b*, 1994; Damasio & Damasio 1994; for details on dispositional knowledge and convergence zone framework.) Dispositional knowledge can be made explicit in (a) motor responses of varied types and complexity (some combinations of which can constitute emotions), and in (b) images. The result of all motor responses, including those that are not generated consciously (i.e. minded), can be represented in images and become minded.
4. that knowledge can be classified as follows:
    A. innate and acquired knowledge concerning bioregulatory processes and body states and actions, including those which are made explicit as emotions.
    B. knowledge about entities, facts (e.g. relations, rules), actions and action-complexes, and stories, which are usually made explicit as images.
    C. knowledge about the linkages between B items and A items, as reflected in individual experience.
    D. knowledge resulting from the categorizations of items in A, B and C.

Specific structures and operations

(i) *Ventromedial prefrontal cortex as a repository of dispositionally recorded linkages between factual knowledge and bioregulatory states*

Structures in ventromedial prefrontal cortex provide the substrate for learning the association between certain classes of complex situation, on the one hand, and the type of bioregulatory state (including emotional state) usually associated with that class of situation in prior individual experience. The ventromedial sector would hold linkages between the facts that compose a given situation, and the emotion previously paired with it in an individual's contingent experience. The linkages are 'dispositional' in the sense that they do not hold the representation of the facts or of the emotional state explicitly, but hold rather the potential to reactivate an emotion by acting on the appropriate cortical or subcortical structures (see Damasio 1989 *a,b*, 1994; Damasio & Damasio 1994; for discussion of the concept of disposition and the convergence zone framework; see also Damasio 1994, 1995*b* for a discussion on the neurobiology of emotion). What I envision here is that the experience we acquire regarding a complex situation and its components—a certain configuration of actors and actions requiring a response; a set of response options; a set of immediate and long-term outcomes for each response option—is processed in sensory imagetic and motor terms and is then recorded in dispositional and categorized form. (The records are maintained in distributed form in large-scale systems which involve many cortices including those in prefrontal sectors other than the ventromedial.) But the experience of some of those components, individually or in sets, has been associated with emotional responses, which were triggered from cortical and subcortical limbic sites that were dispositionally prepared to organize such a response. I propose that the ventromedial prefrontal cortex establishes a simple linkage, a memory in fact, between the disposition for a certain aspect of a situation (for instance, the long-term outcome for a type of response option), and the disposition for the type of emotion that in past experience has been associated with the situation.

(ii) *The reactivation of signals related to previous individual contingencies*
When a situation arises for which some factual aspect has been previously categorized, related dispositions are activated in higher-order association cortices (including in good likelihood some prefrontal cortices). This leads to the recall of pertinently associated facts which will be experienced in imagetic form. Simultaneously, or nearly so, the related ventromedial prefrontal linkages are also activated, and as a consequence, the emotional disposition apparatus is activated too (e.g. in the amygdala). The result of these combined activations is the approximate reconstruction of a previously learned factual-emotional set. In short, when a situation of a given class recurs, factual knowledge pertaining to the situation—possible options of action, outcomes of such actions immediately and at longer term—is evoked in sensory images based on the appropriate sensory cortices. But depending on previous individual contingencies, signals related to some or even many of those images, or even the entire situation, act on the ventromedial prefrontal cortex (which has previously acquired the link between the situation or its components and the class of somatic state), and trigger the re-activation of the somato-sensory pattern that describes the appropriate emotion.

The re-activation described above can be carried out in one of two ways: via a 'body loop', in which the soma actually changes in response to the activation and the ensuing changes are relayed to somatosensory cortices; or via an 'as if body loop', in which the reactivation signals are conveyed to the somatosensory cortices which then adopt the appropriate pattern, the body being bypassed. From both evolutionary and ontogenetic perspectives I believe that the 'body loop' is the original mechanism but has been superseded by the 'as if' body loop and is possibly used less frequently than the 'as if' loop. The results of either 'body loop' or 'as if body loop' may become overt (conscious) or remain covert (non-conscious).

(iii) *A marker role for signals related to previous emotional state contingencies*

The establishment of a somatosensory pattern appropriate to the situation, via the 'body loop' or via the 'as if' loop, either overtly or covertly, is co-displayed with factual evocations pertinent to the situation and, qualifies those factual evocations. In doing so, it operates to constrain the process of reasoning over multiple options and multiple future outcomes. For instance, when the so-matosensory image which defines a certain emotional response is juxtaposed to the images which describe a related scenario of future outcome, and which triggered the emotional response via the ventromedial linkage, the somatosensory pattern marks the scenario as good or bad. In other words, the images of the scenario are 'judged' and marked by the juxtaposed images of the somatic state.

When this process is overt, the somatic state operates as an alarm signal or an incentive signal. The somatic state is alerting you to the goodness or badness of a certain option-outcome pair. The device produces its result at the openly cognitive level. When the process is covert the somatic state constitutes a biasing signal. Using an indirect and non-conscious influence, for instance through a non-specific neurotransmitter system such as dopamine, the device influences cognitive processing.

(iv) *Somatic markers participate in process as well as content*

Certain emotion-related somatosensory patterns also act as boosters in the processes of attention and working memory. In addition to assisting with the process of specific experiential contents (e.g. certain combinations of facts and emotions), I believe they may also assist with response inhibition.

(v) *Somatic markers facilitate logical reasoning*

The operation of logical reasoning is facilitated by steps (iii) and (iv). Certain option-outcome pairs can be rapidly rejected or endorsed and, perti-nent facts can be more effectively processed. The hypothesis thus suggests that somatic markers normally help constrain the decision-making space by making that space manageable for logic-based, cost-benefit analyses. In situations in which there is remarkable uncertainty about the future and in which the decision should be influenced by previous individual experience, such constraints permit the organism to decide efficiently within short time intervals.

In the absence of a somatic marker, options and outcomes become virtually equalized and the process of choosing will depend entirely on logic operations over many option-outcome pairs. The strategy is necessarily slower and may fail to take into account previous experience. This is the pattern of slow and error-prone decision behaviour we often see in ventromedial frontal lobe patients. Random and impulsive decision making is a related pattern.

Whether body states are real or vicarious (what I term 'as if'), the corresponding neural pattern can be made conscious and constitute a feeling. However, although many important choices involve feelings, a number of our daily decisions undoubtedly proceed without feelings. That does not mean that the evaluation that normally leads to a body state has not taken place, or that the body state or its surrogate has not been engaged, or that the dispositional machinery underlying the process has not been activated. It simply means that the body state or its surrogate have not been attended. Without attention, neither will be part of consciousness, although either can be part of a covert action on the mechanisms that govern, without wilful control, our appetitive (approach) or aversive (withdrawal) attitudes toward the world. While the hidden machinery underneath has been activated, we may never know it.

There is yet another mechanism for covert action: it consists of triggering activity in certain neurotransmitter nuclei (e.g. dopamine), which is part of the 'emotional response', a physiological step which will subsequently bias cognitive processes, thus influencing the mode of reasoning and decision making.

4.3 A neural network for somatic markers

Why is it that ventral and medial prefrontal cortices are ideally situated to establish the kind of linkages outlined above? These cortices, judging from what is known of nonhuman primate neuroanatomy, receive projections from all sensory modalities, directly or indirectly (Pandya & Kuypers 1969; Jones & Powell 1970; Chavis & Pandya 1976; Potter & Nauta 1979; Petrides & Pandya 1995; Pandya & Yeterian 1996 and this volume). In turn, they are the only known source of projections from frontal regions toward central autonomic control structures (Nauta 1971), and such projections have a demonstrated physiological influence on visceral control (Hall *et al.* 1977). The ventromedial cortices have extensive bidirectional connections with the hippocampus and amygdala (Van Hoesen *et al.* 1972; Van Hoesen *et al.* 1975; Porrino *et al.* 1981; Amaral & Price 1984; Goldman-Rakic *et al.* 1984;). Moreover, as shown by Rolls and colleagues (Chapter 6), nearby cortices in the orbitofrontal region contain the secondary association areas for taste and olfaction, receive other sensory inputs, namely visual, and are clearly involved in the signalling of reward to perceived stimuli.

This anatomical design is quite compatible with the idea that the ventromedial cortices contain convergence zones which hold a record of temporal
conjunctions of activity in other neural units (e.g. varied sensory, limbic
structures) hailing from both external and internal stimuli. This would be
a record of signals from regions that were active simultaneously and which, as
a set, defined a given situation or salient aspects of it. As noted, when parts of
certain exteroceptive–interoceptive conjunctions are re-processed, consciously
or not, their activation is signalled to ventromedial cortices, which in turn
activate somatic effectors in amygdala, hypothalamus, and brainstem nuclei,
or activate somatosensory structures directly. One might describe this process
as an attempt to reconstitute the kind of somatic state that belonged to the
conjunction in the first place.

The systems network necessary for somatic markers to operate thus includes
the following essential structures: (1) ventromedial frontal cortices which contain convergence zones that record links between (a) the dispositions that
represent categorizations of certain complex situations and their components,
and (b) the dispositions that represent the somatic states that have been pre-
valently associated with the situations referred above; (2) central autonomic
effectors, for example the amygdala, which can activate somatic responses in
viscera, vascular bed, endocrine system and nonspecific neurotransmitter systems; (3) somatosensory cortices (namely insula, SII, and SI) and their inter-
locking projections (especially in the non-dominant hemisphere), which can
receive signals from the soma (or signals from ventromedial cortices prescribing
an 'as if' somatic pattern).

It is possible that structures in basal ganglia are also part of this network and
can mediate responses from ventromedial cortices by acting on somatomotor
structures (Tranel & Damasio 1993).

It is important to note that the evocation of a somatic marker for stimuli that
are unconditioned and basic, for instance, a startling noise or a flash of light,
uses a different and simpler network; that is, a network that can cope with
behaviourally relevant stimuli that do not need the complex informational
processing that social configurations do. The alternate network would bypass
the cerebral cortex altogether and activate autonomic centres (e.g. amygdala
and others) directly from thalamus (Clugnet et al. 1988; Farb et al. 1988). My
formulation predicts a dissociation between responses to complex stimuli which
require cortical processing, and to basic stimuli which do not.

4.4 The nature of the marker

Why should somatic signals be so critical to the process of reasoning and
decision making? My answer is that certain classes of situation, namely those
that concern personal and social matters, are frequently linked to punishment
and reward and thus to pain, pleasure, and the regulation of homeostatic states,
including the part of the regulation that is expressed by emotion and feeling.

The inevitability of somatic participation comes from the fact that all of these bioregulatory phenomena, including emotion, are represented via the somatosensory system.

One may also ask why a signal external to the representations over which one reasons is needed at all. The answer, as suggested above, has to do with the uncertainty of outcomes, the dimension of the logical operations required by deciding under uncertainty, and the advantage of constraining the decision-making space.

The realm of basic survival behaviour provides the right setting to explain the possible origin of somatic markers. Let us assume that the brain has long had available, in evolution, a means to select good responses rather than bad ones in terms of survival. I suspect that the mechanism has been co-opted for behavioural guidance outside the realm of basic survival. Nature would have evolved a highly successful mechanism of guidance to cope with basic problems whose answer might maximize survival. But a very large range of other problems, including those which pertain to the social realm, are indirectly linked to precisely the same framework of survival versus danger, of advantage versus disadvantage, of gain and balance versus loss and disequilibrium. It is plausible that a system geared to produce markers and signposts to guide basic survival, would have been pre-adapted to assist with 'intellectual' decision making. The somatic markers would not necessarily be perceived in the form of 'feelings'. They could act covertly to highlight, in the form of an attentional mechanism, certain components over others, and to direct, in effect, the go, stop, and turn signals necessary for much decision making and planning on even the most abstract of topics. Shallice & Burgess (1993), have also proposed that some form of marker is needed in decision making, although they have not specified the neurobiological nature of the marker and it may be different from what I propose here. Nonetheless my proposal and theirs do share this trait.

In conclusion, in normal individuals, certain situations require high-order composite memories formed by 'facts' and by the 'body states' which usually accompany those facts in an individual's experience. The 'fact' memories are held in dispositional form in the appropriate association cortices. The 'body state' memories do not need to be held permanently, as body states can be re-enacted on demand. Only the memory of the linkage between certain classes of situation and certain body states must be held permanently, and I believe the system necessary for such memories is in ventral and medial prefrontal cortices.

Patients with ventromedial frontal lobe damage fail to evoke part of the composite memory, for a class of situation; the part that describes the association between the class of situation and the somatosensory state linked to the situation. The factual knowledge component of the composite memory can still be evoked, but somatic states cannot be re-enacted, overtly or covertly, relative to those facts. This limitation poses no problem for situations that have minimal somatic state associations in previous experience, but is catastrophic for situations that do.

4.5 Testing the somatic marker hypothesis

We have begun a series of experiments aimed at providing a possible physio-pathological explanation for the defect. Some pertinent results are described below.

Somatic responses to emotionally charged stimuli

In these experiments we tested the hypothesis that patients with bilateral damage in the ventromedial prefrontal cortices would not generate somatic states in response to emotionally charged stimuli. The basic idea was that the processing of stimuli with emotional significance would be affected by the previous experiences the subjects had with those stimuli, and that the ventro-medial prefrontal cortex would be pivotal to reactivate the somatic states that had been usually engendered when those stimuli were experienced.

In order to assess the presence or absence of a change in somatic state we decided to measure a standard autonomic index, the skin conductance response (SCR). We studied 3 groups of subjects. The first was constituted by normal controls, without neurological or psychiatric illness. The second com-prised subjects with lesions located outside the frontal cortices. The third comprised subjects with lesions in the ventromedial frontal cortex. All subjects in the third group had both bilateral damage in the target region and the index condition, that is, acquired defects in decision making in their real life, real time behaviour.

The experimental condition called for the subjects to view two types of visual image. One type was emotionally neutral, for example landscapes or abstract patterns. The other was emotionally charged, for example scenes of social catastrophe, or body mutilation.

The state of responsivity of the autonomic nervous system was assessed in all three groups of subjects by their SCRs to startling stimuli such as loud noises, or to the behaviours that reliably elicit SCRs, for example deep breath. All three groups had normal SCRs in that condition. In the experimental condition, however, while both normal controls and nonfrontal brain damaged groups exhibited standard SCR responses to the emotionally charged stimuli and little or no response to the neutral stimuli, the subjects with ventromedial frontal damage failed to react to the emotionally charged stimuli (Damasio *et al.* 1990; Damasio *et al.* 1991; Tranel 1994; Tranel *et al.* 1995). The findings suggest that patients with bilateral ventromedial frontal damage and decision-making defects in personal and social domain, no longer have a normal ability to generate somatic responses to stimuli with an emotional component.

The gambling experiments

Another approach to the testing of the somatic marker hypothesis relied on a novel card gambling task (Bechara *et al.* 1994). The task is an attempt to create in the laboratory a realistic situation in which subjects gradually learn how to play a card game, to their best advantage, in situations of limited knowledge about the contingencies, and under the control of rewards and penalties. As described in our original publication, the task operates as follows: the subjects sit in front of four decks of cards equal in appearance and size, and are given a $2000 loan of play money (facsimile US dollar bills). They are told that the game requires a series of card selections, one card at a time, from any of the four decks, until they are told to stop. The subjects are also told that (1) the goal of the task is to maximize profit on the loan of play money, (2) they are free to switch from any deck to another, at any time, and as often as wished; but (3) they are not told in advance how many card selections must be made. The task is stopped after 100 card selections. After each card turning, the subjects receive some money. The amount is announced after the turning and varies with the deck. Turning any card from decks A or B yields $100; turning any card from decks C or D yields $50. After turning some cards of any deck, however, the subjects are both given money and asked to pay a penalty. Again the amount is announced after the card is turned and varies with the deck and the position in the deck according to a schedule unknown to the subjects. The ultimate yield of each deck varies because the penalty amounts are higher in the high-paying decks (A and B), and lower in the low-paying decks (C and D). For example, after turning ten cards from deck A, the subjects have earned $1000, but they have also encountered five unexpected punishments bringing their total cost to $1250, and incurring a net loss of $250. They encounter the same problem on deck B. On the other hand, after turning ten cards from decks C or D, the subjects earn $500, but their unpredicted punishments only amount to $250, that is subjects incur a net gain of $250. In short, decks A and B are equivalent in terms of overall net loss over the trials. The difference is that in deck A, the punishment is more frequent, but of smaller magnitude, whereas in deck B, the punishment is less frequent but of higher magnitude. Decks C and D are also equivalent in terms of overall net loss. In deck C, the punishment is more frequent and of smaller magnitude, while in deck D the punishment is less frequent but of higher magnitude. Decks A and B are 'disadvantageous' because they cost the most in the long run, while decks C and D are 'advantageous' because they result in an overall gain in the long run.

The performance of a group of normal control subjects (21 women and 23 men) in this task was compared to those of ventromedial prefrontal subjects (4 men and 2 women). The age range of normal controls was from 20 to 79 years; for ventromedial subjects it was from 43 to 84 years. About half the number of subjects in each group had a high school education, and the other half had a college education.

The results were clear cut. Normals and patients without frontal damage sample from all decks for a while and gradually begin playing more frequently from the good decks than from the bad. About half way through the game they finally adopt this strategy and never abandon it. As a result they come out ahead. Ventromedial frontal lobe patients, on the contrary, continue to play predominantly from the bad decks, in spite of repeated losses. As a result they lose all of their loan and need to borrow money.

Although the gambling task involves a long series of gains and losses, it is not possible for subjects to perform an exact calculation of the net gains or losses generated from each deck as they play. (A group of normal control subjects with superior memory and IQ, whom we asked to think aloud while performing the task and keep track of the magnitudes and frequencies of the various punishments, could not provide figures for the net gains or losses from each deck). The subjects must rely on their ability 'to sense', overtly or not, which decks are risky and which are profitable. The performance profile of ventro-medial patients is comparable to their real-life inability to decide advant-ageously, especially in personal and social matters, a domain for which in life, as in the task, an exact calculation of the future outcomes is not possible and choices must be based on approximations. This task offers, for the first time, the possibility of detecting these patients' elusive impairment in the laboratory.

My colleagues and I have considered several possibilities for why the target patients make choices that have high immediate reward but severe delayed punishment. The first is that patients are so sensitive to reward that the pro-spect of future (delayed) punishment is outweighed by that of immediate gain. The second is that they are insensitive to punishment, and thus the prospect of reward always prevails, even if they are not abnormally sensitive to reward. The third is that they are generally insensitive to future consequences, positive or negative, and thus their behaviour is mostly guided by immediate prospects. We also considered mechanisms behind these three possibilities. For instance, an apparent sensitivity to immediate reward might be caused by defective response inhibition. This would assume that previous learning in comparable situations would have led to a systematic suppression of a prior, more basic drive to reach for reward. There is much in both animal and human studies to support this idea (see, for instance, Diamond 1990 and Chapter 6; Dias et al. 1996). But the complexity of the task, the wealth of knowledge available to the minds of the players, and the length of time over which the result continues to be consistently obtained, makes this mechanism implausible as the sole source of the defect. A change in the task's design (placing punishment up front and using unpredictable reward schedules as the unexpected variable) reveals that the patients continue to behave the same way, which goes against both the possibility of hypersensitivity to reward and insensitivity to punishment (Anderson et al. 1996).

Our preferred account, given evidence from other studies to indicate that these patients retain and access the knowledge necessary to conjure up options of actions and scenarios of future outcomes and yet fail to act on such know-ledge, is that a lack of both covert as well as overt markers for scenarios of future outcome, fails to provide helpful 'positive' signals to guide the perform-ance and thus cannot counteract the influence of 'negative' signals (Bechara et *al.* 1994). It is also possible that the somatic marker failure weakens support processes such as attention and working memory thus rendering unstable the representations of future outcomes that these patients evoke. In other words, the representations would not be held in working memory long enough for attention to enhance them and for reasoning strategies to operate on them. This mechanism invokes a defect along the lines proposed for behavioural domains dependent on dorsolateral prefrontal cortex networks (Goldman-Rakic 1987), also invoked in other accounts of frontal lobe defect (see Fuster 1989; Posner & Petersen 1990; Baddeley 1995).

The psychophysiological dimension of the gambling experiments

In a further test to the somatic marker test hypothesis we undertook a continuous monitoring of SCRS, while normal subjects and patients were engaged in the gambling task (Bechara *et al.* 1996). The most salient result of this study was the finding that, in normal subjects, during the time window that precedes the selection of a card from a given deck—an interval of about four seconds— normal subjects begin to respond with high amplitude skin conductance responses whenever they are about to make a selection from a bad deck. They show no comparable responses when they are about to make a selection from a good deck. As the task unfolds, the SCRS to the bad decks continue to appear systematically and they rise in amplitude. This does not happen for the responses associated with the good decks. Quite remarkably, no such anticipatory responses are seen in the patients with ventromedial frontal damage, who do show, nonetheless, normal SCRS to actual loss of money; that is, SCRS to punishment.

One possible interpretation is that the SCR is part of a very early and automated alarm signal, which is triggered, as proposed in the somatic marker hypothesis, from the ventromedial region. The signal affects further processing of the factual knowledge connected with the situation by marking a particular option-outcome pair with a negative bias. Incidentally, this interpretation holds whether the signal is overt and fully appreciated in consciousness, or covert and entirely operated at an unconscious level.

An alternative interpretation is that normal subjects reason, early on, that certain decks are bad and certain decks are good, and that on the basis of their cognition of 'badness' and 'goodness', they generate a somatic response which is indexed by the SCR. I find the latter interpretation less plausible for reasons that have to do with my perspective on the evolutionary biology and adaptive value of an automated somatic marker device. Moreover, recent studies in our laboratory suggest that normal subjects begin producing their SCRS to bad decks long before they have, according to their testimony, any notion whatsoever of the good or evil nature of each deck and of the design of the game they are playing (Bechara *et al.* 1997).

Acknowledgements

Supported in part by NIH NINDS POl NS19632.

References

Amaral, D. G. & Price, J. L. 1984 Amygdalo-cortical projections in the monkey (*Macaca fascicularis*). *J. Comp. Neurol.* **230**, 465–96.

Anderson, S. W., Bechara, W., Tranel, D., Damasio, H. & Damasio, A. R. 1996 Characterization of the decision-making defect of subjects with ventromedial frontal lobe damage. *Society for Neuroscience Abstracts*, **22**, 1108.

Baddeley, A. 1995 *Handbook of memory disorders* (ed. A. D. Baddeley, B. A. Wilson, & F. N. Watts), pp. 1–26. New York: John Wiley and Sons Ltd.

Bechara, A., Damasio, A. R., Damasio, H. & Anderson, S. W. 1994. Insensitivity to future consequences following damage to human prefrontal cortex. *Cognition* **50**, 7–12.

Bechara, A., Tranel, D., Damasio, H. & Damasio, A. R. 1996 Failure to respond autonomically to anticipated future outcomes following damage to prefrontal cortex. *Cerebral Cortex*, **6**, 215–25.

Bechara, A., Damasio, H., Tranel, D. & Damasio, A. R. 1997 Deciding advantageously before knowing the advantageous strategy. *Science* **275**, 1293–5.

Chavis, D. A. & Pandya, D. N. 1976 Further observations on corticofrontal connections in the rhesus monkey. *Brain Res.* **117**, 369–86.

Clugnet, C., LeDoux, J. E., Morrison, S. F. & Reis, D. J. 1988 Short latency orthodromic action potentials evoked in amygdala and caudate-putamen by stimulation of the medial geniculate body. *Society for Neuroscience Abstracts* **14**: 1227.

Damasio, A. R. 1979 The frontal lobes. In *Clinical neuropsychology* (ed. K. M. Heilman & E. Valenstein), pp. 360–412. New York: Oxford University Press.

Damasio, A. R. 1989*a* The brain binds entities and events by multiregional activation from convergence zones. *Neural Computation* **1**, 123–32.

Damasio, A. R. 1989*b* Time-locked multiregional retroactivation: A systems level proposal for the neural substrates of recall and recognition. *Cognition* **33**, 25–62.

Damasio, A. R. 1994 *Descartes' error: emotion, reason, and the human brain*. New York: Grosset/Putnam.

Damasio, A. R. 1995*a* On some functions of the human prefrontal cortex. In *Structure and functions of the human prefrontal cortex* (ed. K. Holyoak). *Proc. N.Y. Acad. Sci.* **769**, 241–51.

Damasio, A. R. 1995*b* Toward a neurobiology of emotion and feeling: operational concepts and hypotheses. *The Neuroscientist* **1**, 19–25.

Damasio, A. R. & Damasio, H. 1994 Cortical systems for retrieval of concrete knowledge: the convergence zone framework. In *Large-scale neuronal theories of the brain* (ed. C. Koch), pp. 61–74. Cambridge, MA: MIT Press.

Damasio, A. R., Tranel, D. & Damasio, H. 1990 Individuals with sociopathic behavior caused by frontal damage fail to respond autonomically to social stimuli. *Beh. Brain Res.* **41**, 81.

Damasio, A. R., Tranel, D. & Damasio, H. 1991 Somatic markers and the guidance of behavior: theory and preliminary testing. In *Frontal lobe function and dysfunction* (ed.

H. S. Levin, H. M. Eisenberg & A. L. Benton), pp. 217–29. New York: Oxford University Press.

Diamond, A. 1990 Developmental time course in human infants and infant monkeys, and the neural bases of inhibitory control in reaching. In *The development and neural bases of higher cognitive functions* (ed. A. Diamond), pp. 637–69. New York: Annals New York Academy of Sciences.

Dias, R., Robbins, T. W. & Roberts, A. C. 1996 Dissociation in prefrontal cortex of affective and attentional shifts. *Nature, Lond.* **380**, 69–72.

Farb, C. F., Ruggiero, D. A. & LeDoux, J. E. 1988 Projections from the acoustic thalamus terminate in the lateral but not central amygdala. *Society for Neuroscience Abstracts* **14**, 1227.

Fuster, J. M. 1989 *The prefrontal cortex: anatomy, physiology and neuropsychology of the frontal lobe*, 2nd edn. New York: Raven Press.

Goldman-Rakic, P. S. 1987 Circuitry of primate prefrontal cortex and regulation of behavior by representational memory. In *Handbook of physiology: the nervous system* (ed. F. Plum & V. Mountcastle), **5**, 373–401. Bethesda, MD: The American Physiological Society.

Goldman-Rakic, P. S., Selemon, L. D. & Schwartz, M. L. 1984 Dual pathways connecting the dorsolateral prefrontal cortex with the hippocampal formation and para-hippocampal cortex in the rhesus monkey. *Neuroscience* **12**, 719–43.

Hall, R. E., Livingston, R. B. & Bloor, C. M. 1977 Orbital cortical influences on cardiovascular dynamics and myocardial structure in conscious monkeys. *J. Neurosurg.* **46**, 638–47.

Jones, E. G. & Powell, T. P. S. 1970 An anatomical study of converging sensory pathways within the cerebral cortex of the monkey. *Brain* **93**, 793–820.

Milner, B. 1963 Effects of different brain lesions on card sorting. *Arch. Neurol.* **9**, 90–100.

Milner, B. 1964 Some effects of frontal lobectomy in man. In *The frontal granular cortex and behavior* (ed. J. M. Warren & K. Akert). New York: McGraw-Hill.

Milner, B., Petrides, M. & Smith, M. L. 1985 Frontal lobes and the temporal organization of memory. *Human Neurobiology* **4**, 137–42.

Nauta, W. J. H. 1971 The problem of the frontal lobe: a reinterpretation. *J. Psychiatr. Res.* **8**, 167–87.

Pandya, D. N. & Kuypers, H. G. J. M. 1969 Corticocortical connections in the rhesus monkey. *Brain Res.* **13**, 13–36.

Pandya, D. N. & Yeterian E. H. 1996 Morphological correlations of human and monkey frontal lobe. In *Neurobiology of decision making* (ed. A. R. Damasio, H. Damasio & Y. Christen), pp. 13–46. New York: Springer Verlag.

Petrides, M. & Milner, B. 1982 Deficits on subject-ordered tasks after frontal and temporal lobe lesions in man. *Neuropsychologia* **20**, 249–62.

Petrides, M. & Pandya, D. N. 1995 Comparative architectonic analysis of the human and macaque frontal cortex. In *Handbook of neuropsychology* (ed. J. Grafman & F. Boller). Amsterdam: Elsevier Science Publishers BV.

Porrino, L. J., Crane, A. M. & Goldman-Rakic, P. S. 1981 Direct and indirect pathways from the amygdala to the frontal lobe in rhesus monkeys. *J. Comp. Neurol.* **198**, 121–36.

Posner, M. I. & Petersen, S. E. 1990 The attention system of the human brain. *Ann. Rev. Neurosci.* **13**, 25–42.

Potter, H. & Nauta, W. J. H. 1979 A note on the problem of olfactory associations of the orbitofrontal cortex in the monkey. *Neuroscience* **4**, 316–67.

Saver, J. L. & Damasio, A. R. 1991 Preserved access and processing of social knowledge in a patient with acquired sociopathy due to ventromedial frontal damage. *Neuropsychologia* **29**, 1241–49.

Shallice, T. & Burgess, P. W. 1993 Supervisory control of action and thought selection. In *Attention: selection, awareness, and control: a tribute to Donald Broadbent* (ed. A. Baddeley & L. Weiskrantz), pp. 171–87. Oxford: Clarendon Press.

Shallice, T. & Evans, M. E. 1978 The involvement of the frontal lobes in cognitive estimation. *Cortex* **14**, 294–303.

Tranel, D. 1994 'Acquired sociopathy': the development of sociopathic behavior following focal brain damage. In *Progress in experimental personality and psychopathology research* (ed. D. C. Fowles, P. Sutker & S. H. Goodman), **17**, 285–311. New York: Springer.

Tranel, D. & Damasio, A. R. 1993 The covert learning of affective valence does not require structures in hippocampal system or amygdala. *J. Cog. Neurosci.* **5**, 79–88.

Tranel, D., Damasio, H. & Damasio, A. R. 1995 Double dissociation between overt and covert face recognition. *J. Cog. Neurosci.* **7**, 425–32.

Van Hoesen, G. W., Pandya, D. N. & Butters, N. 1972 Cortical afferents to the entorhinal cortex of the rhesus monkey. *Science, Wash.* **175**, 1471–73.

Van Hoesen, G. W., Pandya, D. N. & Butters, N. 1975 Some connections of the entorhinal (area 28) and perirhinal (area 35) cortices of the rhesus monkey: II. Frontal lobe afferents. *Brain Res.* **95**, 25–38.

5

Comparison of prefrontal architecture and connections

D. N. Pandya and E. H. Yeterian

5.1 Introduction

The various areas of the prefrontal cortex (PFC) seem to contribute to specific and differential functions. In the human, on the basis of clinical syndromes as well as brain imaging studies, it has been suggested that whereas the ventro-medial PFC is involved in decision-making processes, the lateral portion has a role in working memory, planning and sequencing of behaviour, language, and attention. Likewise, in non-human primates, experimental studies have shown that the ventrolateral PFC has a role in response inhibition, whereas the dorsolateral PFC is implicated in spatial processes, working memory and sequencing of behaviour. The caudal PFC is reported to be involved in atten-tional mechanisms (e.g. Goldberg & Bruce 1985). Some of these functions are limited to one or two specific architectonic areas (e.g. Fuster 1989; Damasio & Anderson 1993; Wilson *et al.* 1993).

The areal designations in architectonic maps of PFC in monkeys and humans do not coincide in certain cases. Thus, it becomes difficult to relate results obtained from animal experimentation to findings in humans. To address this problem, Petrides & Pandya (1994) reanalysed and compared the architecture of PFC in human and monkey brains. Their results show that there is overall correspondence among all PFC areas in these brains. To facilitate such com-parison, existing numbering schemas have to be modified, albeit maintaining common nomenclature in the two species.

The functional role of a given cortical area *per se* in either human or monkey brains can be revealed by using imaging techniques or by experimental approaches. However, to understand more fully the contributions of a given cortical region to specific processes, it is important to know how that region is connected with other cerebral cortical areas. Substantial connectional data have been gathered by several investigators during the past three decades in non-human primates. Evidence of architectonic areal correspondence as described below allows one to extrapolate connectional relationships from monkeys to humans. We will describe connectional information from experiments in monkeys specifically designed to reveal afferent connectivity of prefrontal regions, and will briefly discuss functional implications.

5.2 Architectonics

Several investigators have developed architectonic maps of PFC in humans and monkeys (Brodmann 1905, 1909; Vogt & Vogt 1919; Economo & Koskinas 1925; Walker 1940; Bonin & Bailey 1947; Sarkissov et al. 1955; Barbas & Pandya 1989; Preuss & Goldman-Rakic 1991). An examination of Brodmann's (1905, 1909) maps (figures 5.1 a, b) reveals correspondence in nomenclature and location only for certain areas, namely 24, 25 and 32. Walker (1940; figure 5.1c) reinvestigated the architectonic organization of PFC in macaque monkeys,

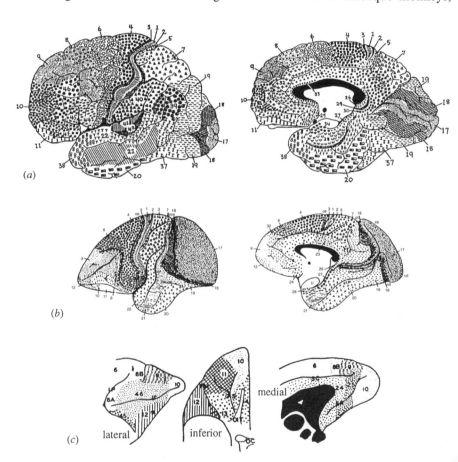

Fig. 5.1 (a) Cytoarchitectonic map of the human cerebral cortex by Brodmann (1909); (b) cytoarchitectonic maps of the cerebral cortex in monkeys by Brodmann (1905); (c) cytoarchitectonic maps of the prefrontal cortex in monkeys by Walker (1940).

with the intent of resolving some of the differences in nomenclature and location of areas with regard to Brodmann's human map. For example, consistent with Brodmann's map of the human brain, Walker localized area 10 in the monkey to the medial and lateral aspects of the frontal pole. However, the locations of other areas in Walker's map differ significantly from those of Brodmann. For example, Walker designated area 12 in the ventrolateral prefrontal region. In contrast, Brodmann termed a corresponding region in the human brain as area 47. Moreover, the relative size and extent of Walker's areas 9, 8 and 46 were different compared to areas of the same names designated by Brodmann in humans. The locations of areas 14, 13 and 11 were also inconsistent in Brodmann's human and Walker's monkey maps. Our maps, based on a reanalysis of architectonic features of PFC, attempt to resolve these differences (figure 5.2). We will provide only a brief summary of comparative architectonic descriptions below. A detailed presentation has been given elsewhere (Petrides & Pandya 1994).

(a) Area 44

In the human brain, this area is located in the pars opercularis, and constitutes the major portion of Broca's area. Architectonically, area 44 appears dysgranular, with large pyramidal neurons in deep layer III. Although well documented in humans, this area has not been delineated previously in monkeys (figure 5.1). According to our findings, an area with architectonic features corresponding to area 44 in the human brain is found in the caudal bank of the lower limb of the arcuate sulcus in monkeys (figure 5.2b). We have designated this cortical subregion in the monkey as area 44.

(b) Area 8

In both humans and monkeys, area 8 lies on the dorsolateral PFC, caudal to area 9 and rostral to area 6. Walker (1940) specified two subdivisions of this area, 8A in the concavity of the arcuate sulcus, and 8B located dorsally and extending toward midline (figure 5.1c). Although historically in the human brain this area has been delineated as a single entity, our findings indicate that it comprises two major subdivisions as in the monkey, designated 8A and 8B, based on architectonic features. Moreover, in both species, area 8A can be divided into dorsal (8Ad) and ventral (8Av) sectors (figure 5.2).

(c) Area 45

In the human brain, this area is located in the pars triangularis, in the inferior frontal gyrus. Walker (1940) placed area 45 in the monkey mainly within the rostral bank of the lower limb of the arcuate sulcus (figure 5.1c). According to our findings, area 45 is located not only within the sulcus, but also extends further rostrally on to the inferior prefrontal convexity. Moreover, on the basis

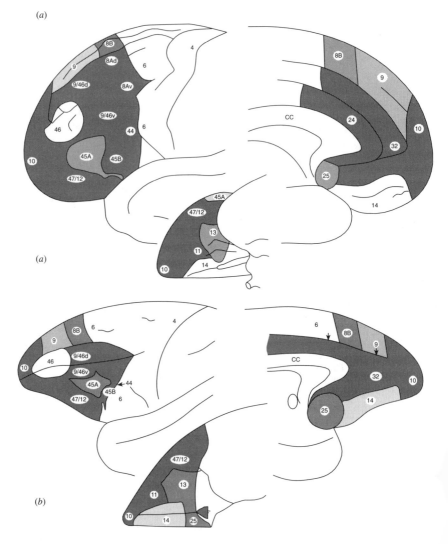

Fig. 5.2 Cytoarchitectonic maps of the lateral, medial, and ventral surfaces of the cerebral cortex of the human (*a*) and monkey (*b*) brain by Petrides & Pandya (1994).

of architectonic differences, we have divided this area into two sectors, 45A rostrally and 45B caudally, as in the human brain (figure 5.2).

(d) Areas 9 and 46

In both humans and monkeys, these areas occupy the mid- dorsolateral sector of the PFC. In the monkey brain, they appear to have a simple topographic relationship to one another, with area 9 dorsal to area 46 (figure 5.1*c*). In contrast, in the human brain, area 9 has been shown to encircle area 46, except for the rostral portion of the latter area (figure 5.1a). In the monkey, area 46 has been localized in and around the principal sulcus, and has been reported to have further subdivisions (Barbas & Pandya 1989; Preuss & Goldman-Rakic 1991). According to our analysis, area 9 in both the human and the monkey brain is located dorsal to area 46, and extends medially to the cingulate region. In the human brain, the part of area 9 caudal and ventral to area 46 has architectonic characteristics similar to caudal area 46 of the monkey. Therefore, this region previously delineated as ventral area 9 in the human brain and as caudal area 46 in the monkey brain has been designated as area 9/46 in both species (figure 5.2). Furthermore, we have subdivided area 9/46 into dorsal and ventral divisions, areas 9/46d and 9/46v, respectively.

(e) Areas 47 and 12

Brodmann (1909) described area 47 in the human brain as a region located ventral to area 45 and caudal to area 10, extending on to the lateral orbital surface (figure 5.1a). In the monkey, Walker (1940) outlined a topographically similar region, but designated it as area 12 (figure 5.1c). On the basis of their topographic as well as architectonic similarity, we have labelled these regions as area 47/12 in both species (figure 5.2).

(f) Area 13

Although Walker (1940) identified this area in the monkey as occupying the caudal part of the orbitofrontal cortex, in the human brain it has been subsumed within area 47 (figures 5.1a,c). According to our observations, this caudal orbital region has common architectonic features in both species. Therefore, on the basis of similar topography as well as morphology, we have labelled this region area 13 in the human brain (figure 5.2).

(g) Area 11

In the monkey, area 11 occupies a location between areas 13 and 10 on the orbital surface (figure 5.1c). In the human, in contrast, the region designated as area 11 has been localized within the gyrus rectus on the ventromedial surface of the hemisphere by Brodmann (1909; figure 5.1a). We have identified a region in the human brain with similar architectonic characteristics as area 11 in the monkey, located between areas 10 and 13 on the orbital surface, and have designated it as area 11 (figure 5.2).

(h) Area 14

This area in the monkey has been shown to occupy the gyrus rectus, and to be bordered by area 10 rostrally and area 25 caudally (figure 5.1c). In the human as mentioned above, the cortex in the area of the gyrus rectus has been delineated as areas 11 and 12. On the basis of topographic and architectonic similarities, we have designated this cortical region as area 14 in both species (figure 5.2).

5.3 Corticocortical connections

One approach that can be used to support the existence of discrete architectonic areas is to establish specific patterns of cortical connectivity for those areas. As a number of investigators have outlined the connections of PFC on the basis of earlier maps, we will restrict our discussion to differential inputs to some of the newly defined prefrontal areas, as revealed by the fluorescent retrograde tracing method.

(a) Dorsal prefrontal areas

In case 1, a fluorescent tracer (diamidino yellow, DY) was placed in dorsal area 6, rostral to the superior precentral dimple (figure 5.3). The retrograde labelling revealed a unique overall pattern of cortical inputs, both locally within the frontal lobe as well as distally from the post-Rolandic cortex. Thus, this area receives projections from areas 8B and 9 rostrally, and dorsal areas 6 and 4 caudally. Other inputs arise from the supplementary motor area (MII), the cortex in the depths of the cingulate sulcus corresponding to cingulate motor regions (e.g. He et al. 1995; Morecraft & Van Hoesen 1993) and area 24. This area receives post-Rolandic projections from the medial parietal region, including areas 31 and the supplementary sensory area (Murray & Coulter 1981). Another source of input is the caudal superior parietal lobule, and area 7A of the inferior parietal lobule (IPL).

In case 2, a retrograde tracer (Fast Blue, FB) was injected in area 8Ad in the dorsal concavity of the arcuate sulcus (figure 5.3). Local connections to this region are derived from areas 8B, 9, 9/46 and 45. Distant projections arise from area 31 on the medial surface and the caudal part of the lower bank of the intraparietal sulcus (IPS). Significant input to area 8Ad seems to come from the caudal superior temporal gyrus (STG), and from the caudal superior temporal sulcus (STS), including the multimodal area of the STS (MM-STS) and area MST.

An injection (FB) in area 8B revealed local connections from areas 8Ad, 9/46d, 9, and 6 (case 3, figure 5.4). This region also receives projections from areas 45, 47/12 and 46v, as well as area 11 on the orbital surface. From the medial surface, inputs are derived from areas 8B and 9, as well as from rostral area 24. Distant projections to this prefrontal region arise from caudal area 23, area 31 and the rostral part of medial area 19. Area 8B also receives input from the caudal IPL, rostral insular cortex, MM-STS and area TH of the parahippocampal gyrus.

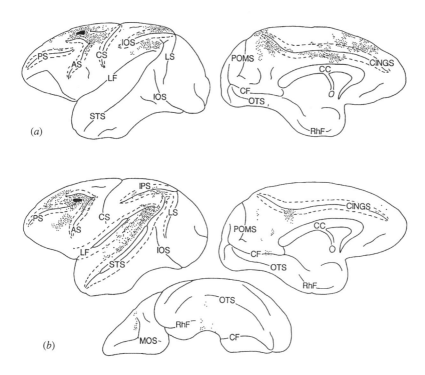

Fig. 5.3 Diagrammatic representations of the injection sites (shown in black) in (*a*) case 1 and (*b*) case 2, and the distribution of retrogradely labelled cells (shown as dots) on the lateral, medial, and ventral surfaces of the cerebral hemispheres. (Abbreviations in this and subsequent figures: AS, arcuate sulcus; CC, corpus callosum; CF, calcarine fissure; CING S, cingulate sulcus; CS, central sulcus; IOS, inferior occipital sulcus; IPS, intra-parietal sulcus; LF, lateral fissure; LS, lunate sulcus; MOS, medial orbital sulcus; OTS, occipitotemporal sulcus; POMS, medial parieto-occipital sulcus; PS, principal sulcus; RhF, rhinal fissure; STS, superior temporal sulcus.)

An injection (DY) in lateral area 9 demonstrated local connections from rostral area 9, area 8B, dorsal area 6 and area 8Ad (case 4, figure 5.4). Within the frontal lobe, areas 47/12, 11, 14, 13 and orbital area Pro (proisocortex) also project to lateral area 9. Substantial input is derived from the adjacent medial surface, including areas 8B, 9, 32 and rostral area 24. Distant projections originate from caudal area 23, retrosplenial cortex, rostral MM-STS and rostral STG. Finally, lateral area 9 receives input from area TH.

In case 5, an injection (FB) was placed in dorsal area 9/46 (figure 5.7). The basic pattern of afferent projections to this region was similar to that of the preceding case, with some minor variations. Thus, local projections originate rostrally from area 46, and caudally from areas 8B, 8Ad and 6. Other frontal afferents arise from the orbital surface, mainly from area 11. On the medial

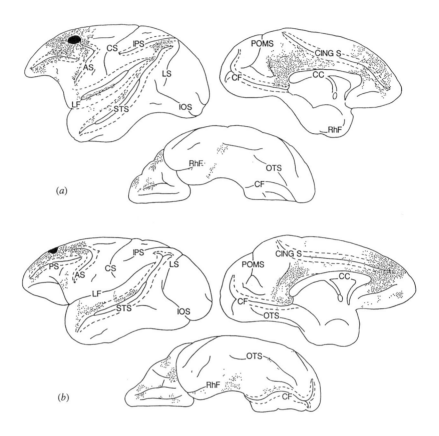

Fig. 5.4 Diagrammatic representations of the injection sites in (*a*) case 3 and (*b*) case 4, and the distribution of retrogradely labelled cells.

surface, areas 9, 32 and 24 send projections to dorsal area 9/46. Distant inputs to this region arise from area 23, retrosplenial cortex, the ventral part of the medial parietal region and medial area 19. Some projections also are derived from rostral MM-STS, rostral STG, and area TH.

(b) Ventral prefrontal areas

In case 6, an injection (DY) was placed in area 44 of the caudal bank of the inferior limb of the arcuate sulcus (figure 5.5). Local projections to this region arise from areas 9/46v, 47/12, 13, orbital area Pro and ventral area 6. Area 44 also receives input from the dorsal part of area MII, the cingulate motor region and caudal area 24. Distant projections are derived from the dorsal Sylvian opercular cortex including areas proM and SII, and from the rostral insula. Substantial connections also arise from the rostral and

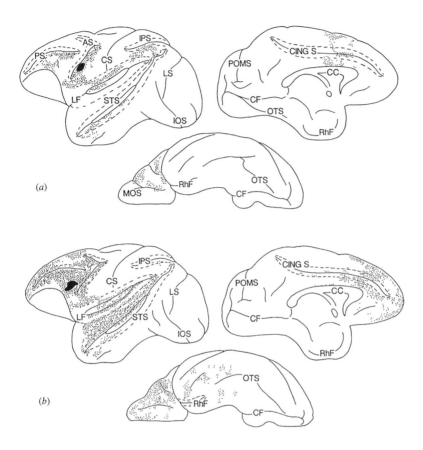

Fig 5.5   Diagrammatic representations of the injection sites in (*a*) case 6 and (*b*) case 7, and the distribution of retrogradely labelled cells.

middle IPL. Some projections are derived from the rostral part of the lower bank of the STS.

In case 7, an injection (FB) was placed in area 45 (figure 5.5). This area receives projections from virtually all divisions of the prefrontal cortex, with the exception of most of area 9/46d. Unlike the preceding case, a significant amount of input is derived from the entire STG, and the cortex of the circular sulcus. Area proM and the precentral portions of areas 2 and 1 also seem to give rise to projections to this region. A notable amount of input is derived from the caudal insular cortex, the entire extent of MM-STS and area MST. Other connections originate from the rostral inferotemporal region, and from the rostral parahippocampal gyrus, mainly area TL (Rosene & Pandya 1983).

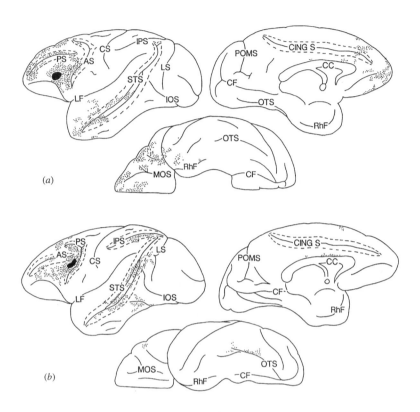

Fig 5.6 Diagrammatic representations of the injection sites in (*a*) case 8 and (*b*) case 9, and the distribution of retrogradely labelled cells.

An injection (DY) in area 47/12 (case 8, figure 5.6) revealed local projections arising from areas 45 and 9/46v caudally, and from area 10 rostrally. Area 47/12 also receives input from dorsal area 46 and from area 9. Distinct foci within areas 14, 10, 11 and 13 on the orbital surface, and areas 14, 32 and 9 on the medial surface, send projections to this area. Distant connections arise from the rostral temporal lobe, including rostral area TL, the inferotemporal region, rostral MM- STS, and rostral STG.

An injection (FB) was placed in area 8Av in the lower bank of the arcuate sulcus (case 9, figure 5.6). Local afferent projections are relatively sparse and are derived from areas 8Ad and 8B dorsally, and 45, 47/12 and 46 rostrally. Distant projections originate from the lower bank of IPS, the lower bank and depths of STS and caudal MM-STS. Other connections arise from the caudal inferotemporal area and from lateral area V4.

Finally, an injection (DY) was placed in area 9/46v (case 10, figure 5.7). Local projections are derived from rostroventral area 46, and areas 47/12, 11 and 13

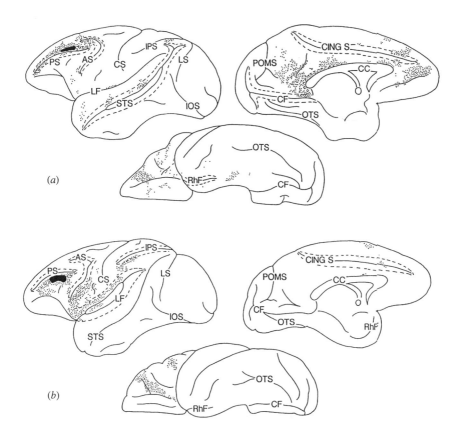

Fig. 5.7 Diagrammatic representations of the injection sites in (*a*) case 5 and (*b*) case 10, and the distribution of retrogradely labelled cells.

Distant connections arise from ventral area 6, area proM, opercular area SII, rostral IPL and rostral insula.

5.4 Conclusion

The architectonic areas that have been redesignated to correspond to each other in the monkey and the human brain appear to have common morphological features. It should be emphasized that although there are common patterns of laminar distribution of neurons for any pair of corresponding areas in the human and the monkey brain, this should not be construed as implying that these areas have identical cellular composition.

Each architectonically distinct prefrontal region, as studied in the monkey brain, has been shown to have a distinctive overall pattern of cortical connectivity. In regard to local (intrinsic prefrontal) connections, areas above the principal sulcus tend to have input mainly from dorsal and medial prefrontal regions, whereas those below the principal sulcus have input predominantly from ventrolateral and orbital cortices. There is evidence for certain prefrontal areas having much more diverse local afferents, e.g. area 45 receives significant input from dorsal and medial as well as ventrolateral and orbital prefrontal regions. Likewise, dorsal areas 9 and 9/46 have significant connections from various orbital regions.

With regard to post-Rolandic inputs to PFC, architectonically distinct areas have differential connectional relationships. For example, dorsal area 6 has inputs predominantly from sensory-motor regions (frontal, parietal and cingulate), as well as from area 7A involved in visuospatial functions, and limbic input from area 24. In contrast, lateral area 9 has a different pattern of afferent connectivity. Thus, this region has its main inputs from limbic-related areas, such as area 32, rostral area 24, area 23, caudal orbitofrontal cortex, retrosplenial cortex and parahippocampal gyrus, as well as from multimodal cortex (MM-STS). Area 9/46d has a pattern of afferent connections basically similar to that of lateral area 9, except that it has much stronger inputs from orbitofrontal area 11, from retrosplenial cortex and from medial area 19 (visuospatial input).

On the basis of architectonic studies, three subdivisions have been demarcated for area 8 in both the human and the monkey brain. In terms of connections, area 8B, which is situated between area 6 caudally and area 9 rostrally, has different inputs compared to both adjoining areas as well as other subdivisions of area 8. Thus, major inputs to area 8B are derived from limbic regions such as rostral area 24, area 23, retrosplenial cortex, parahippocampal gyrus and rostral insula. Area 8B receives other inputs of a visuospatial nature from medial area 19 and caudal IPL, as well as inputs from MM-STS. Area 8Ad, like area 8B, receives projections from visuospatial regions, namely caudal IPL. However, it receives little input from limbic related areas. Additionally, area 8Ad has significant afferents from auditory-related areas of STG, visually-related area MST and caudal MM-STS. In contrast to the other divisions of area 8, area 8Av has inputs mainly from visually-related cortices, in the lower bank of IPS and in STS, and in the lateral extrastriate and caudal inferotemporal regions. In short, area 8B has preferential connections from limbic-related areas, 8Ad from visuospatial and audiospatial areas, and 8Av from areas relating to central as well as peripheral vision. It should be pointed out that in a recent review, Paus (1996) has challenged the notion that area 8 in the human brain represents the location of the frontal eye field, although such a relationship appears to be the case in monkeys. Therefore, further studies are needed to address the functional role of area 8 in humans.

Within the ventral prefrontal region, there appear to be different overall patterns of afferent inputs to areas 44, 45 and 47/12. Connections to area 44, the homologue of Broca's area pars opercularis in humans, arise mainly from somatosensory-related regions in the Sylvian operculum—area SII, as well as rostral IPL corresponding to the supramarginal gyrus. Area 44 receives only minor projections from the visually related areas of the inferotemporal region. In contrast, input to area 45, the homologue of Broca's area pars triangularis in the human brain, is derived mainly from auditory association areas of STG and the cortex of the circular sulcus, and from MM-STS. Area 45 has minor connections from the somatosensory cortices of the rostral Sylvian operculum, and from visual areas of the rostral inferotemporal region. Finally, this area receives connections from limbic regions—area 24, insular cortex and area TL. Area 47/12 also is considered to belong to the rostral part of Broca's area, pars orbitalis, in the human brain. Inputs to this region are derived from somato-sensory area SII and from visual inferotemporal areas. Area 47/12 has only minor inputs from limbic-related cortices. Finally, inputs to area 9/46v, com-pared to those of Broca's related areas, are derived predominantly from soma-tosensory regions of the Sylvian operculum and from rostral IPL. Thus, each architectonically distinct area below the principal sulcus has a unique overall pattern of cortical connectivity.

The overall executive role of PFC undoubtedly depends on the integrated activity of diverse architectonic regions. Nevertheless, a consideration of con-nectional relationships of various morphologically distinct prefrontal areas suggests the existence of two broad categories. In general, prefrontal areas above the principal sulcus are related preferentially to post-Rolandic cortices located on the medial surface as well as dorsolaterally. In contrast, prefrontal areas below the principal sulcus are linked strongly with post-Rolandic regions located ventrolaterally and ventromedially. Within each of these categories of frontal regions, there seem to be differing patterns of cortical connectivity as one progresses farther rostrally within PFC. The caudolateral frontal region above the principal sulcus (areas 6 and 8Ad) receives input mainly from somatomotor association areas relating to the trunk and limbs, and from areas involved in visuospatial and audiospatial processes. In contrast, more rostral areas (9 and 9/46d) receive input predominantly from limbic regions and multimodal areas. Consistent with their morphological and con-nectional specificity, these dorsal frontal regions appear to have different over-all functional roles. Thus, whereas caudal regions are involved in conditional response tasks and in attentional processes, more rostral regions have a role in spatial functions and in working memory (e.g. Goldman-Rakic 1987; Petrides 1987, 1991; Wilson *et al* 1993)

Similar differential anatomical and functional correlations can be observed for frontal regions below the principal sulcus. Thus, the caudal region receives input mainly from modality-specific regions—area 44 from somatomotor asso-ciation areas relating to the head, neck and face, as well as from inferior parietal association areas, and area 8Av from areas relating to central vision. Function-ally, area 44 has been shown to have a role in higher-order programming of orofacial movement, whereas area 8Av is involved in visual attentional pro-cesses regarding objects (Suzuki 1985; Rizzolatti *et al.* 1988). In contrast, area 47/12 receives its main input from the rostral inferotemporal area, and appears to be involved in a number of functions, including response inhibition and the appreciation of the behavioural significance of stimuli (e.g. Iversen & Mishkin 1970; Suzuki & Azuma 1977). Area 9/46v has inputs predominantly from area SII and from insular and somatomotor association areas, and has been proposed to have a role in working memory for orofacial functions (Preuss & Goldman-Rakic 1989). Finally, area 45 has a distinctive pattern of connections, and receives significant input from auditory association areas, as well as from somatomotor and visual regions. This area also receives substantial projections from multimodal areas and from the insula. Although the precise functional nature of this region in monkeys is not well understood, area 45 corresponds to the pars triangularis of Broca's area in the human brain, which is known to have a role in language function. The fact that area 45 in the monkey receives strong input from the superior temporal region is suggestive of involvement in non-verbal communication.

Exactly how discrete prefrontal architectonic regions and their differential connections contribute to the executive role of the frontal lobe remains to be determined. Nevertheless, processes such as attention, working memory and response inhibition can be viewed as key components of a general capacity for effecting appropriate behaviour. To that end, our results are consistent with an overall dichotomy between dorsal and ventral frontal regions, with the former involved in spatial functions and the latter in processes in which specific stimuli are the focus of behaviour (e.g. Fuster 1989; Wilson *et al.* 1993). Alternatively, Petrides (1994, 1995) has suggested that ventrolateral PFC areas play a role in active encoding and retrieval of specific information held in visual, auditory and somatosensory association areas with which they are connected. This would allow for selection, comparison and decision processes regarding information held in short- and long-term memory. The mid-dorsolateral PFC, in contrast, is thought to be involved when information that has been retrieved must be monitored and manipulated in the planning and execution of behaviour. It may be the combination of these various processes that underlies the full executive function of PFC.

References

Barbas, H. & Pandya, D. N. 1989 Architecture and intrinsic connections of the prefrontal cortex in the rhesus monkey. *J. Comp. Neurol.* **286**, 353–75.

Bonin, G. von & Bailey, P. 1947 *The neocortex of the Macaca mulatta.* Urbana, IL: University of Illinois Press.

Brodmann, K. 1905 Beitraege zur histologischen Lokalisation der Grosshirnrinde: III. Mitteilung. Die Rindenfelder der niederen Affen. *J. Psychol. Neurol.* **4**, 177–206.

Brodmann, K. 1909 *Vergleichende Lokalisationslehre der Grosshirnrinde in ihren Prinzipien dargestellt auf Grund des Zellenbaues.* Leipzig: Barth.

Damasio, A. R. & Anderson, S. W. 1993 The frontal lobes. In *Clinical neuropsychology* 3rd edn (ed. K. M. Heilman & E. Valenstein), pp. 409–60. New York: Oxford University Press.

Economo, C. von & Koskinas, G. N. 1925 *Die Cytoarchitektonik der Hirnrinde des erwachsenen Menschen*. Berlin: Springer.

Fuster, J. M. 1989 *The prefrontal cortex*, 2nd edn (*Anatomy, physiology, and neuropsychology of the frontal lobe*). New York: Raven Press.

Goldberg, M. E., & Bruce, C. J. 1985 Cerebral cortical activity associated with the orientation of visual attention in the rhesus monkey. *Vision Res.* **25**, 471–81.

Goldman-Rakic, P. S. 1987 Circuitry of primate prefrontal cortex and regulation of behavior by representational memory. In *Handbook of physiology*, vol. 5, pt *1* (ed. V. B. Mountcastle & F. Plum), pp. 373–417. Bethesda, MD: American Physiological Society.

He, S., Dum, R. P. & Strick, P. L. 1995 Topographic organization of corticospinal projections from the frontal lobe: motor areas on the medial surface of the hemisphere. *J. Neurosci.* **15**, 3284–306.

Iversen, S. D. & Mishkin, M. 1970 Perseverative interference in monkeys following selective lesions of the inferior prefrontal convexity. *Exp. Brain Res.* **11**, 376–86.

Morecraft, R. J. & Van Hoesen, G. W. 1993 Frontal granular cortex input to the cingulate (M3), supplementary (M2) and primary (M1) motor cortices in the rhesus monkey. *J. Comp. Neurol.* **337**, 669–89.

Murray, E. A. & Coulter, J. D. 1981 Supplementary sensory area: The medial parietal cortex in the monkey. In *Cortical sensory organization*, vol. 1 (*Multiple somatic areas*) (ed. C. N. Woolsey), pp. 167–95. Clifton, NJ: Humana Press.

Paus, T. 1996 Location and function of the human frontal eye- field: a selective review. *Neuropsychologia* **34**, 475–83.

Petrides, M. 1987 Conditional learning and the primate frontal cortex. In *The frontal lobes revisited*. (ed. E. Perecman), pp. 91–108. New York: The IRBN Press.

Petrides, M. 1991 Functional specialization within the dorsolateral frontal cortex for serial order memory. *Proc. R. Soc. Lond.* B **246**, 299–306.

Petrides, M. 1994 Frontal lobes and working memory. In *Handbook of neuropsychology*, vol. 9 (ed. F. Boller & J. Grafman), pp. 59–82. Amsterdam: Elsevier Science B.V.

Petrides, M. 1995 Functional organization of the human frontal cortex for mnemonic processing: Evidence from neuroimaging studies. *Ann. N.Y. Acad. Sci.* **769**, 85–96.

Petrides, M. & Pandya, D. N. 1994 Comparative architectonic analysis of the human and macaque frontal cortex. In *Handbook of neuropsychology*, vol. 9 (ed. F. Boller & J. Grafman), pp. 17–58. Amsterdam: Elsevier Science B.V.

Preuss, T. M. & Goldman-Rakic, P. S. 1989 Connections of the ventral granular frontal cortex of macaques with perisylvian premotor and somatosensory areas: anatomical evidence for somatic representation in primate frontal association cortex. *J. Comp. Neurol.* **282**, 293–316.

Preuss, T. M. & Goldman-Rakic, P. S. 1991 Myelo-and cytoarchitecture of the granular frontal cortex and surrounding regions in the strepsirhine primate *Galago* and the anthropoid primate *Macaca*. *J. Comp. Neurol.* **310**, 429–74.

Rizzolatti, G., Camarda, R., Fogassi, L., Gentilucci, M., Luppino, G. & Matelli, M. 1988 Functional organization of inferior area 6 in the macaque monkey: II. Area F5 and the control of distal movements. *Exp. Brain Res.* **71**, 491–507.

Rosene, D. L. & Pandya, D. N. 1983 Architectonics and connections of the posterior parahippocampal gyrus in the rhesus monkey. *Soc. Neurosci. Abstr.* **9**, 222.

Sarkissov, S. A., Filimonoff, I. N., Kononowa, E. P. & Preobraschenskaja, I. S. 1955 *Atlas of the cytoarchitectonics of the human cerebral cortex*. Moscow: Medgiz.

Suzuki, H. 1985 Distribution and organization of visual and auditory neurons in the monkey prefrontal cortex. *Vision Res.* **25**, 465–69.

Suzuki, H. & Azuma, M. 1977 Prefrontal unit activity during gazing at a light spot in the monkey. *Brain Res.* **126**, 497–508.

Vogt, C. & Vogt, O. 1919 Allgemeinere Ergebnisse unserer Hirnforschung. *J. Psychol. Neurol.* **25**, 279–462.

Walker, A. E. 1940 A cytoarchitectural study of the prefrontal area of the macaque monkey. *J. Comp. Neurol.* **73**, 59–86.

Wilson, F. A. W., Scalhaide, S. P. O. & Goldman-Rakic, P. S. 1993 Dissociation of object and spatial processing domains in primate prefrontal cortex. *Science* **260**, 1955–58.

6

The orbitofrontal cortex

Edmund T. Rolls

6.1 Introduction

The prefrontal cortex is the cortex that receives projections from the medio-dorsal nucleus of the thalamus and is situated in front of the motor and premotor cortices (Areas 4 and 6) in the frontal lobe. Based on the divisions of the mediodorsal nucleus, the prefrontal cortex may be divided into three main regions (Fuster 1989). First, the magnocellular, medial, part of the me-diodorsal nucleus projects to the orbital (ventral) surface of the prefrontal cortex (which includes Areas 13 and 12). It is called the orbitofrontal cortex, and receives information from the ventral or object-processing visual stream, and taste, olfactory and somatosensory inputs. Second, the parvocellular, lateral, part of the mediodorsal nucleus projects to the dorsolateral prefrontal cortex. This part of the prefrontal cortex receives inputs from the parietal cortex, and is involved in tasks such as spatial short-term memory tasks (Rosenkilde 1979; Fuster 1989). Third, the pars paralamellaris (most lateral) part of the mediodorsal nucleus projects to the frontal eye fields (Area 8) in the anterior bank of the arcuate sulcus.

The orbitofrontal cortex is considered in this paper. The cortex on the orbital surface of the frontal lobe includes Area 13 caudally, and Area 14 medially, and the cortex on the inferior convexity includes Area 12 caudally and Area 11 anteriorly (see figure 6.1 and Carmichael & Price 1994; Petrides & Pandya 1995). This brain region is poorly developed in rodents, but well developed in primates including humans. To understand the function of this brain region in humans, the majority of the studies described were therefore performed with macaques or with humans.

6.2 Connections

Rolls *et al.* (1990) discovered a taste area in the lateral part of the orbitofrontal cortex, and showed that this was the secondary taste cortex in that it receives a major projection from the primary taste cortex (Baylis *et al.* 1994). More medially, there is an olfactory area (Rolls & Baylis 1994). Anatomically, there are direct connections from the primary olfactory cortex, pyriform cortex, to

area 13a of the posterior orbitofrontal cortex, which in turn has onward
projections to a middle part of the orbitofrontal cortex (area 11) (Price *et al.*
1991; Morecraft *et al.* 1992; Barbas 1993; Carmichael *et al.* 1994) (see figures
6.1 and 6.2). Visual inputs reach the orbitofrontal cortex directly from the
inferior temporal cortex, the cortex in the superior temporal sulcus, and the
temporal pole (Jones & Powell 1970; Barbas 1988, 1993; Petrides & Pandya,
1988; Seltzer & Pandya 1989; Barbas & Pandya 1989; Morecraft *et al.* 1992;
Barbas 1995). There are corresponding auditory inputs (Barbas 1988, 1993),
and somatosensory inputs from somatosensory cortical areas 1, 2 and SII in the
frontal and pericentral operculum, and from the insula (Barbas 1988; Preuss &
Goldman-Rakic 1989). The caudal orbitofrontal cortex receives strong inputs
from the amygdala (e.g. Price *et al.* 1991). The orbitofrontal cortex also receives
inputs via the mediodorsal nucleus of the thalamus, pars magnocellularis,
which itself receives afferents from temporal lobe structures such as the prepyri-
form (olfactory) cortex, amygdala and inferior temporal cortex (Nauta 1972;
Krettek & Price 1974, 1977). The orbitofrontal cortex projects back to temporal
lobe areas such as the inferior temporal cortex, and, in addition, to the entorhinal cortex (or 'gateway to the hippocampus') and cingulate cortex (Nauta

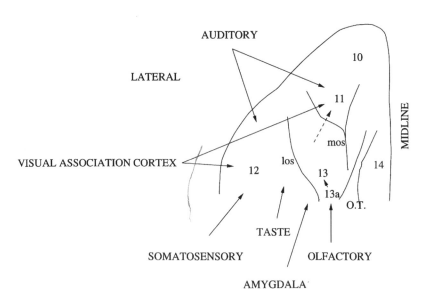

Fig. 6.1 Ventral view of the macaque orbitofrontal cortex. The midline is on the left of
the diagram, and the inferior convexity is laterally, on the right. Subdivisions (after
Barbas & Pandya 1989) and some afferents to the orbitofrontal cortex are shown, mos
medial orbital sulcus; los lateral orbital sulcus.

1964; Insausti *et al.* 1987). The orbitofrontal cortex also projects to the preoptic region and lateral hypothalamus, to the ventral tegmental area (Nauta 1964; Johnson *et al.* 1968), and to the head of the caudate nucleus (Kemp & Powell 1970). Reviews of the cytoarchitecture and connections of the orbitofrontal cortex are provided by Carmichael & Price (1994), Barbas (1995), Petrides & Pandya (1995) and Pandya & Yeterian (1996).

6.3 Effects of lesions of the orbitofrontal cortex

Macaques with lesions of the orbitofrontal cortex are impaired at tasks which involve learning about which stimuli are rewarding and which are not, and especially in altering behaviour when reinforcement contingencies change. The monkeys may respond when responses are inappropriate for example they are no longer rewarded, or may respond to a non-rewarded stimulus. For example, monkeys with orbitofrontal damage are impaired on go–no go task performance, in that they go on the no go trials (Iversen & Mishkin, 1970), in an object reversal task in that they respond to the object which was formerly rewarded with food, and in extinction in that they continue to respond to an object which is no longer rewarded (Butter 1969; Jones & Mishkin 1972). There is some evidence for dissociation of function within the orbitofrontal cortex, in that lesions to the inferior convexity produce the go–no go and object reversal deficits, whereas damage to the caudal orbitofrontal cortex, area 13, produces the extinction deficit (Rosenkilde 1979).

Lesions more laterally, in for example the inferior convexity, can influence tasks in which objects must be remembered for short periods, for example delayed matching to sample and delayed matching to non-sample tasks (Passingham 1975; Mishkin & Manning 1978; Kowalska *et al.* 1991), and neurons in this region may help to implement this visual object short term memory by holding the representation active during the delay period (Rosenkilde *et al.* 1981; Wilson *et al.* 1993). Whether this inferior convexity area is specifically involved in a short term object memory is not yet clear, and a medial part of the frontal cortex may also contribute to this function (Kowalska *et al.* 1991). It should be noted that this short term memory system for objects (which receives inputs from the temporal lobe visual cortical areas in which objects are represented) is different to the short term memory system in the dorsolateral part of the prefrontal cortex, which is concerned with spatial short term memories, consistent with its inputs from the parietal cortex (see e.g. Williams *et al.* 1993).

Damage to the caudal orbitofrontal cortex in the monkey also produces emotional changes (e.g. decreased aggression to humans and to stimuli such as a snake and a doll), and a reduced tendency to reject foods such as meat (Butter *et al.* 1969; Butter *et al.* 1970; Butter & Snyder, 1972) or to display the normal preference ranking for different foods (Baylis & Gaffan 1991). In the human, euphoria, irresponsibility, and lack of affect can follow frontal lobe damage (see Kolb & Whishaw 1990; Damasio 1994), particularly orbito-frontal damage (Rolls *et al.* 1994).

6.4 Neurophysiology of the orbitofrontal cortex

(a) Taste

One of the recent discoveries that has helped us to understand the functions of the orbitofrontal cortex in behaviour is that it contains a major cortical representation of taste (see Rolls 1989, 1995*a*; cf. figure 6.2). Given that taste can act as a primary reinforcer, that is, without learning as a reward or punishment, we now have the start for a fundamental understanding of the function of the orbitofrontal cortex in stimulus-reinforcement association learning. We know how one class of primary reinforcers reaches and is represented in the orbito-frontal cortex. A representation of primary reinforcers is essential for a system that is involved in learning associations between previously neutral stimuli and primary reinforcers, for example between the sight of an object, and its taste.

The representation (shown by analysing the responses of single neurons in macaques) of taste in the orbitofrontal cortex includes robust representations of the prototypical tastes sweet, salt, bitter and sour (Rolls *et al.* 1990), but also separate representations of the taste of water (Rolls *et al.* 1990), of protein or

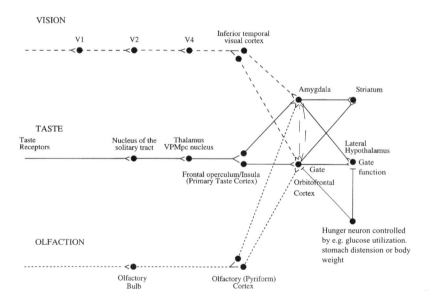

Fig. 6.2 Schematic diagram showing some of the gustatory, olfactory, and visual pathways to the orbitofrontal cortex, and some of the outputs of the orbitofrontal cortex. The secondary taste cortex, and the secondary olfactory cortex, are within the orbitofrontal cortex. VI—primary visual cortex. V4—visual cortical area V4.

umami as exemplified by monosodium glutamate (Baylis & Rolls 1991) and inosine monophosphate (Rolls *et al.* 1996*a*), and of astringency as exemplified by tannic acid (Critchley & Rolls 1996*c*).

The nature of the representation of taste in the orbitofrontal cortex is that the reward value of the taste is represented. The evidence for this is that the responses of orbitofrontal taste neurons are modulated by hunger (as is the reward value or palatability of a taste). In particular, it has been shown that orbitofrontal cortex taste neurons stop responding to the taste of a food with which the monkey is fed to satiety (Rolls *et al.* 1989). In contrast, the representation of taste in the primary taste cortex (Scott *et al.* 1986; Yaxley *et al.* 1990) is not modulated by hunger (Rolls *et al.* 1988; Yaxley *et al.* 1988). Thus in the primary taste cortex, the reward value of taste is not represented, and instead the identity of the taste is represented. Additional evidence that the reward value of food is represented in the orbitofrontal cortex is that monkeys work for electrical stimulation of this brain region if they are hungry, but not if they are satiated (Mora *et al.* 1979). Further, neurons in the orbitofrontal cortex are activated from many brain-stimulation reward sites (Mora *et al.* 1980; Rolls *et al.* 1980). Thus there is clear evidence that it is the reward value of taste that is represented in the orbitofrontal cortex.

The secondary taste cortex is in the caudolateral part of the orbitofrontal cortex, as defined anatomically (Baylis *et al.* 1994). This region projects on to other regions in the orbitofrontal cortex (Baylis *et al.* 1994), and neurons with taste responses (in what can be considered as a tertiary gustatory cortical area) can be found in many regions of the orbitofrontal cortex (see Rolls *et al.* 1990; Rolls & Baylis 1994; Rolls *et al.* 1996*a*).

(b) Convergence of taste and olfactory inputs in the orbitofrontal cortex: the representation of flavour

In these further parts of the orbitofrontal cortex, not only unimodal taste neurons, but also unimodal olfactory neurons are found. In addition some single neurons respond to both gustatory and olfactory stimuli, often with correspondence between the two modalities (Rolls & Baylis 1994; cf. figure 6.2). It is probably here in the orbitofrontal cortex of primates that these two modalities converge to produce the representation of flavour (Rolls & Baylis 1994). Evidence will soon be described that indicates that these representations are built by olfactory–gustatory association learning, an example of stimulus-reinforcement association learning.

(c) An olfactory representation in the orbitofrontal cortex

Takagi, Tanabe and colleagues (see Takagi 1991) described single neurons in the macaque orbitofrontal cortex that were activated by odours. A ventral frontal region has been implicated in olfactory processing in humans (Jones-Gotman & Zatorre 1988; Zatorre & Jones-Gotman 1991; Zatorre *et al.* 1992).

Rolls and colleagues have analysed the rules by which orbitofrontal olfactory representations are formed and operate in primates. For 65% of neurons in the orbitofrontal olfactory areas, Critchley & Rolls (1996a) showed that the representation of the olfactory stimulus was independent of its association with taste reward (analysed in an olfactory discrimination task with taste reward). For the remaining 35% of the neurons, the odours to which a neuron responded were influenced by the taste (glucose or saline) with which the odour was associated. Thus the odour representation for 35% of orbitofrontal neurons appeared to be built by olfactory to taste association learning. This possibility was confirmed by reversing the taste with which an odour was associated in the reversal of an olfactory discrimination task. It was found that 73% of the sample of neurons analysed altered the way in which they responded to odour when the taste reinforcement association of the odour was reversed (Rolls *et al.* 1996a) (25% showed reversal, and 48% no longer discriminated after the reversal. The olfactory to taste reversal was quite slow, both neurophysiologically and behaviourally, often requiring 20–80 trials, consistent with the need for some stability of flavour representations. The relatively high proportion of neurons with modification of responsiveness by taste association in the set of neurons in this experiment was probably related to the fact that the neurons were preselected to show differential responses to the odours associated with different tastes in the olfactory discrimination task.) Thus the rule according to which the orbitofrontal olfactory representation was formed was for some neurons by association learning with taste.

To analyse the nature of the olfactory representation in the orbitofrontal cortex, Critchley & Rolls (1996b) measured the responses of olfactory neurons that responded to food while they fed the monkey to satiety. They found that the majority of orbitofrontal olfactory neurons decreased their responses to the odour of the food with which the monkey was fed to satiety. Thus for these neurons, the reward value of the odour is what is represented in the orbitofrontal cortex. We do not yet know whether this is the first stage of processing at which reward value is represented in the olfactory system (although in rodents the influence of reward association learning appears to be present in some neurons in the pyriform cortex (Schoenbaum & Eichenbaum 1995).

Although individual neurons do not encode large amounts of information about which of 7–9 odours has been presented, we have shown that the information does increase linearly with the number of neurons in the sample (Rolls *et al.* 1996b). This ensemble encoding does result in useful amounts of information about which odour has been presented being provided by orbitofrontal olfactory neurons.

(d) Visual inputs to the orbitofrontal cortex, and visual stimulus—reinforcement association learning and reversal

We have been able to show that there is a major visual input to many neurons in the orbitofrontal cortex, and that what is represented by these neurons is, in many cases, the reinforcement association of visual stimuli. The visual input is from the ventral, temporal lobe, visual stream concerned with 'what' object is being seen, in that orbitofrontal visual neurons frequently respond differentially to objects or images depending on their reward association (Thorpe *et al.* 1983; Rolls *et al.* 1996*a*). The primary reinforcer that has been used is taste. Many of these neurons show visual-taste reversal in one or a very few trials (see example in figure 6.3). (In a visual discrimination task, they will reverse the stimulus to which they respond, from e.g. a triangle to a square, in one trial when the taste delivered to a response to that stimulus is reversed.) This reversal learning probably occurs in the orbitofrontal cortex, for it does not occur one synapse earlier in the visual inferior temporal cortex (Rolls *et al.* 1977), and it is in the orbitofrontal cortex that there is convergence of visual and taste pathways onto the same neurons (Thorpe *et al.* 1983; Rolls *et al.* 1996). The probable mechanism for this learning is Hebbian modification of synapses conveying visual input onto taste-responsive neurons, implementing a pattern association network (Rolls & Treves 1990).

In addition to these neurons that encode the reward association of visual stimuli, other neurons in the orbitofrontal cortex detect non-reward, in that they respond for example, when an expected reward is not obtained when a visual discrimination task is reversed (Thorpe *et al.* 1983). Different populations of such neurons respond to other types of non-reward, including the removal of a formerly approaching taste reward, and the termination of a taste reward (Thorpe *et al.* 1983). The presence of these neurons is fully consistent with the hypothesis that they are part of the mechanism by which the orbitofrontal cortex enables very rapid reversal of behaviour by stimulus-reinforcement association relearning when the association of stimuli with reinforcers is altered or reversed (see Rolls 1989*a*, 1990). Different orbitofrontal cortex neurons respond to different types of non-reward (Thorpe *et al.* 1983), potentially enabling task or context-specific reversal to occur.

Another type of information represented in the orbitofrontal cortex is information about faces. There is a population of orbitofrontal neurons which respond in many ways similar to those in the temporal cortical visual areas (see Rolls 1984*a*, 1992*a*, 1994*a*, 1995*b*, 1996 for a description of their properties). The orbitofrontal face responsive neurons, first observed by Thorpe *et al.* (1983), then by Rolls *et al.* (1983), and then by Rolls *et al.* (unpublished data), tend to respond with longer latencies than temporal lobe neurons (140–200 ms typically, compared to 80–100 ms); also convey information about which face is being seen, by having different responses to different faces; and are typically rather harder to activate strongly than temporal cortical face-selective neurons, in that many of them respond much better to real faces than to two-dimensional images of faces on a video monitor (see Rolls & Baylis, 1986). Some of the orbitofrontal face-selective neurons are responsive to face gesture or movement. The findings are consistent with the likelihood that these neurons are activated via the inputs from the temporal cortical visual areas in which face-selective neurons are found (see figure 6.2). The significance of the neurons

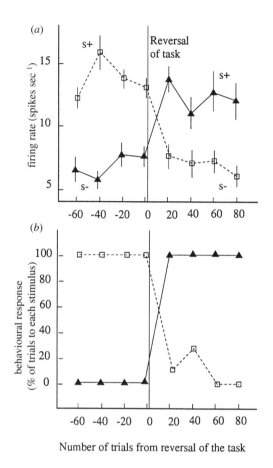

Fig. 6.3 Visual discrimination reversal of the responses of a single neuron in the macaque orbitofrontal cortex when the taste with which the two visual stimuli (a triangle and a square) were associated was reversed. Each point is the mean poststimulus firing rate measured in a 0.5 s period over approximately 10 trials to each of the stimuli. Before reversal, the neuron fired most to the square when it indicated (S+) that the monkey could lick to obtain a taste of glucose. After reversal, the neuron responded most to the triangle when it indicated that the monkey could lick to obtain glucose. The response was low to the stimuli when they indicated (S –) that if the monkey licked then aversive saline would be obtained. In (b) the behavioural response to the triangle and the square is shown, and indicates that the monkey reversed rapidly. (After Rolls, *et al.* 1996a.)

is likely to be related to the fact that faces convey information that is important in social reinforcement, both by conveying face expression (see Hasselmo *et al.* 1989), which can indicate reinforcement; and by encoding information about which individual is present, also important in evaluating and utilizing reinforcing inputs in social situations.

6.5 A neurophysiological basis for stimulus-reinforcement learning and reversal in the orbitofrontal cortex

The neurophysiological and lesion evidence described suggests that one function implemented by the orbitofrontal cortex is rapid stimulus-reinforcement association learning, and the correction of these associations when reinforcement contingencies in the environment change. To implement this, the orbitofrontal cortex has the necessary representation of primary reinforcers, such as taste, as described above (see figure 6.2), but also somatosensory inputs, as described elsewhere (Critchley *et al.* 1993). It also receives information about objects, for example visual information, and can associate this very rapidly at the neuronal level with primary reinforcers such as taste, and reverse these associations. Another type of stimulus which can be conditioned in this way in the orbitofrontal cortex is olfactory, although here the learning is slower. It is likely that auditory stimuli can be associated with primary reinforcers in the orbitofrontal cortex, though there is less direct evidence of this yet. The orbitofrontal cortex also has neurons which detect non-reward, and which are likely to be used in behavioural extinction and reversal. They may do this not only by helping to reset the reinforcement association of neurons in the orbitofrontal cortex, but also by sending a signal to the striatum which could be routed by the striatum to produce appropriate behaviours for non-reward (Rolls & Johnstone 1992; Williams *et al.* 1993; Rolls 1994*b*). Indeed, it is via this route, the striatal, that the orbitofrontal cortex may directly influence behaviour when the orbitofrontal cortex is decoding reinforcement contingencies in the environment, and is altering behaviour in response to altering reinforcement contingencies. Some of the evidence for this is that neurons which reflect these orbitofrontal neuronal responses are found in the ventral part of the head of the caudate nucleus and the ventral striatum, which receive from the orbitofrontal cortex (Rolls *et al.* 1983*b*; Williams *et al.* 1993); and lesions of the ventral part of the head of the caudate nucleus impair visual discrimination reversal (Divac *et al.* 1967).

Decoding the reinforcement value of stimuli, which involves for previously neutral (e.g. visual) stimuli learning their association with a primary reinforcer, often rapidly, and which may involve not only rapid learning but also rapid relearning and alteration of responses when reinforcement contingencies change, is then a function proposed for the orbitofrontal cortex. This way of producing behavioural responses would be important in for example motivational and emotional behaviour. It would be important for example in motivational behaviour such as feeding and drinking by enabling primates to learn rapidly about the food reinforcement to be expected from visual stimuli (see Rolls 1994*c*). This is important, for primates frequently eat more than 100 varieties of food; vision by visual-taste association learning can be used to identify when foods are ripe; and during the course of a meal, the pleasantness of the sight of a food eaten in the meal decreases in a sensory-specific way (Rolls *et al.* 1983*a*), a function that is probably implemented by the sensory-specific satiety-related responses of orbitofrontal visual neurons (Critchley & Rolls 1996*b*).

With respect to emotional behaviour, decoding and rapidly readjusting the reinforcement value of visual signals is likely to be crucial, for emotions can be described as responses elicited by reinforcing signals (For the purposes of this paper, a positive reinforcer or reward can be defined as a stimulus which the animal will work to obtain, and a negative reinforcer or punishment as a stimulus that an animal will work to avoid or escape (see further Rolls 1986*a*, *b*, 1990, 1995*b*). The ability to perform this learning very rapidly is probably very important in social situations in primates, in which reinforcing stimuli are continually being exchanged, and the reinforcement value of these must be continually updated (relearned), based on the actual reinforcers received and given. Although the operation of reinforcers such as taste, smell, and faces are best understood in terms of orbitofrontal cortex operation, there are tactile inputs that are likely to be concerned with reward evaluation, and in humans the rewards processed in the orbitofrontal cortex include quite general rewards such as working for 'points', as will be described shortly.

Although the amygdala is concerned with some of the same functions as the orbitofrontal cortex, and receives similar inputs (see figure 6.2), there is evidence that it may function less effectively in the very rapid learning and reversal of stimulus-reinforcement associations, as indicated by the greater difficulty in obtaining reversal from amygdala neurons (see e.g. Rolls 1992*b*), and by the greater effect of orbitofrontal lesions in leading to continuing behavioural responses to previously rewarded stimuli (Jones & Mishkin 1972). In primates, the necessity for very rapid stimulus-reinforcement re-evaluation, and the development of powerful cortical learning systems, may result in the orbitofrontal cortex effectively taking over this aspect of amygdala functions (see Rolls 1992*b*).

6.6 The human orbitofrontal cortex

It is of interest that a number of the symptoms of frontal lobe damage in humans appear to be related to this type of function, of altering behaviour when stimulus-reinforcement associations alter, as described next. Thus, humans with frontal lobe damage can show impairments in a number of tasks in which an alteration of behavioural strategy is required in response to a change in environmental reinforcement contingencies (see Goodglass & Kaplan 1979; Jouandet & Gazzaniga 1979; Kolb & Whishaw 1990). For example, Milner (1963) showed that in the Wisconsin Card Sort Test (in which cards are to be sorted according to the colour shape, or number of items on each card depending on whether the examiner says 'right' or 'wrong' to each placement), frontal patients either had difficulty in determining the first sorting principle, or in shifting to a second principle when required to. Also, in stylus mazes, frontal patients have difficulty in changing direction when a sound indicates that the correct path has been left (see Milner 1982). It is of interest that, in both types of test, frontal patients may be able to verbalize the correct rules, yet may be unable to correct their *behavioural*, or strategies appropriately. Some of the personality changes that can follow frontal lobe damage may be related to a similar type of dysfunction. For example, the euphoria, irresponsibility, lack of affect, and lack of concern for the present or future which can follow frontal lobe damage (see Hecaen & Albert 1978) may also be related to a dysfunction in altering behaviour appropriately in response to a change in reinforcement contingencies. Indeed, in so far as the orbitofrontal cortex is involved in the disconnection of stimulus reinforcement associations, and such associations are important in learned emotional responses (see above), then it follows that the orbitofrontal cortex is involved in emotional responses by correcting stimulus-reinforcement associations when they become inappropriate.

These hypotheses, and the role in particular of the orbitofrontal cortex in human behaviour, have been investigated in recent studies in humans with damage to the ventral parts of the frontal lobe. (The description ventral is given to indicate that there was pathology in the orbitofrontal or related parts of the frontal lobe, and not in the more dorso-lateral parts of the frontal lobe.) A task which was directed at assessing the rapid alteration of stimulus-reinforcement associations was used, because the findings above indicate that the orbitofrontal cortex is involved in this type of learning. This was used instead of the Wisconsin Card Sort Test, which requires patients to shift from category (or dimension) to category, for example from colour to shape. The task used was visual discrimination reversal, in which patients could learn to obtain points by touching one stimulus when it appeared on a video monitor, but had to withhold a response when a different visual stimulus appeared, otherwise a point was lost. After the subjects had acquired the visual discrimination, the reinforcement contingencies unexpectedly reversed. The patients with ventral frontal lesions made more errors in the reversal (or in a similar extinction) task, and completed fewer reversals, than control patients with damage elsewhere in the frontal lobes or in other brain regions (Rolls *et al.* 1994). The impairment correlated highly with the socially inappropriate or disinhibited behaviour of the patients, and also with their subjective evaluation of the changes in their emotional state since the brain damage. The patients were not impaired at other types of memory task, such as paired associate learning. The findings are being extended in current research by Hornak, Rolls & Wade in which visual discrimination acquisition and reversal are also found to be impaired in a visual discrimination task in which two stimuli are always present on the video monitor, and the patient obtains points by touching the correct stimulus, and loses points by touching the incorrect stimulus. It is of interest that the patients can often verbalize the correct response, yet commit the incorrect action. This is consistent with the hypothesis that the orbitofrontal cortex is normally involved in executing behaviour when the behaviour is performed by evaluating the reinforcement associations of environmental stimuli (see below). The orbitofrontal cortex appears to be involved in this in both humans and non-human primates, when the learning must be performed rapidly, in, for example, acquisition, and during reversal.

To investigate the possible significance of face-related inputs to orbitofrontal visual neurons described above, we also tested the responses of these patients to faces. We included tests of face (and also voice) expression decoding, because these are ways in which the reinforcing quality of individuals is often indicated. Impairments in the identification of facial and vocal emotional expression were demonstrated in a group of patients with ventral frontal lobe damage who had socially inappropriate behaviour (Hornak *et al.* 1996). The expression identification impairments could occur independently of perceptual impairments in facial recognition, voice discrimination, or environmental sound recognition. The face and voice expression problems did not necessarily occur together in the same patients, providing an indication of separate processing. Poor performance on both expression tests was correlated with the degree of alteration of emotional experience reported by the patients. There was also a strong positive correlation between the degree of altered emotional experience and the severity of the behavioural problems (e.g. disinhibition) found in these patients. A comparison group of patients with brain damage outside the ventral frontal lobe region, without these behavioural problems, was unimpaired on the face expression identification test, was significantly less impaired at vocal expression identification, and reported little subjective emotional change (Hornak *et al.* 1996). In current studies, these findings are being extended, and it is being found that patients with face expression decoding problems do not necessarily have impairments at visual discrimination reversal, and vice versa. This is consistent with some topography in the orbitofrontal cortex (see e.g. Rolls & Baylis 1994).

6.7 Executive functions of the orbitofrontal cortex

The research described indicates that the orbitofrontal cortex is involved in the execution of behavioural responses when these are computed by reward or punishment association learning, a function for which the orbitofrontal cortex is specialized, in terms of representations of primary (unlearned) reinforcers, and in rapidly learning and readjusting associations of stimuli with these primary reinforcers. The fact that patients with ventral frontal lesions often can express verbally what the correct responses should be, yet cannot follow what previously obtained rewards and punishments indicate is appropriate behaviour, is an indication that when primates (including humans) normally execute behavioural responses on the basis of reinforcement evaluation, they do so using the orbitofrontal cortex. Eliciting behaviour on the basis of rewards and punishments obtained previously in similar situations is of course a simple and adaptive way to control behavioural responses that has been studied and accepted for very many years (see e.g. the history of psychology; and in terms of brain mechanisms, see e.g. Rolls 1975, 1986a, b, 1990, 1994b, 1995b, 1998), and has been recently emphasized by Damasio (1994). The particular utility of one of the alternative routes to behaviour (there are of course many routes to behaviour) made possible by language is that this enables long-term planning, where the plan involves many syntactic arrangements of symbols (e.g. many if...then statements). It is suggested that when this linguistic (in terms of syntactic manipulation of symbols) system needs correction, being able to think about the plans (higher order thoughts), enables the plans to be corrected, and that this process is closely related to explicit, conscious, processing (Rolls 1995b, 1997; see also Rosenthal 1993). It follows that the functions performed by the orbitofrontal cortex need not be performed with explicit (conscious) processing, but can be performed with implicit processing. It is in this way that the orbitofrontal cortex is suggested to be involved in some, but certainly not all, types of executive function.

In that the orbitofrontal cortex may retain as a result of synaptic modification in a pattern associator (see Rolls & Treves 1990) the most recent reinforcement association for large numbers of different stimuli, it could perhaps be fitted into a view that the frontal cortical areas are in general concerned with different types of working memory. However, the term working memory is normally used in neurophysiology to refer to a memory in which the memoranda are held in the memory by continuing neuronal activity, as in an autoassociator or attractor network (see e.g. Treves & Rolls 1991). It should be realised that although there may be a functional similarity between such a working memory and the ability of the orbitofrontal cortex to retain the most recent reinforcement association of many stimuli, the implementations are very different. The different implementations do in fact have strong functional consequences: it is difficult to retain more than a few items active in an autoassociative memory, and hence in practice individual items are retained typically only for short periods in such working memories; whereas in pattern associators, because synaptic modification has taken place, the last reinforcement association of a very large number of stimuli can be stored for long periods, and recalled whenever each stimulus is seen again in the future, without any neuronal firing to hold the representation active (see e.g. Rolls & Treves 1997).

It is perhaps useful to note how the orbitofrontal cortex may link to output systems to control behaviour, for the occasions when the orbitofrontal cortex does control behaviour. Rolls has proposed elsewhere (Rolls 1984b, 1994b; Rolls & Johnstone 1992) the outline of a theory of striatal function, according to which all areas of the cerebral cortex gain access to the striatum, compete within the striatum and rest of the basal ganglia system for behavioural output depending on how strongly each part of the cerebral cortex is calling for output, and the striatum maps (as a result of slow previous habit or stimulus-response learning) each particular type of input to the striatum to the appropriate behavioural output (implemented via the return basal ganglia connections to premotor/prefrontal parts of the cerebral cortex). This is one of the ways in which reinforcing stimuli can exert their influence relatively directly on behavioural output. The importance of this route is attested to by the fact that restricted striatal lesions impair functions implemented by the part of the cortex which projects to the lesioned part of the striatum (see Rolls 1984b, 1994b; Rolls & Johnstone 1992). This hypothesis is very different from that of Damasio (1994), who has effectively tried to resurrect a weakened version of the James–Lange theory of emotion from the last century, by arguing with his somatic marker hypothesis that after reinforcers have been evaluated, a bodily response ('somatic marker') normally occurs, then this leads to a bodily feeling, which in turn is appreciated by the organism to then make a contribution to the decision-making process. (In the James–Lange theory, it was emotional feelings that depend on peripheral feedback; for Damasio, it is the decision of which behavioural response to make that is normally influenced by the peripheral feedback.) The James–Lange theory has a number of major weaknesses, including the evidence that inactivation of peripheral feedback does little to abolish feelings or behaviour to emotion-provoking (reinforcing) stimuli (see Grossman (1967) for an extensive review of this literature; Schachter & Singer (1962), who could alter the magnitude but not the quality of experienced emotion by artificially inducing peripheral feedback; and Reisenzein (1983), who produced by pharmacological blockers little reduction of emotion); does not in any case account for the fundamental question analysed here of how it is that some stimuli produce emotional responses and others do not (see Rolls 1990), that is the decoding of whether a stimulus is associated with reinforcement that must be performed according to both the direct and peripheral hypotheses; and does not take account of the fact that once an information processor has determined that a response should be made or inhibited based on reinforcement association, a function attributed here in part to the orbitofrontal cortex, it would be very inefficient and noisy to place in the execution route a peripheral response, and transducers to attempt to measure that peripheral response, itself a notoriously difficult procedure (see e.g. Grossman 1967). Even if Damasio were to argue that the peripheral somatic marker and its feedback can be bypassed using conditioning of a representation in for example, the somatosensory cortex to the ventral prefrontal command signal, he apparently would still wish to argue that the activity in the somatosensory cortex is important for the emotion to be appreciated or to influence behaviour. (Without this, the somatic marker hypothesis would vanish.) The prediction would apparently be that if an emotional response were produced to a visual stimulus, then this would necessarily involve activity in the somatosensory cortex or other brain region in which the 'somatic marker' would be represented. This prediction could be tested (for example in patients with somatosensory cortex damage), but it seems most unlikely that an emotion produced by a visual reinforcer would require activity in the somatosensory cortex. The alternative view proposed here (and by Rolls 1990) is that where the reinforcement value of the visual stimulus is decoded, namely in the orbitofrontal cortex and the amygdala, is the appropriate part of the brain for outputs to influence behaviour (via e.g. the orbitofrontal-to-striatal connections), and that the orbitofrontal cortex is the likely place where neuronal activity is directly related to the felt emotion (see further Rolls 1997).

The fact that ventral prefrontal lesions block autonomic responses to learned reinforcers (Damasio 1994) (actually known since at least the 1950s, e.g. Elithorn *et al.* 1955 in humans; Grueninger *et al.* 1965 in macaques) is of course consistent with the hypothesis that learned reinforcers elicit autonomic responses via the orbitofrontal cortex and amygdala (see e.g. Rolls 1986*a, b*, 1990); but does not prove the hypothesis that behavioural responses elicited by conditioned reinforcers are mediated via peripheral changes, themselves used as 'somatic markers' to determine which response to make. Instead, the much more direct neural route from the orbitofrontal cortex and amygdala to the basal ganglia provides a pathway which is much more efficient, and is directly implicated in producing, the behavioural responses to learned incentives (Rolls 1994*b*; Williams *et al.* 1993; Everitt & Robbins 1992; Divac *et al.* 1967).

Acknowledgements

The author has worked on some of the experiments described here with L. L. Baylis, G. C. Baylis, H. Critchley, M. E. Hasselmo, J. Hornak, C. M. Leonard, F. Mora, D. I. Perrett, T. R. Scott, S. J. Thorpe, E. A. Wakeman and F. A. W. Wilson, and their collaboration is sincerely acknowledged. Some of the research described was supported by the Medical Research Council, PG8513790.

References

Barbas, H. 1988 Anatomic organization of basoventral and mediodorsal visual recipient prefrontal regions in the rhesus monkey. *J. Comp. Neurol.* **276**, 313–42.

Barbas, H. 1993 Organization of cortical afferent input to the orbitofrontal area in the rhesus monkey. *Neuroscience* **56**, 841–64.

Barbas, H. 1995 Anatomic basis of cognitive-emotional interactions in the primate prefrontal cortex. *Neurosci. Biobehav. Rev.* **19**, 499–510.

Barbas, H. & Pandya, D. N. 1989 Architecture and intrinsic connections of the prefrontal cortex in the rhesus monkey. *J. Comp. Neurol.* **286**, 353–75.

Baylis, L. L. & Gaffan, D. 1991 Amygdalectomy and ventromedial prefrontal ablation produce similar deficits in food choice and in simple object discrimination learning for an unseen reward. *Exp. Brain Res.* **86**, 617–22.

Baylis, L. L. & Rolls, E. T. 1991 Responses of neurons in the primate taste cortex to glutamate. *Physiol. Behav.* **49**, 973–79.

Baylis, L. L., Rolls, E. T. & Baylis, G. C. 1994 Afferent connections of the orbitofrontal cortex taste area of the primate. *Neuroscience* **64**, 801–12.

Butter, C. M. 1969 Perseveration in extinction and in discrimination reversal tasks following selective prefrontal ablations in Macaca mulatta. *Physiol. Behav.* **4**, 163–71.

Butter, C. M., McDonald, J. A. & Snyder, D. R. 1969 Orality, preference behavior, and reinforcement value of non-food objects in monkeys with orbital frontal lesions. *Science* **164**, 1306–07.

Butter, C. M. & Snyder, D. R. 1972 Alterations in aversive and aggressive behaviors following orbitofrontal lesions in rhesus monkeys. *Acta Neurobiol. Exp.* **32**, 525–65.

Butter, C. M., Snyder, D. R. & McDonald, J. A. 1970 Effects of orbitofrontal lesions on aversive and aggressive behaviors in rhesus monkeys. *J. Comp. Physiol. Psychol.* **72**, 132–44.

Carmichael, S. T., Clugnet, M. C. & Price, J. L. 1994 Central olfactory connections in the macaque monkey. *J. Comp. Neurol.* **346**, 403–34.

Carmichael, S. T. & Price, J. L. 1994 Architectonic subdivision of the orbital and medial prefrontal cortex in the macaque monkey. *J. Comp. Neurol.* **346**, 366–402.

Critchley, H. D., Rolls, E. T. & Wakeman, E. A. 1993 Orbitofrontal cortex responses to the texture, taste, smell and sight of food. *Appetite* **21**, 170.

Critchley, H. D. & Rolls, E. T. 1996a Olfactory neuronal responses in the primate orbitofrontal cortex: analysis in an olfactory discrimination task. *J. Neurophysiol.* **75**, 1659–72.

Critchley, H. D. & Rolls, E. T. 1996b Hunger and satiety modify the responses of olfactory and visual neurons in the primate orbitofrontal cortex. *J. Neurophysiol.* **75**, 1673–86.

Critchley, H. D. & Rolls, E. T. 1996c Responses of primate taste cortex neurons to the astringent tastant tannic acid. *Chem. Senses* **21**, 135–45.

Damasio, A. R. 1994 *Descartes' error.* New York: Putnam. Divac, I., Rosvold, H. E., Szwarcbart, M. K. 1967 Behavioral effects of selective ablation of the caudate nucleus. *J. Comp. Physiol. Psych.* **63**, 184–90.

Elithorn, A., Piercy, M. F. & Crosskey, M. A. 1955 Prefrontal leucotomy and the anticipation of pain. *J. Neurol. Neurosurg. Psychiat.* **18**, 34–43.

Everitt, B. J. & Robbins, T. W. 1992 Amygdala-ventral striatal interactions and reward-related processes. In *The amygdala* (ed. J. P. Aggleton), pp. 401–30. Chichester: Wiley.

Fuster, J. M. 1989 *The prefrontal cortex*, second edition. New York: Raven Press.

Goodglass, H. & Kaplan, E. 1979 Assessment of cognitive deficit in brain-injured patient. In *Handbook of behavioral neurobiology. Vol 2 Neuropsychology* (ed. M. S. Gazzaniga), pp. 3–22. New York: Plenum.

Grossman, S.. 1967 *A textbook of physiological psychology.* New York: Wiley.

Grueninger, W. E., Kimble, D. P., Grueninger, J. & Levine, S. 1965 GSR and corticosteroid response in monkeys with frontal ablations. *Neuropsychologia* **3**, 205–16.

Hasselmo, M. E., Rolls, E. T. & Baylis, G. C. 1989 The role of expression and identity in the face-selective responses of neurons in the temporal visual cortex of the monkey. *Behav. Brain Res.* **32**, 203–18.

Hecaen, H. & Albert, M. L. 1978 *Human neuropsychology.* New York: Wiley.

Hornak, J., Rolls, E. T. & Wade, D. 1996 Face and voice expression identification in patients with emotional and behavioural changes following ventral frontal lobe damage. *Neuropsychologia* **34**, 247–61.

Insausti, R., Amaral, D. G. & Cowan, W. M. 1987 The entorhinal cortex of the monkey. II. Cortical afferents. *J. Comp. Neurol.* **264**, 356–95.

Iversen, S. D. & Mishkin, M. 1970 Perseverative interference in monkey following selective lesions of the inferior prefrontal convexity. *Exptl. Brain Res.* **11**, 376–86.

Johnson, T. N., Rosvold, H. E. & Mishkin, M. 1968 Projections from behaviorally defined sectors of the prefrontal cortex to the basal ganglia, septum and diencephalon of the monkey. *Exptl. Neurol.* **21**, 20–34.

Jones, B. & Mishkin, M. 1972 Limbic lesions and the problem of stimulus-reinforcement associations. *Exptl. Neurol.* **36**, 362–77.

Jones, E. G. & Powell, T. P. S. 1970 An anatomical study of converging sensory pathways within the cerebral cortex of the monkey. *Brain*, **93**, 793–820.

Jones-Gotman, M. & Zatorre, R. J. 1988 Olfactory identification in patients with focal cerebral excision. *Neuropsychologia*, **26**, 387–400.

Jouandet, M. & Gazzaniga, M. S. 1979 The frontal lobes. In *Handbook of behavioral neurobiology. Vol 2, Neuropsychology* (ed. M. S. Gazzaniga), pp. 25–59. New York: Plenum.

Kemp, J. M. & Powell, T. P. S. 1970 The cortico-striate projections in the monkey. *Brain* **93**, 525–46.

Kolb, B. & Whishaw, I. W. 1990 *Fundamentals of human neuropsychology*, 3rd edn. New York: Freeman.

Kowalska, D-M., Bachevalier, J. & Mishkin, M. 191 The role of the inferior prefrontal convexity in performance of delayed nonmatching-to-sample. *Neuropsychologia* **29**, 583–600.

Krettek, J. E. & Price, J. L. 1974 A direct input from the amygdala to the thalamus and the cerebral cortex. *Brain Res.* **67**, 169–74.

Krettek, J. E. & Price, J. L. 1977 The cortical projections of the mediodorsal nucleus and adjacent thalamic nuclei in the rat. *J. Comp. Neurol.* **171**, 157–92.

Milner, B. 1963 Effects of different brain lesions on card sorting. *Arch. Neurol.* **9**, 90–100.

Milner, B. 1982 Some cognitive effects of frontal-lobe lesions in man. *Phil. Trans. R. Soc. Lond.* **B 298**, 211–26.

Mishkin, M. & Manning, F. J. 1978 Non-spatial memory after selective prefrontal lesions in monkeys. *Brain Res.* **143**, 313–24.

Mora, F., Avrith, D. B., Phillips, A. G. & Rolls, E. T. 1979 Effects of satiety on self-stimulation of the orbitofrontal cortex in the monkey. *Neuroscience Letters* **13**, 141–45.

Mora, F., Avrith, D. B. & Rolls, E. T. 1980 An electro-physiological and behavioural study of self-stimulation in the orbitofrontal cortex of the rhesus monkey. *Brain Res. Bull.* **5**, 111–15.

Morecraft, R. J., Geula, C., & Mesulam, M.-M. 1992 Cytoarchitecture and neural afferents of orbitofrontal cortex in the brain of the monkey. *J. Comp. Neurol.* **323**, 341–58.

Nauta, W. J. H. 1964 Some efferent connections of the prefrontal cortex in the monkey. In *The frontal granular cortex and behavior* (ed. J. M. Warren & K. Akert), pp. 3907–407. New York: McGraw Hill.

Nauta, W. J. H. 1972 Neural associations of the frontal cortex. *Acta. Neurobiol. Exp.* **32**, 125–40.

Norgren, R. 1984 Central neural mechanisms of taste. In *Handbook of physiology – The nervous system III, Sensory processes 1*. (I. Darien-Smith, editor; Section Editors, J. Brookhart and V. B. Mountcastle), pp. 1087–128. Washington, DC: American Physiological Society.

Passingham, R. 1975 Delayed matching after selective prefrontal lesions in monkeys (*Macaca mulatta*). *Brain Res.* **92**, 89–102.

Petrides, M. & Pandya, D. N. 1988 Association fiber pathways to the frontal cortex from the superior temporal region in the rhesus monkey. *J. Comp. Neurol.* **273**, 52–66.

Petrides, M. & Pandya, D. N. 1995 Comparative architectonic analysis of the human and macaque frontal cortex. In *Handbook of neuropsychology* (ed. J. Grafman & F. Boller) Elsevier Science Publishers, Amsterdam.

Preuss, T. M. & Goldman-Rakic, P. S. 1989 Connections of the ventral granular frontal cortex of macaques with perisylvian premotor and somatosensory areas: anatomical evidence for somatic representation in primate frontal association cortex. *J. Comp. Neurol.* **282**, 293–316.

Price, J. L., Carmichael, S. T., Carnes, K. M., Clugnet, M.-C., Kuroda, M. & Ray, J. O. 1991 Olfactory input to the prefrontal cortex. In *Olfaction: a model system for computational neuroscience* (ed. J. L. Davis & H. Eichenbaum), pp. 101–20: Cambridge, MA: MIT Press.

Reisenzein, R. 1983 The Schachter theory of emotion: two decades later. *Psychol. Bull.* **94**, 239–64.

Rolls, E. T. 1975 *The brain and reward*. Oxford: Pergamon.

Rolls, E. T. 1984a Neurons in the cortex of the temporal lobe and in the amygdala of the monkey with responses selective for faces. *Hum. Neurobiol.* **3**, 209–22.

Rolls, E. T. 1984b Activity of neurons in different regions of the striatum of the monkey. In *The basal ganglia: structure and function* (ed. J. S. McKenzie, R. E. Kemm & L. N. Wilcox), pp. 467–93 New York: Plenum.

Rolls, E. T. 1986a A theory of emotion, and its application to understanding the neural basis of emotion. In *Emotions. neural and chemical control* (ed. Y. Oomura), pp. 325–44. Tokyo: Japan Scientific Societies Press, and Karger: Basel.

Rolls, E. T. 1986b Neural systems involved in emotion in primates. In *Emotion: theory, research, and experience*. Volume 3: *Biological foundations of emotion* (ed. R. Plutchik & H. Kellerman), pp. 125–43. New York: Academic Press.

Rolls, E. T. 1989 Information processing in the taste system of primates. *J. Exptl. Biol.* **146**, 141–64.

Rolls, E. T. 1990 A theory of emotion, and its application to understanding the neural basis of emotion. *Cog. Emot.* **4**, 161–90.

Rolls, E. T. 1992a Neurophysiological mechanisms underlying face processing within and beyond the temporal cortical visual areas. *Phil. Trans. R. Soc. Lond.* **B 335**, 11–21.

Rolls, E. T. 1992b Neurophysiology and functions of the primate amygdala. In *The amygdala* (ed. J. P. Aggleton), ch. 5, pp. 143–65, New York: Wiley-Liss.

Rolls, E. T. 1994a Brain mechanisms for invariant visual recognition and learning. *Behav. Proc.* **33**, 113–38.

Rolls, E. T. 1994b Neurophysiology and cognitive functions of the striatum. *Revue Neurologique* (*Paris*) **150**, 648–60.

Rolls, E. T. 1994c Neural processing related to feeding in primates. In *Appetite: neural and behavioural bases* (ed. C. R. Legg & D. A. Booth), ch. 2, pp. 11–53, Oxford: Oxford University Press.

Rolls, E. T. 1995a Central taste anatomy and neurophysiology. In *Handbook of olfaction and gustation* (ed. R. L. Doty), ch. 24, pp. 549–73, New York: Dekker.

Rolls, E. T. 1995b A theory of emotion and consciousness, and its application to understanding the neural basis of emotion. In *The cognitive neurosciences* (ed. M. S. Gazzaniga), ch. 72, pp. 1091–06. Cambridge, MA: MIT Press.

Rolls, E. T. 1997 A neurophysiological and computational approach to the functions of the temporal lobe cortical visual areas in invariant object recognition. In *Computational and biological mechanisms of visual coding* (ed. L. Harris & M. Jenkin), pp. 184–220, Cambridge: Cambridge University Press.

Rolls, E. T. 1997 Brain mechanisms of vision, memory and consciousness. In *Cognition, computation, and consciousness* (ed. M. Ito, Y. Miyashita & E. T. Rolls), pp.81–120, Oxford: Oxford University Press.

Rolls, E. T. *The brain and emotion*. Oxford: Oxford University Press. (In press.)

Rolls, E. T. & Baylis, G. C. 1986 Size and contrast have only small effects on the responses to faces of neurons in the cortex of the superior temporal sulcus of the monkey. *Expl. Brain Res.* **65**, 38–48.

Rolls, E. T. & Baylis, L. L. 1994 Gustatory, olfactory and visual convergence within the primate orbitofrontal cortex. *J. Neurosci.* **14**, 5437–52.

Rolls, E. T., Burton, M. J. & Mora, F. 1980 Neurophysiological analysis of brain-stimulation reward in the monkey. *Brain Res.* **194**, 339–57.

Rolls, E. T., Critchley, H., Mason, R. & Wakeman, E. A. 1996a Orbitofrontal cortex neurons: role in olfactory and visual association learning. *J. Neurophysiol.* **75**, 1970–81.

Rolls, E. T., Critchley, H. D. & Treves, A. 1996b The representation of olfactory information in the primate orbitofrontal cortex. *J. Neurophysiol.* **75**, 1982–96.

Rolls, E. T., Critchley, H., Wakeman, E. A. & Mason, R. 1996c Responses of neurons in the primate taste cortex to the glutamate ion and to inosine 5′-monophosphate. *Physiol. Behav.* **59**, 991–1000.

Rolls, E. T., Hornak, J., Wade, D. & McGrath, J. 1994 Emotion-related learning in patients with social and emotional changes associated with frontal lobe damage. *J. Neurol. Neurosurg. Psychiat.* **57**, 1518–24.

Rolls, E. T. & Johnstone, S. 1992 Neurophysiological analysis of striatal function. In *Neuropsychological disorders associated with subcortical lesions* (ed. G. Vallar, S. F. Cappa & C. W. Wallesch), ch. 3, pp. 61–97, Oxford: Oxford University Press.

Rolls, E. T., Judge, S. J. & Sanghera, M. 1977 Activity of neurons in the inferotemporal cortex of the alert monkey. *Brain Res.* **130**, 229–38.

Rolls, E. T., Rolls, B. J. & Rowe, E. A. 1983a Sensory-specific and motivation-specific satiety for the sight and taste of food and water in man. *Physiol. Behav.* **30**, 185–92.

Rolls, E. T., Scott, T. R., Sienkiewicz, Z. J. & Yaxley, S. 1988 The responsiveness of neurones in the frontal opercular gustatory cortex of the macaque monkey is independent of hunger. *J. Physiol.* **397**, 1–12.

Rolls, E. T., Sienkiewicz, Z. J. & Yaxley, S. 1989 Hunger modulates the responses to gustatory stimuli of single neurons in the caudolateral orbitofrontal cortex of the macaque monkey. *European J. Neurosci.* **1**, 53–60.

Rolls, E. T., Thorpe, S. J. & Maddison, S. P. 1983b Responses of striatal neurons in the behaving monkey. 1. Head of the caudate nucleus. *Behav. Brain Res.* **7**, 179–210.

Rolls, E. T. & Treves, A. 1990 The relative advantages of sparse versus distributed encoding for associative neuronal networks in the brain. *Network* **1**, 407–21.

Rolls, E. T. & Treves, A. 1998 *Neuronal networks and brain function*, Oxford, Oxford University Press.

Rolls, E. T., Yaxley, S. & Sienkiewicz, Z. J. 1990 Gustatory responses of single neurons in the orbitofrontal cortex of the macaque monkey. *J. Neurophysiol.* **64**, 1055–66.

Rosenkilde, C. E. 1979 Functional heterogeneity of the prefrontal cortex in the monkey: a review. *Behav. Neural Biol.* **25**, 301–45.

Rosenkilde, C. E., Bauer, R. H. & Fuster, J. M. 1981 Single unit activity in ventral prefrontal cortex in behaving monkeys, *Brain Res.* **209**, 375–94.

Rosenthal, D. M. 1993 Thinking that one thinks. In *Consciousness* (ed. M. Davies & G. W. Humphreys), ch. 10, pp. 197–223, Oxford: Blackwell.

Schachter, S. & Singer, J. 1962 Cognitive, social and physiological determinants of emotional state. *Phsychol. Rev.* **69**, 378–99.

Schoenbaum, G. & Eichenbaum, H. 1995 Information encoding in the rodent prefrontal cortex. I. Single-neuron activity in orbitofrontal cortex compared with that in pyriform cortex. *J. Neurophysiol.* **74**, 733–50.

Scott, T. R., Yaxley, S., Sienkiewicz, Z. J. & Rolls, E. T. 1986 Gustatory responses in the frontal opercular cortex of the alert cynomolgus monkey. *J. Neurophysiol.* **56**, 876–90.

Seltzer, B. & Pandya, D. N. 1989 Frontal lobe connections of the superior temporal sulcus in the rhesus monkey. *J. Comp. Neurol.* **281**, 97–113.

Takagi, S. F. 1991 Olfactory frontal cortex and multiple olfactory processing in primates. In *Cerebral cortex.* vol. 9 (ed. A. Peters & E. G. Jones), pp. 133–52. New York: Plenum Press.

Thorpe, S. J., Rolls, E. T. & Maddison, S. 1983 Neuronal activity in the orbitofrontal cortex of the behaving monkey. *Exptl. Brain Res.* **49**, 93–115.

Treves, A. & Rolls, E. T. 1991 What determines the capacity of autoassociative memories in the brain? *Network* **2**, 371–97.

Williams, G. V., Rolls, E. T., Leonard, C. M. & Stern, C. 1993 Neuronal responses in the ventral striatum of the behaving monkey. *Behav. Brain Res.* **55**, 243–52.

Wilson, F. A. W., Scalaidhe, S. P. O. & Goldman-Rakic, P. S. 1993 Dissociation of object and spatial processing domains in primate prefrontal cortex. *Science* **260**, 1955–58.

Yaxley, S., Rolls, E. T. & Sienkiewicz, Z. J. 1988 The responsiveness of neurones in the insular gustatory cortex of the macaque monkey is independent of hunger. *Physiol. Behav.* **42**, 223–29.

Yaxley, S., Rolls, E. T. & Sienkiewicz, Z. J. 1990 Gustatory responses of single neurons in the insula of the macaque monkey. *J. Neurophysiol.* **63**, 689–700.

Zatorre, R. J. & Jones-Gotman, M. 1991 Human olfactory discrimination after unilateral frontal or temporal lobectomy. *Brain,* **114**, 71–84.

Zatorre, R. J., Jones-Gotman, M., Evans, A. C. & Meyer, E. 1992 Functional localization of human olfactory cortex. *Nature,* **360**, 339–40.

7

The prefrontal landscape: implications of functional architecture for understanding human mentation and the central executive

P. S. Goldman-Rakic

7.1 Introduction

The prefrontal cortex is the area of the brain most often associated with executive processes in humans. Concerning this venerated organ of mind, two points are rarely contested: first, that this large expanse of neocortex has a compartment organization based on its cytoarchitectonic subdivisions; and second, that injury to this cortex in humans and animals results in a diversity of behavioural abnormalities. One of the major questions confronted by our field is that of how function maps onto structure in association cortex. Do the different regions carry out distinctive functions, e.g. inhibitory control, motor planning and spatial memory, as argued at different times by numerous contributors to the prefrontal literature (e.g. Fulton 1950; Mishkin 1964; Brutkowski 1965; Fuster 1980; Pribram 1987)? Is there a hierarchical relationship between superior and inferior dorsolateral cortex as recently proposed by Owen *et al.* (1996)? Or is the prefrontal cortex organized into subregions according to informational domain with the different domains sharing a common specialization that can uniquely be identified with prefrontal cortex (Goldman-Rakic 1987)? According to this latter view, content, not function, is mapped onto major cytoarchitectonic fields. It would be premature to draw strong conclusions and firm answers to the questions that will be raised here. However, a field advances when discrete hypotheses can be generated, compared and eventually some of them falsified. Furthermore, an understanding of the 'functional map' in prefrontal cortex has direct implications for the nature and existence of a general purpose central executive (Baddeley & Hitch 1974; Baddeley 1986) and/ or a supervisory attentional system (Shallice 1982), as well as for defining the concept of polymodal cortex, the nature of consciousness and the organization of mind. This essay addresses the landscape of prefrontal cortex anatomically and functionally, based on the premise that structure and function are inextricably related. And I would argue further, that every theory of cortical function should be integrated with knowledge of regional circuitry and physiology. The Discussion Meeting has provided an opportunity to review different organizational schemes and suggest ways they may be harmonized and/or tested in future research.

7.2 Tradition of functional duality

A major organizing principle of prefrontal function since mid-century has been that of a duality between the dorsolateral and orbital cortices. An early example of this partition can be found in the Salmon Lecture delivered by John Fulton (1950). Fulton subdivided the prefrontal cortex into mesopallium—posterior areas 13 and 14 of Walker—and neopallium—Walker's areas 9, 10, 11 and 12, 46 and 8. The mesopallium was part of the visceral brain involved in emotion and affect while the neopallium was considered important for intellectual functions. The trend for orbital lesions, particularly posterior or mesopallial areas to produce selective impairments on tasks which evoke emotional or appetitive responses and for lateral lesions of the convexity to produce impairments on tests requiring integration of information has persisted in one form or another to the present day. The caudal regions of the orbital cortex have long been associated with the interoceptive and palpable senses (Fulton 1950) and anatomical evidence is accumulating to show that the orbital areas subserving these functions are definable in terms of the relevant afferent inputs (e.g. Baylis *et al.* 1995; Carmichael & Price 1995). Dias *et al.* (1996) have shown deficits in reversing stimulus-reward associations following orbital lesions in the marmoset presumably attributable to connections with limbic areas. Finally, clinical studies reveal an autonomic pattern of deficits associated with orbital lesions (Damasio *et al.* 1991), although cognitive deficits have also been observed (Eslinger & Damasio 1985; Freedman & Oscar-Berman 1986).

The neopallium or dorsolateral convexity in turn can also be further differentiated into functional territories. In an influential 1964 essay, Mishkin introduced a division of labour between dorsal and ventral portions of the neopallium according to which the dorsolateral convexity represented by the principal sulcus was concerned with spatial function, while the ventral part, or the inferior prefrontal convexity (including the cortex of the lateral orbital cortex) was associated with the maintenance of what was termed 'central sets' (Mishkin 1964). Although then, as now, impairment on delayed-response tasks defined the dorsolateral contribution, emphasis was placed more on its spatial nature and less in terms of the immediate memory process. The tradition of functional diversity was further elaborated by Fuster (1989) who expanded duality of function into the functional trinity of preparatory set, retrospective provisional memory and suppression of external and internal influences. In Fuster's system, the first two functions were associated with the dorsal prefrontal convexity; the last mentioned with the orbital prefrontal cortex

Importantly, however, these three functions were considered subordinate to the synthetic role of prefrontal cortex in 'the formation of temporal structures of behavior with a unifying purpose or goal' (Fuster 1980, p. 126). With respect to memory, Fuster & Alexander (1971), Pribram and Tubbs (1967) and Goldman & Rosvold (1970) all placed emphasis on the temporal structuring of delayed-response tasks, considering their spatial properties as subsidiary. Further, Fuster considered the memory function of prefrontal cortex to be highly localized to one subarea of cortex which subserved both non-spatial as well as spatial processing. Depression of activity in the principal sulcus region by cooling produced both non-spatial and spatial impairments (Bauer & Fuster 1976). On the other hand, surgical removals of the dorsolateral and inferior convexity portions of the dorsolateral cortex have yielded evidence of dissociation between the spatial and non-spatial memory systems of the prefrontal cortex. Passingham (1975), for one, found deficits on delayed colour matching task following inferior convexity lesions; delayed alternation was unimpaired by the same lesion. Conversely, lesions of the principal sulcus produce impairments on spatial delayed-response tasks and rarely on a non-spatial task (for review, see Goldman-Rakic 1987). Nevertheless, the interpretation often given to this dissociation is that the inferior convexity plays a role in inhibiting or overcoming incorrect or prepotent response tendencies while the dorsolateral prefrontal cortex, exemplified by the salient delayed-response deficits, is central to the memorial programming of appropriate motor programmes.

More recent studies have offered additional views of prefrontal functional architecture. Petrides has advanced the idea of a two-stage hierarchical organization of prefrontal cortex according to which the midfrontal areas 9 and 46 carry out sequential processing and self-monitoring functions while the inferior convexity areas 45 and 47 (in humans) are engaged in a lower level function entailing 'comparison between stimuli in short-term memory as well as the active organization of sequences of responses based on conscious explicit retrieval of information from posterior cortical association systems'. In the Petrides model, each level can operate on either spatial or non-spatial information.

This brief review of the literature is intended to make one point—how widespread and deeply rooted is the view that the prefrontal cortex is a composite of functionally distinct or hierarchically arranged areas engaged respectively with the cardinal psychological processes of attention, affect, emotion, memory and motor aspects of behaviour. In this paper I will expand on another view that (1) the dorsolateral prefrontal cortex as a whole has a generic function—'on-line' processing of information or working memory in the service of a wide range of cognitive functions; (2) that this process is iteratively represented throughout several and possibly many subdivisions of the prefrontal neopallium, and (3) that each autonomous subdivision integrates attentional, memorial, motor and possibly affective dimensions of behaviour by virtue of network connectivity with relevant sensory, motor and limbic areas of brain. This view is compatible with the diversity of behavioural deficits described for frontal lobe patients and animals with experimental lesions, and differs mainly with interpretations of data rather than with the data itself, which, in my view, is remarkably consistent (reviewed in Goldman-Rakic 1987).

7.3 Working memory and 'on-line' processing

The tissue surrounding the caudal half of the principal sulcus (Walker's area 46; Brodmann's area 9) including portions of the frontal eye field (area 8) in the rhesus monkey qualifies as a mental sketch pad and central processor of visuo-spatial information. Lesions restricted to this region have been shown repeatedly to impair performance on spatial delayed-response tasks which tax an animal's working memory ability, i.e. to hold an item of information 'in mind' for a short period of time and to update information from moment to moment. The impairments are selective in two critical respects; performance on tasks which engage memory for objects such as visual discrimination object reversal, learning set, match-to-sample is not affected by the same lesions nor do these lesions impair performance which relies on associative memory (e.g. Jacobsen 1936; Goldman *et al.* 1971; Passingham 1975; Mishkin & Manning 1978) or sensory-guided responses (e.g. Funahashi *et al.* 1993a; Sawaguchi & Goldman-Rakic 1993; Chafee & Goldman-Rakic 1994). In general, neither the consistent rules of a task nor its sensorimotor requirements cause a problem for the prefrontally lesioned animal. The monkey's difficulty lies in recalling information and using it to guide a correct response. Thus, on the basis of neuropsychological evidence, I have suggested that the brain obeys the distinction between working and associative memory, and that prefrontal cortex is pre-eminently involved in the former while other areas of the neopallium and hippocampus are likely the necessary critical substrates of memory consolidation and long-term storage (Goldman-Rakic 1987).

Single neuron recording has been used extensively to dissect the neuronal elements involved in working memory processes. This approach also can provide fresh insights into issues of functional allocation as well as deliver convergent validation of their essential nature. In the oculomotor delayed response paradigm utilized for this purpose, briefly presented visuospatial stimuli are remembered in order to provide guidance *from memory* for subsequent saccadic eye movements (figure 7.1a). The essential feature of this task is that the item to be recalled (in this case, the location of an object) has to be updated on every trial as in the moment-to-moment process of human mentation. The prefrontal cortex contains classes of neurons engaged respectively in registering the sensory cue, in holding the cued information 'on line', and in releasing the motor responses in the course of task performance whether the task is conducted in the manual (Fuster & Alexander 1971) or oculomotor (Goldman-Rakic *et al.* 1991) mode. In aggregate, dorsolateral prefrontal cortex contains a local circuit that encompasses the entire range of subfunctions necessary to carry out an integrated response: sensory input, through retention in short-term memory, to motor response. Thus, attentional, memorial and response control mechanisms

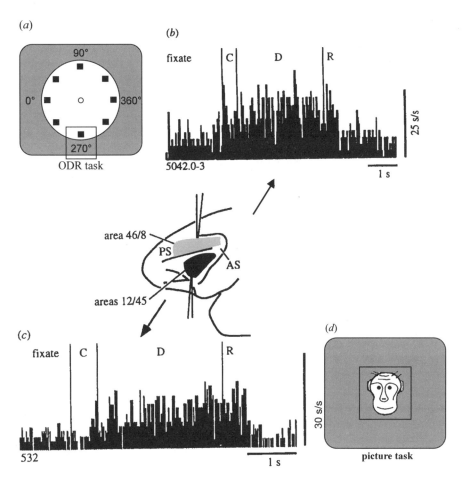

Fig. 7.1 Multiple memory domains are illustrated in this diagram of the monkey prefrontal cortex. The dorsolateral area around the principal sulcus and anterior arcuate is important for spatial working memory; that for features or attributes of objects, in the inferior convexity of the prefrontal cortex. (*a*) Diagram of ODR task; (*b*) activity of a neuron recorded from area 46 during the ODR task. The neuron shown was activated in the delay whenever the monkey had to recall the target presented at the 270° location and at no other location; (*c*) a neuron activated in the delay whenever the stimulus to be recalled was a picture of a particular face during a picture working memory task; the same neuron was unresponsive to other memoranda or in relation to direction of response. (*d*) Diagram of picture working memory task. These results illustrate that prefrontal neurons can code selective aspects of or selected images in working memory. Modified from Funahashi *et al.* 1989 and Wilson *et al.* 1993.

exist within this one area of prefrontal cortex and need not be allocated to separate architectonic regions. Much remains to be learned about a dedicated area like the principal sulcus, including whether it has further functional sub-specializations that have yet to be delineated.

Prefrontal neurons that express 'memory fields' are particularly relevant to this discussion (see figure 7.1*b*). The concept of a 'memory field' is based on the finding that the same neuron appears to always code the same location and different neurons code different locations. Consequently, individual neurons capable of holding specific visuospatial coordinates 'on line' appear to be aggregated into a working memory system within an area of the prefrontal cortex. These aggregates likely form modular or columnar units defined by common visual–spatial coordinates but with the specialized subfunctions of cue registration, maintenance of the mnemonic trace and response preparedness allocated to different neurons within a column (Goldman-Rakic 1984). Again, much remains to be learned about these modules but, even at a microarchitectural level of cortical function, sensory, memorial and motor subfunctions are represented in the circuitry of the module. We have demonstrated that temporary inactivation of one or a few modules results in loss of 'on-line' memory for particular target locations (Sawaguchi & Goldman-Rakic 1991). Further, in instances where the memory field of a neuron is not maintained throughout the delay and the activity falters, the animal is highly likely to make an error (Funahashi *et al.* 1989). The finding that neuronal firing is content-specific and directly associated with accurate recall provides a dramatic example of a compartmentalized and constrained architecture for memory processing equivalent to that observed in sensory systems. Additionally, it has been shown that prefrontal neurons can code the direction of an impending response iconically, i.e. without reference to the direction of the response (Funahashi *et al.* 1993*b*). These and other results provide strong evidence at a cellular level for the theorized role of prefrontal neurons in working memory, i.e. maintenance of representational information in the *absence* of the stimulus that was initially present. Knowledge of these neuronal properties helps to provide an explanation for the observation that monkeys and humans with prefrontal lesions have little difficulty in moving their eyes to a visible target or reaching for a desired object; rather their problem is organizing and directing these same motor responses to *remembered* targets and objects. In the same vein, damage to the prefrontal cortex does not impair knowledge about the world or long-term memory; it impairs only the ability to bring this knowledge to mind and utilize it to guide behaviour.

7.4 Working memory, mental processing and perseveration

Two issues have dominated thinking in the area of prefrontal localization. One already mentioned is the degree of dissociation between areas subserving motor control, disinhibition and perseveration on the one hand and memory processes on the other. Another related issue is the separate location of a temporary storage component and a processing component of working memory (Just & Carpenter 1985; Baddeley 1986). Both issues can be addressed in non-human primates to some degree with an anti-saccade task in which monkeys are trained to suppress the automatic or prepotent tendency to respond in the direction of a remembered cue and instead respond in the opposite direction, a transformation that is not particularly easy for human subjects (Guitton *et al.* 1985). The anti-saccade task could be viewed as a member of a class of tasks like the Stroop test, which require prepotent response tendencies to be overridden by opponent or unlike responses. In our experiment with monkeys (Funahasi *et al.* 1993), we implemented a compound delayed-response paradigm, in which, on some trials, the monkey learned to make deferred eye movements to the same direction signalled by a brief visual cue (standard oculomotor delayed-response (ODR) task), and on other trials, cued by a change in the colour of the fixation spot, to suppress that response and direct its gaze to the opposite direction (delayed anti-saccade task, DAS). The monkeys succeeded in learning this difficult task at high (85% and above) levels of accuracy, in itself an indication that monkeys are capable of holding 'in mind' two sequentially presented items of information—the colour of the fixation point and the location of a spatial cue and transforming the direction of response from left to right (or the reverse) based on a mental synthesis of that information. Approximately one-third of the task-related population coded the direction of the impending response, showing a pattern of activation in the delay period that presaged rightward or leftward responses. However, the majority (approximately 60%) of prefrontal neurons were iconic, i.e. their activity in the delay period reflected the location of the cue, whether the intended movement was toward or away from the designated target. These results, together with numerous other single unit studies of prefrontal neurons, establish the following two major points: (1) the same area of cortex harbours sensory, mnemonic and response coding mechanisms, thus supporting an integral localization of the functions of attention, memory and motor response; and (2) the very same neuron involved in commanding an oculomotor response is also engaged when opposing responses are suppressed and/or redirected. Thus prefrontal neurons engaged in directing a response from memory are at the same time part of the mechanism engaged to inhibit the immediate or prepotent tendency to respond. Based on these findings, we would interpret the common association of verbal fluency and Stroop-like deficits discussed in the recent study by Burgess & Shallice (1996) as a failure to suppress a prepotent response (naming the word) due to an inability to use working memory to initiate the correct response (naming the colour of the word based on recent instruction). Perseveration and disinhibition may be the inevitable result of a loss of the neural substrate necessary to generate the correct response.

7.5 Multiple working memory domains

According to the working memory analysis of prefrontal function, a working memory function should be demonstrable in more than one area of the prefrontal cortex and in more than one knowledge domain. Thus, different areas within prefrontal cortex will share in a common process—working memory; however, each will process different types of information. Thus, informational domain, not process, will be mapped across prefrontal cortex. Evidence on this point has recently been obtained in our laboratory from studies of non-spatial memory systems in areas on the inferior convexity of the prefrontal cortex (O Scalaidhe *et al.* 1992; Wilson *et al.* 1992; Wilson *et al.* 1993). In particular, we explored the hypothesis that the inferior convexity of the prefrontal cortex comprising Walker's areas 12 and 45 may contain specialized circuits for recalling the attributes of stimuli and holding them in short-term memory—thus processing non-spatial information in a manner analogous to the mechanism by which the principal sulcus mediates memory of visuospatial information. The inferior convexity cortex lying below and adjacent to the principal sulcus is a likely candidate for processing non-spatial—colour and form—information, in that lesions of this area produce deficits on tasks requiring memory for the colour or patterns of stimuli (e.g. Passingham 1975; Mishkin & Manning 1978) and the receptive fields of the neurons in this area, unlike those in area 46 on the dorsolateral cortex above, represent the fovea (Mikami *et al.* 1982; Suzuki & Azuma 1983) the region of the retina specialized for the analysis of fine detail and colour—stimulus attributes important for the recognition of objects.

We recorded from the inferior convexity region in monkeys trained to perform delayed-response tasks in which spatial or feature *memoranda* had to be recalled on independent, randomly interwoven trials. For the spatial delayed-response trials (SDR), stimuli were presented 13° to the left or right of fixation while the monkeys gazed at a fixation point on a video monitor. After a delay of 2500 ms, the fixation point disappeared, instructing the animal to direct its gaze to the location where the stimulus appeared before the delay. For the picture delayed-response (PDR) trials, various patterns were presented in the centre of the screen (figure 7.1 *d*); one stimulus indicated that a left-directed and the other a right-directed response would be rewarded at the end of the delay. Thus, both spatial and feature trials required exactly the same eye movements at the end of the delay; but differed in the nature of the mnemonic representation that guided those responses.

We found that neurons were responsive to events in both delayed response tasks. However, a given neuron was generally responsive to the spatial aspects or the feature aspects and not both (Wilson *et al.* 1993). Thus, the majority of the neurons examined in both tasks were active in the delay period when the monkey was recalling a stimulus pattern which required a 13° response to the right *or* left. The same neurons did not respond above baseline during the delay preceding an identical rightward or leftward response on the PDR trials. Neurons exhibiting selective neuronal activity for patterned memoranda were almost exclusively found in or around area 12 on the inferior convexity of the prefrontal cortex, beneath the principal sulcus, while neurons that responded selectively in the SDR were rarely observed in this region, appearing instead in the dorsolateral cortical regions where spatial processing has been localized in our previous studies. In addition, we discovered that the neurons in the inferior convexity were highly responsive to complex stimuli, such as pictures of faces or specific objects. We subsequently used pictures of monkey or human faces as memoranda in a working memory task and demonstrated that such stimuli could indeed serve as memoranda in memory tasks (figure 7.1 *a*, *c*). The same cells are unresponsive on trials when the monkey has to remember a different face or pattern nor do they code the direction of an impending response (Wilson *et al.* 1993). Finally, we have shown that the areas from which face or object selective neurons are recorded are connected directly with area TE in the inferotemporal cortex which is a major relay of the ventral pathway for object vision (Mishkin *et al.* 1982) and an area rich in cells that respond to the features of visual stimuli, including faces (e.g. Rolls & Baylis 1986; Tanaka *et al.* 1991). Together with the evidence for dissociation of inferior prefrontal and dorsolateral prefrontal lesions *vis-à-vis* object processing (reviewed in Goldman-Rakic 1987), these several results establish that non-spatial attributes of an object or stimulus may be processed separately from those dedicated to the analysis of spatial location and vice versa. Furthermore, within inferior prefrontal cortex, different features appear to be encoded by different neurons (Wilson *et al.* 1993; and in preparation). Thus, feature and spatial memory— what and where an object is—are dissociable not only at the areal level but at the cellular level as well. Altogether these findings support the prediction that different prefrontal subdivisions represent different informational domains rather than different processes and thus, more than one working memory domain exists in the prefrontal cortex—one in and around the caudal principal sulcus concerned with spatial information and another on the caudal inferior convexity concerned with object information. If the inferior prefrontal cortex carries out temporal integration of information analogous to the spatial processing of the dorsolateral region, as we have proposed, then it will surely be engaged in 'comparison between stimuli in short-term memory as well as the active organization of sequences of responses based on conscious explicit retrieval of information from posterior cortical association systems' as formulated by Petrides and colleagues (Owen *et al.* 1996). The question to be decided in future research is whether this function is at a lower level of a hierarchical processing than the 'monitoring' function proposed by the same authors for superior prefrontal cortical areas. To decide this, the performance of monkeys with cortical lesions in superior areas will have to be directly compared to that of monkeys with inferior convexity lesions on the same set of tasks.

The functional architecture suggested by physiological and lesion studies in monkeys appear to be supported by findings from positron emission tomography and magnetic resonance imaging in humans. Thus, the middle frontal gyrus where area 46 is located are consistently activated as human subjects access visuo-spatial information from long-term storage and/or immediate experience through representation-based action (e.g. McCarthy *et al.* 1994; Nichelli *et al.* 1994; Baker *et al.* 1996; Gold *et al.* 1996; Goldberg *et al.* 1996; Owen *et al.* 1996; Smith *et al.* 1996; Sweeney *et al.* 1996). In contrast, working memory for the features of objects or faces engages anatomically more lateral and inferior prefrontal regions (Adcock *et al.* 1996; Cohen *et al.* 1994; Courtney *et al.* 1996; McCarthy *et al.* 1996) and semantic encoding and retrieval as well as other verbal processes engages still more inferior, insular and/or anterior prefrontal regions (Paulesu *et al.* 1993; Raichle *et al.* 1994; Demb *et al.* 1995; Fiez *et al.* 1996; Price *et al.* 1996). The superior to inferior localization of spatial, object and linguistic processing in imaging studies of human cognition support a multiple domain hypothesis of prefrontal functional architecture and indicate that there may be a common bauplan for their network organization.

As to the remaining expanse of prefrontal areas, less is known. The evidence from recent studies of the orbital surface indicate that this general region of the frontal lobe may be similarly compartmentalized as to informational domain, though it is not yet clear that these regions have domain-specific 'on-line' memory functions. However, Rolls (see Chapter 6) has mapped a taste area in the caudolateral orbitofrontal cortex near an area concerned with olfaction (Tanabe *et al.* 1974), together providing sensory definition to the mesopallial map. Certainly, the studies of Rolls and others (Tanabe *et al.* 1974; Baylis *et al.* 1995; Carmichael & Price 1995) clearly define gustatory and olfactory regions in the mesopallial areas. What lies in between these and the dorsolateral regions—in the ventromedial and ventrolateral expanse of the orbital cortex—remains to be explored as do the dorsomedial and medial areas of the prefrontal cortex. Studies of orbital lesions in humans have revealed an autonomic pattern of deficits (Damasio *et al.* 1991) as well as subtle executive deficits in real world social contexts (Grattan *et al.* 1994; Eslinger *et al.* 1995).

7.6 Levels of processing: distributed networks subserve sensory, motor, limbic and mnemonic components constrained by informational domain

Although the prefrontal cortex has a pre-eminent role in working memory functions, it does so as part of an integrated network of areas, each dedicated to carrying out specialized functions. Each working memory domain is embedded in and supported by a distinct and essentially independent network of cortical areas; thus networks are functionally integrated by domain. For example, the prefrontal areas engaged in spatial working memory are interconnected with portions of posterior parietal cortex (Cavada & Goldman-Rakic 1989), while the feature working memory areas of the inferior prefrontal cortex are interconnected with area TE in the temporal lobe (Barbas 1988, 1993; Bates *et al.* 1994; Rodman 1994; Webster *et al.* 1994; Carmichael & Price 1995). A network is composed of sensory association (temporal and parietal), premotor (cingulate motor areas, pre-SMA) and limbic (retrosplenial cingulate, parahippo-campal or perirhinal) areas at a minimum and virtually all of the connections within a network are reciprocal (Selemon & Goldman-Rakic

1985). Thus, this model of prefrontal network organization contrasts with other theories of prefrontal organization which distribute attention, affect, memory and motor action among the different cytoarchitectonic regions of the prefrontal cortex. The multiple domain model distributes these functions among the cortical areas within networks defined by informational domain.

Allocation of function within a widespread cortical network is a subject currently under examination by a number of laboratories. Here I give two examples from our own work with respect to the spatial cognition network (Selemon & Goldman-Rakic 1988). Posterior parietal regions carry directionally specific information in all phases of the delayed response task (cue, delay and response) and thus, neurons in posterior parietal cortex mirror those in prefrontal cortex (Chafee *et al.* 1989; Chafee & Goldman-Rakic 1994). In contrast to the parietal cortex, neuronal activity in posterior cingulate cortex is, in general, not directionally tuned but rather posterior cingulate neurons appear to be engaged in a non-specific form of activation related to response anticipation (figure 7.2; Carlson *et al.* 1993). Both the single unit studies described here and a series of 2-deoxyglucose metabolic imaging studies in the literature (e.g. Friedman & Goldman-Rakic 1994) indicate that when spatial memories are activated, parietal, cingulate and prefrontal components of the spatial cognition network are coactivated, though each area may be essential for different aspects of the task in question.

7.7 The supervisory attentional system, the central executive and the domain-specific slave systems

One of the most powerful and influential ideas in cognitive psychology is Baddeley's working memory model (Baddeley 1986). This tripartite model of cognitive architecture invokes a supervisory controlling system called the 'central executive' and two slave systems, the 'articulatory loop' and the 'visuospatial scratch pad' or 'sketch pad', specialized for language and spatial material, respectively (figure 2). The model recognizes the separation of informational domains for lower level tasks handled by the 'slave' systems but retains the traditional notion of a general purpose, panmodal processor in the central executive that manages control and selection processes, similar to the supervisory attentional system of Shallice (1982). The findings reviewed above provide an alternative model in which the expression of central executive processing is a result of the interaction of multiple independent information processing modules each with its own sensory, mnemonic and motor control features. This multiple domain model reduces but does not necessarily eliminate 'the residual area of ignorance' called the central executive but it does open the question of how these independent systems cooperate to result in an integrated behavioural script.

Our view is that the central executive may be composed of multiple segregated special purpose processing domains rather than one central processor served

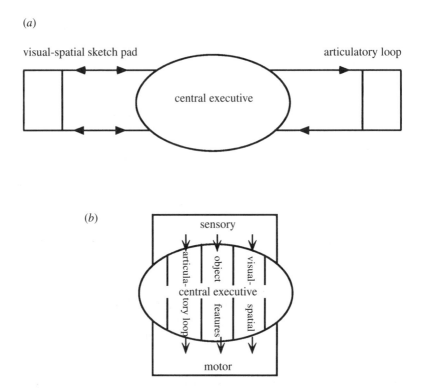

Fig. 7.2 (*a*) Diagram of the central executive (psychologically based; Baddeley 1989). The model consists of a central executive and two slave systems—the phonological loop and the visuospatial sketchpad. The slave systems and central processor are presumed to be localized in separated regions of the cortex. (*b*) Model of the 'central executive' based on functional architecture elucidated in studies of non-human primates (Goldman-Rakic 1996). According to this neurologically based model, the central executive may be considered an emergent property of coactivated multiple domain-specific processors located in prefrontal cortex but interconnected both with the domain-relevant long-term storage sites in posterior regions of the cortex (sensory) and with appropriate motor pathways.

by slave systems converging to a central processor; and that each specialized domain consists of local and extrinsic networks with sensory, mnemonic, motor and motivational control elements (figure 2; Goldman-Rakic 1987). This process-oriented view explains the dysexecutive syndrome—disorganization, perseveration and distractibility—as a default in one or more independent working memory domains. The working memory specialization of the prefrontal cortex is especially suited to retrieve information from long-term memory and process it 'on line'. It is possible to view the coactivation of multiple working memory domains and their associated cortical networks as a well designed parallel processing architecture for the brain's highest level cognition.

References

Adcock, R. A., Constable, R. T., Gore, J. C. & Goldman-Rakic, P. 1996 Functional magnetic resonance imaging of frontal cortex during performance of non-spatial memory tasks. *Neuroimage* **3**, 552.

Baddeley, A. 1986 *Working memory*. Oxford University Press.

Baddeley, A. D. & Hitch, G. 1974 Working memory. In *The psychology of learning and motivation. Advances in research and theory* (ed. G. H. Bower), pp. 47–89. New York: Academic Press.

Baker, S. C., Frith, C. D., Frackowiak, R. S. J. & Dolan, R. J. 1996 Active representation of shape and spatial location in man. *Cereb. Cortex.* **6**, 612–17.

Barbas, H. 1988 Anatomic organization of basoventral and mediodorsal visual recipient prefrontal regions in the rhesus monkey. *J. Comp. Neurol.* **276**, 313–42.

Bates, J. F., Wilson, F. A. W., O Scalaidhe, S. P. & Gold-man-Rakic, P. S. 1994 Area TE connections with inferior prefrontal regions responsive to complex objects and faces. *Soc. Neurosci. Abstr.* **20**, 434.10.

Bauer, R. H. & Fuster, J. M. 1976 Delayed matching and delayed-response deficit from cooling dorsolateral prefrontal cortex in monkeys. *J. Comp. Physiol. Psychol.* **90**, 293–302.

Baylis, L. L., Rolls, E. T. & Baylis, G. C. 1995 Afferent connections of the caudolateral orbitofrontal cortex taste area of the primate. *Neurosci.* **64**, 801–12.

Brutkowski, S. 1965 Functions of prefrontal cortex in animals. *Physiol. Rev.* **45**, 721–46.

Burgess, P. W. & Shallice, T. 1996 Response suppression, initiation and strategy use following frontal lobe lesions. *Neuropsychologia* **34**, 263–73.

Carlson, S., Mikami, A. & Goldman-Rakic, P. S. 1993 Omnidirectional delay activity in the monkey posterior cingulate cortex during the performance of an oculomotor delayed response task. *Soc. Neurosci. Abstr.* **19**, 800.

Carmichael, S. T. & Price, J. L. 1995 Sensory and premotor connections of the orbital and medial prefrontal cortex of macaque monkeys. *J. Comp. Neurol.* **363**, 642–64.

Cavada, C. & Goldman-Rakic, P. S. 1989 Posterior parietal cortex in rhesus monkey: II. Evidence for segretated corticocortical networks linking sensory and limbic areas with the frontal lobe. *J. Comp. Neurol.* **287**, 422–45.

Chafee, M. & Goldman-Rakic, P. S. 1994 Prefrontal cooling dissociates memory-and sensory-guided oculo-motor delayed response functions. *Soc. Neurosci. Abstr.* **20**, 335.1.

Chafee, M., Funahashi, S. & Goldman-Rakic, P. S. 1989 Unit activity in the primate posterior parietal cortex during delayed response performance. *Soc. Neurosci. Abstr.* **15**, 786.

Cohen, J. D., Forman, S. D, Braver, T. S., Casey, B. J., Servan-Schreiber, D. & Noll, D. C. 1994 Activation of the prefrontal cortex in a nonspatial working memory task with functional MRI. *Hum. Brain Map* **1**, 293–304.

Courtney, S. M., Ungerleider, L. G., Keil, K. & Haxby, J. V. 1996 Object and spatial visual working memory activate separate neural systems in human cortex. *Cereb. Cortex* **6**, 39–49.

Damasio, A. R., Tranel, D. & Damasio, H. C. 1991 Somatic markers and the guidance of behavior: Theory and preliminary testing. In *Frontal lobe function and dysfunction* (ed. H. S. Levin, H. M. Eisenberg, & A. L. Benton), pp. 217–29. New York: Oxford University Press.

Demb, J. B., Desmond, J. E., Wagner, A. D., Vaidya, C. J., Glover, G. H. & Gabrieli, J. D. E. 1995 Semantic encoding and retrieval in the left inferior prefrontal cortex:

A functional MRI study of task difficult and process specificity. *J. Neurosci.* **15**, 5870–78.

Dias, R., Robbins, T. W. & Roberts, A. C. 1996 Dissociation in prefrontal cortex of affective and attentional shifts. *Nature* **380**, 69–72.

Eslinger, P. J. & Damasio, A. R. 1985 Severe disturbance of higher cognition after bilateral frontal lobe ablation: Patient EVR. *Neurology* **35**, 1731–41.

Eslinger, P. J., Grattan, L. M. & Geder, L. 1995 Impact of frontal lobe lesions on rehabilitation and recovery from acute brain injury. *NeuroRehabilitation* **5**, 161–82.

Fiez, J. A., Raife, E. A., Balota, D. A., Schwarz, J. P., Raichle, M. E. & Petersen, S. E. 1996 A position emission tomography study of the short-term maintenance of verbal information. *J. Neurosci.* **16**, 808–22.

Freedman, M. & Oscar-Berman, M. 1986 Bilateral frontal lobe disease and selective delayed response deficits in humans. *Behav. Neurosci.* **100**, 337–42.

Fulton, J. F. 1950 *Frontal lobotomy and affective behavior.* New York: Norton.

Funahashi, S., Bruce, C. J. & Goldman-Rakic, P. S. 1989 Mnemonic coding of visual space in the monkey's dorsolateral prefrontal cortex. *J. Neurophysiol.* **61**, 1–19.

Funahashi, S., Bruce, C. J. & Goldman-Rakic, P. S. 1993*a* Dorsolateral prefrontal lesions and oculomotor delayed-response performance: Evidence for mnemonic scotomas. *J. Neurosci.* **13**, 1479–97.

Funahashi, S., Chafee, M. V. & Goldman-Rakic, P. S. 1993*b* Prefrontal neuronal activity in rhesus monkeys performing a delayed anti-saccade task. *Nature* **365**, 753–56.

Fuster, J. M. 1980 *The prefrontal cortex.* New York: Raven Press.

Fuster, J. M. 1989 *The prefrontal cortex.* 2nd edn. New York: Raven Press.

Fuster, J. M. & Alexander, G. E. 1971 Neuron activity related to short-term memory. *Science* **173**, 652–54.

Gold, J. M., Berman, K. F., Randolph, C., Goldberg, T. E. & Weinberger, D. R. 1966 PET validation and clinical application of a novel prefrontal task. *Neuropsychology* **10**, 3–10.

Goldberg, T. E., Berman, K. F., Randolph, C., Gold, J. M. & Weinberger, D. R. 1996 Isolating the mnemonic component in spatial delayed response: A controlled PET 0–15 water regional cerebral blood flow study in normal humans. *Neuroimage.* (In the press.)

Goldman, P. S. & Rosvold, H. E. 1970 Localization of function within the dorsolateral prefrontal cortex of the rhesus monkey. *Experimental Neurology* **27**, 291–304.

Goldman, P. S., Rosvold, H. E., Vest, B. & Galkin, T. W. 1971 Analysis of the delayed-alternation deficit produced by dorsolateral prefrontal lesions in the rhesus monkey. *J. Comp. Physiol. Psychol.* **77**, 212–20.

Goldman-Rakic, P. S. 1984 The frontal lobes: Uncharted provinces of the brain. *TINS* **7**, 425–29.

Goldman-Rakic, P. S. 1987 Circuitry of primate prefrontal cortex and regulation of behavior by representational memory. In *Handbook of physiology, the nervous system, higher functions of the brain* (ed. F. Plum), sect. I, vol. V, pp. 373–417. Bethesda, MD: American Physiological Society.

Goldman-Rakic, P. S., Funahashi, S. & Bruce, C. J. 1991 Neocortical memory circuits. *Q. J. Quantitative Biology* **55**, 1025–38.

Grattan, L. M., Bloomer, R. H., Archambault, F. X. & Eslinger, P. J. 1994 Cognitive flexibility and empathy after frontal lobe lesion. *Neuropsychiat. Neuropsychol. Behav. Neurol.* **7**, 251–59.

Guitton, D, Buchtel, H. A. & Douglas, R. M. 1985 Frontal lobe lesions in man cause difficulties in suppressing reflexive glances and in generating goal-directed saccades. *Exp. Brain Res.* **58**, 455–72.

Jacobsen, C. F. 1936 Studies of cerebral function in primates. *Comp. Psychol. Monogr.* **13**, 1–8.

Just, M. A. & Carpenter, P. A. 1985 Cognitive coordinate systems: Accounts of mental rotation and individual differences in spatial ability. *Psych. Rev.* **92**, 137–72.

McCarthy, G., Blamire, A. M., Puce, A. *et al.* 1994 Functional magnetic resonance imaging of human prefrontal cortex activation during a spatial working memory task. *Proc. Natl. Acad. Sci. U.S.A.* **91**, 8690–94.

McCarthy, G., Puce, A., Constable, R. T., Krystal, J. H., Gore, J. C. & Goldman-Rakic, P. S. 1996 Activation of human prefrontal cortex during spatial and nonspatial working memory tasks measured by functional MRI. *Cereb. Cortex.* **6**, 600–10.

Mikami, A., Ito, S. & Kubota, K. 1982 Visual response properties of dorsolateral prefrontal neurons during a visual fixation task. *J. Neurophysiol.* **47**, 593–605.

Mishkin, M. 1964 Perseveration of central sets after frontal lesions in monkeys. In *The frontal granular cortex and behavior* (ed. J. M. Warren & K. Akert), pp. 219–41. New York: McGraw-Hill.

Mishkin, M. & Manning, F. J. 1978 Non-spatial memory after selective prefrontal lesions in monkeys. *Brain Res.* **143**, 313–23.

Mishkin, M., Ungerleider, L. G. & Macko, K. A. 1982. Object vision and spatial vision: Two cortical pathways. *TINS* **6**, 414–17.

Nichelli, P. Grafman, J., Pietrini, P., Alway, D., Carton, J. C. & Miletich, R. 1994 Brain activity in chess playing. *Nature* **369**, 191.

O Scalaidhe, S. P., Wilson, F. A. W. & Goldman-Rakic, P. S. 1992 Neurons in the prefrontal cortex of the macaque selective for faces. *Soc. Neurosci. Abstr.* **18**, 705.

Owen, A. M., Evans, A. C. & Petrides, M. 1996 Evidence for a two-stage model of spatial working memory processing with the lateral frontal cortex: A position emission tomography study. *Cereb. Cortex* **6**, 31–38.

Passingham, R. E. 1975 Delayed matching after selective prefrontal lesions in monkeys (*Macaca mulatta*). *Brain Res.* **92**, 89–102.

Paulescu, E., Frith, C. D., & Frackowiak, R. S. J. 1993. Localization of a human system for sustained attention by positron emission tomography. *Nature* **362**, 342–45.

Pribram, K. H. 1987 The subdivisions of the frontal cortex revisited. In *The frontal lobes revisited* (ed. E. Perecman), pp. 11–39. New York: The IRBN Press.

Pribram, K. H. & Tubbs, W. E. 1967 Short-term memory, parsing and the primate frontal cortex. *Science* **156**, 1765–67.

Price, C. J., Wise, R. J. S. & Frackowiak, R. S. J. 1996 Demonstrating the implicit processing of visually presented words and pseudowords. *Cereb. Cortex* **6**, 62–70.

Raichle, M. E., Fiez, J. A., Videen, T. O. *et al.* 1994 Practice-related changes in human brain functional anatomy during non-motor learning. *Cereb. Cortex* **4**, 8–26.

Rodman, H. R. 1994 Development of inferior temporal cortex in the monkey. *Cereb. Cortex* **4**, 484–98.

Rolls, E. T. & Baylis, G. C. 1986 Size and contrast have only small effects on the responses to faces of neurons in the cortex of the superior temporal sulcus of the monkey. *Exp. Brain Res.* **65**, 38–48.

Sawaguchi, T. & Goldman-Rakic, P. S. 1991 D1 dopamine receptors in prefrontal cortex: involvement in working memory. *Science* **251**, 947–50.

Sawaguchi, T. & Goldman-Rakic, P. S. 1993 The role of D1-dopamine receptor in working memory: Local injections of dopamine antagonists into the prefrontal cortex of rhesus monkeys performing an oculomotor delayed-response task. *J. Neurophysiol.* **71**, 515–28.

Selemon, L. D. & Goldman-Rakic, P. S. 1985 Longitudinal topography and interdigitation of corticostriatal projections in the rhesus monkey. *J. Neuroscience*, **5**, 776–94.

Selemon, L. D. & Goldman-Rakic, P. S. 1988 Common cortical and subcortical target areas of the dorsolateral prefrontal and posterior parietal cortices in the rhesus monkey: Evidence for a distributed neural network subserving spatially guided behavior. *J. Neuroscience* **8**, 4049–68.

Shallice, T. 1982 Specific impairments in planning. *Proc. Roy. Soc.* **298**, 199–209.

Smith, E. E., Jonides, J. & Koeppe, R. A. 1996 Dissociating verbal and spatial working memory using PET. *Cereb. Cortex* **6**, 11–20.

Suzuki, H. & Azuma, M. 1983 Topographic studies on visual neurons in the dorsolateral prefrontal cortex of the monkey. *Exp. Brain Res.* **53**, 47–58.

Sweeney, J. A., Mintun, M. A., Kwee, M. B. *et al.* 1996 Positron emission tomography study of voluntary saccadic eye movements and spatial working memory. *J. Neurophsyiol.* **75**, 454–68.

Tanabe, T., Ooshima, Y. & Takagi, S. F. 1974 An olfactory area in the prefrontal lobe. *Brain Res.* **80**, 127–30.

Tanaka, K., Saito, H., Fukada, Y. & Moriya, M. 1991. Coding visual images of objects in the inferotemporal cortex of the macaque monkey. *J. Neurophysiol.* **66**, 170–89.

Webster, M. J., Bachevalier, J. & Ungerleider, L. G. 1994 Connections of inferior temporal areas TEO and TE with parietal and frontal cortex in macaque monkeys. *Cereb. Cortex* **4**, 470–83.

Wilson, F. A. W., O Scalaidhe, S. P. & Goldman-Rakic, P. S. 1992 Areal and cellular segregation of spatial and of feature processing by prefrontal neurons. *Soc. Neurosci. Abstr.* **18**, 705.

Wilson, F. A. W., O Scalaidhe, S. P. & Goldman-Rakic, P. S. 1993 Dissociation of object and spatial processing domains in primate prefrontal cortex. *Science* **260**, 1955–58.

8

Specialized systems for the processing of mnemonic information within the primate frontal cortex

Michael Petrides

8.1 Introduction

What is the role in mnemonic processing of the large region of the lateral frontal cortex that, in the primate brain, extends in front of the precentral motor cortex as far as the frontal pole? Patients with damage to this lateral prefrontal cortical region perform well on several tests that are sensitive indicators of the memory disorder that follows damage to the limbic structures of the medial temporal region. Performance on these standard tests of memory, such as recognition and story recall, can be normal even when the lesions are bilateral, as several studies of patients who had undergone frontal lobotomies have clearly demonstrated (see Petrides 1989 for a review). In cases where a severe memory disorder has been reported after frontal lesions, there was involvement of the caudal orbito-medial limbic region of the frontal lobe and the immediately adjacent basal forebrain region (e.g. septal area, nucleus basalis of Meynert, etc.) or there has been significant damage outside the frontal cortex (see Petrides 1989 for a review). Indeed, there has never been a case of amnesia reported after lesions demonstrated to be restricted to the lateral frontal cortex.

Although damage to the lateral frontal cortex in both the human and the monkey brain does not result in a generalized memory disorder, mnemonic performance can be severely impaired under certain conditions of testing. In the monkey, a long line of studies that had its origin in the now classic demonstration by Jacobsen (1936) that lesions of the frontal cortex impair performance on the delayed response tasks has clearly established the involvement of the lateral frontal cortex in working memory (e.g. Mishkin 1957; Gross & Weiskrantz 1962; Butters & Pandya 1969; Mishkin *et al.* 1969; Goldman & Rosvold 1970; Goldman *et al.* 1971; Passingham 1975; Mishkin & Manning 1978; Funahashi *et al.* 1993). A precise characterization of the nature of this involvement has, however, proved elusive.

In the late 1970s, as part of our effort to capture the essential nature of the specific contribution of the human lateral frontal cortex to mnemonic processing, we developed a working memory task in which subjects were required to monitor their recent selections from a set of stimuli (Petrides & Milner 1982). Thus, in this self-ordered task, short-term memory was combined with one aspect of executive processing, namely monitoring. Patients with lateral frontal excisions were severely impaired on the self-ordered task, although they could perform well on several other memory tests, such as recognition memory and the digit span.

In the self-ordered task, the subjects are presented with different arrangements of the same set of stimuli and have to select a different stimulus, on each trial, until all the stimuli are selected. As soon as they start responding, the subjects must therefore be constantly comparing the responses that they have already made with those still remaining to be carried out, i.e. events in working memory must be closely monitored. Monitoring refers to the fact that each selection must be marked in the subject's mind and simultaneously considered in relation to the others that still remain to be selected. Monitoring within working memory must not be confused with simple attention to a stimulus held in memory. For instance, there are many situations (e.g. recognition memory) in which a particular stimulus in memory is attended to and the other stimuli are not in the centre of current awareness. These situations do not challenge monitoring within working memory in the sense used here, although they demand attention to the stimulus that is being remembered (see Petrides 1995a).

8.2 Mid-dorsolateral frontal cortex is critical for monitoring of events in working memory

In work with the monkey, where lesions can be restricted with precision within particular regions of the brain, it has now been shown that damage to the mid-dorsolateral part of the frontal cortex (i.e. the dorsal part of area 46 and area 9; figure 8.1) will result in a severe impairment on the self-ordered and the related externally ordered nonspatial working memory tasks (Petrides 1991, 1995b). Even more important, however, is the fact that it has been possible to analyse the nature of the impairment after lesions of this cortical region in isolation from the potentially additive/interactive effects of damage to other frontal areas. It is now clear that the impairment on the self-ordered and externally ordered working memory tasks after mid-dorsolateral frontal lesions occurs against a background of normal basic mnemonic processing. For instance, monkeys with such lesions (Petrides 1991, 1995b) or even larger dorsolateral frontal lesions (Bachevalier & Mishkin 1986) are able to perform normally on recognition memory tasks in which they have to identify the novel from the familiar stimuli. In addition, monkeys with dorsolateral frontal lesions perform well on delayed matching-to-sample tasks in which they have to recognize

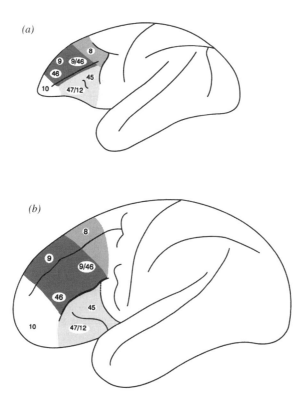

Fig. 8.1 Lateral surface of the macaque monkey (*a*) and the human (*b*) frontal cortex illustrating the mid-dorsolateral frontal region (areas 46, 9, 9/46) and the mid-ventro-lateral frontal region (areas 45 and 47/12). The term mid-dorsolateral frontal cortex is used to distinguish, in the rostrocaudal direction, this region from the frontopolar cortex (i.e. area 10) and the posterior dorsolateral frontal cortex (i.e. area 8 and rostral area 6). In the human brain, the mid-dorsolateral frontal cortex occupies the middle parts of the superior and middle frontal gyri. In the human brain, the ventrolateral frontal cortical areas 45 and 47/12 occupy the pars triangularis and pars orbitalis of the inferior frontal gyrus, respectively. In the macaque monkey brain, the ventrolateral frontal cortex lies below the sulcus principalis, occupying the inferior frontal convexity. It comprises architectonic areas 47/12 and 45. The term area 47/12 is used in both the human and the monkey brain to acknowledge the architectonic correspondence between the part of area 47 that lies on the pars orbitalis of the human inferior frontal gyrus and a large part of Walker's area 12 that occupies the inferior convexity of the macaque monkey (see Petrides & Pandya 1994).

which one of two constantly recurring stimuli was most recently presented (Passingham 1975), as well as on the delayed object alternation task in which they have to alternate their responses between two stimuli (Mishkin *et al.* 1969; Petrides 1995*b*). In other words, mnemonic judgements based on the relative recency or primacy of stimuli need not be affected by dorsolateral frontal damage. This basic mnemonic processing, however, can quickly prove inadequate to sustain normal performance on more challenging non-spatial working memory tasks, such as the self-ordered and the externally ordered tasks.

The fundamental problem of animals with mid-dorsolateral frontal lesions on the self-ordered and on the externally ordered working memory tasks has been shown to stem from the monitoring requirements of the tasks, i.e. the number of stimuli that must be considered as responses are being made (Petrides 1995 b). In one experiment, monkeys with lesions of the mid-dorsolateral frontal cortex were severely impaired when they were required to monitor which one of three possible stimuli they had previously selected, but they were not impaired in remembering which one of two stimuli was chosen, even when a long intertrial interval (60 s) was imposed (see Petrides 1995b, experiments 4 & 5). Thus, the number of possible alternative choices that must be considered (i.e. monitored) within working memory, and not the passage of time *per se*, is the critical factor determining whether or not an impairment will follow mid-dorsolateral frontal lesions.

The mid-dorsolateral part of the frontal cortex appears to be a specialized area of the cerebral cortex in which information can be held on-line for monitoring (in the sense described above) and manipulation of stimuli. It has been argued that it constitutes a specialized neural system where stimuli or events that are first interpreted and maintained in posterior association cortical areas can be recoded for the purpose of planned action or the monitoring of expected acts or events (Petrides 1994). It is a system for the on-line maintenance and monitoring of cognitive representations of intended acts (e.g. self-generated choices) and the occurrence of events from a given set. These specific functional contributions of the mid-dorsolateral frontal cortex, a region that is very well developed in the primate brain, make possible high-level planning and organization of behaviour.

8.3 A two-level hypothesis of the involvement of the lateral frontal cortex in memory

It has been known for a long time that lesions restricted to the cortex lining the sulcus principalis in the monkey lateral frontal lobe result in severe impairments on certain spatial memory tasks, such as the classical delayed response and delayed alternation tasks (e.g. Mishkin 1957; Gross & Weiskrantz 1962; Butters & Pandya 1969; Goldman & Rosvold 1970). But lesions that spare the sulcus principalis and involve only the mid-dorsolateral frontal cortex that lies above it do not yield impairments on these standard spatial delayed response tasks (e.g. Mishkin 1957; Goldman & Rosvold 1970; Goldman et al. 1971) or on non-spatial analogues of these tasks (Mishkin et al. 1969). Performance on the latter non-spatial tasks is severely affected by lesions of the ventrolateral frontal cortex that extends below the sulcus principalis (Passingham 1975; Mishkin & Manning 1978).

The above evidence has often been taken to imply a dichotomy between the mnemonic processing of spatial information in the dorsolateral frontal cortex and non-spatial mnemonic processing in the ventrolateral frontal cortex. There are, however, a number of problems with this distinction. First, the recent demonstration of a severe impairment on the non-spatial self-ordered and externally ordered working memory tasks after lesions of the mid-dorsal part of the lateral frontal cortex (dorsal area 46 and area 9) of the monkey indicates that, at least for this part of the frontal cortex, the mnemonic demands of the task, rather than the modality of the material to be processed, determine whether an impairment will be observed after the lesions (Petrides 1991, 1995b). Second, it must be pointed out that lesions of the ventrolateral frontal cortex (areas 45 and 47/12) of the monkey impair severely performance of both the spatial and the non-spatial versions of the delayed alternation task (Mishkin et al. 1969). The above findings question the idea that the fundamental difference in the functional contribution of the mid-dorsolateral and the mid-ventrolateral frontal cortex can be adequately described as one of modality specificity, namely spatial for the dorsolateral and nonspatial visual for the ventrolateral frontal cortex.

An alternative hypothesis has recently been suggested that views the fundamental difference between the mid-dorsolateral and the mid-ventrolateral frontal cortex as one of distinct levels of involvement in memory rather than simply the result of modality specificity (Petrides 1994). According to this two-level hypothesis, the mid-ventrolateral frontal cortex, in interaction with posterior cortical association areas, subserves the expression within memory of various first-order executive processes, such as active selection, comparison and judgement of stimuli held in short-term and long-term memory (see Petrides 1994 for details; figure 8.2). This type of interaction is necessary for active (explicit) encoding and retrieval of information, i.e. processes initiated under conscious effort by the subject and guided by the subject's plans and intentions. The mid-dorsolateral frontal cortex (areas 9 and 46), on the other hand, constitutes another level of interaction and is involved when several pieces of information in working memory need to be monitored and manipulated on the basis of the requirements of the task or the subject's current plans. It must be emphasized that the two levels of mnemonic executive processing posited above are likely to be involved in several tasks and often simultaneously. The successful demonstration of the specific contribution of the different areas will therefore depend on selective lesion studies (e.g. in non-human primates) in which impaired performance on certain mnemonic tasks is contrasted with normal performance on other similar tasks and on neuroimaging studies with normal human subjects in which experimental tasks are differentially loaded with requirements thought to involve one or the other area.

It should be pointed out here that the two-level hypothesis is fundamentally different from another current theoretical position which suggests that the various prefrontal areas perform a similar role in working memory, but that each will process different types of information (Goldman-Rakic 1995).

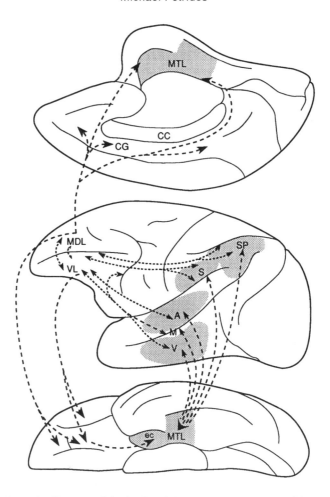

Fig. 8.2 Schematic diagram of the brain of the macaque monkey to illustrate some of the functional interactions postulated by the two-level hypothesis of the role of the lateral frontal cortex to mnemonic processing. Somatosensory (S), spatial (SP), auditory (A), visual (V) and some aspects of multimodal (M) information are processed in posterior temporal and parietal association cortex. In the human brain, linguistic information is processed, primarily in the left hemisphere in the region of the parieto-temporal junction, i.e. supramarginal gyrus in parietal cortex and middle and posterior temporal cortex. Processing in these posterior association cortical areas is assumed by the present model to underlie not only perception and long-term storage, but also transient maintenance of information for further processing. These areas interact with ventrolateral (VL) frontal cortical areas when executive processing, such as decision making, comparison, or active retrieval of information held in memory, is involved. The mid-dorsolateral (MDL) frontal cortex, which is connected with the ventrolateral frontal cortex and with the memory system of the medial temporal lobe (MTL), both directly and indirectly, exercises a higher-order control of mnemonic processing when monitoring and manipulation of information in working memory is required. CC: corpus callosum; CG: cingulate gyrus; ec: entorhinal cortex.

8.4 Functional activation of the human mid-dorsolateral frontal cortex

In studies with positron emission tomography (PET) it has been possible to extend to the human brain the demonstration from the animal work that the mid-dorsolateral frontal cortex constitutes a specialized region for the monitoring, within working memory, of self-ordered and externally ordered responses (Petrides *et al.* 1993*a, b*). In one study, the distribution of cerebral blood flow (i.e. a marker of local neuronal activity) was measured in normal volunteer subjects as they performed a non-spatial visual self-ordered task, a visual matching control task and a visual conditional task (Petrides *et al.* 1993*a*). The same eight visual stimuli (abstract designs) were used in all three tasks and these stimuli were presented in a different random arrangement on each trial. The subjects were required to indicate their response by pointing to particular stimuli. Thus, the only difference between the three tasks lay in their cognitive requirements. In the self-ordered task, the subjects were required to select a different stimulus on each trial until all had been selected. The subjects were therefore required to consider actively (i.e. monitor) their earlier selections as they were preparing their next response. In the matching control task, the subjects had to search and find the same stimulus on each trial. This task therefore involved the same visual stimuli and searching behaviour as the self-ordered task, but did not require that the subjects consider their earlier responses in relation to the current one. In the conditional task, the subjects had learned, prior to scanning, associations between the stimuli and particular colour cues. During scanning, they were required to select the stimulus that was appropriate for the colour cue presented. Thus, the searching among the stimuli was the same as in the self-ordered task, but since the stimulus to be selected, on each trial, was completely determined by the colour cue presented, no monitoring within working memory of prior selections was required. Performance of the self-ordered task, in comparison with either the matching control or the conditional task, resulted in significantly greater activity within the mid-dorsolateral frontal cortex (areas 46 and 9), particularly within the right hemisphere. There was no activation in this region when cerebral blood flow in the conditional task was compared with that of the control task, although there was now significant activity within the posterior dorsolateral frontal cortex in area 8, a region that is known to be critical for visual conditional learning. The contrast in the activation patterns between the self-ordered and the conditional tasks emphasizes the specificity of activation within the mid-dorsolateral frontal cortex in relation to the monitoring requirements of the self-ordered task.

A related study demonstrated bilateral activation of the mid-dorsolateral frontal cortex in relation to the performance of a verbal self-ordered task and a verbal externally ordered task (Petrides *et al.* 1993*b*). With regard to spatial working memory, activation of either the ventrolateral frontal cortex (area 47/12; Jonides *et al.* 1993) or the mid-dorsolateral frontal cortical area

46 (McCarthy *et al.* 1994) has been reported. We have also observed activation of the mid-dorsolateral or the mid-ventrolateral frontal cortex or both, depending on whether the monitoring or the retrieval of specific information from spatial working memory was taxed (Owen *et al.* 1996). When the task required the execution of a sequence of moves previously shown, the ventrolateral frontal cortex was activated. When, however, the task required in addition active monitoring and manipulation of spatial information within working memory, activation was also observed in the mid-dorsolateral frontal cortex.

8.5 Functional contribution of the mid-ventrolateral frontal region: involvement in active retrieval but not automatic retrieval

The two-level hypothesis presented above makes a distinction between active (strategic) retrieval, which requires ventrolateral frontal cortex, and automatic retrieval which does not (Petrides 1994, 1995a). According to this hypothesis, automatic retrieval is the by-product of the triggering of stored representations in posterior cortical association regions either by incoming sensory input that matches pre-existing representations or by recalled events that trigger stored representations of related information on the basis of strong pre-existing associations or other relations, such as thematic context. This kind of automatic retrieval occurs as long as the connections between the posterior temporal and parietal association areas, where sensory processing is carried out, and subcortical structures are intact. The ventrolateral frontal cortex interacts with posterior temporal and parietal association cortex (via strong bi-directional connections) when active retrieval of specific information held in these posterior association areas is required. Active retrieval implies conscious (i.e. willed) effort to retrieve a specific piece of information guided by the subject's intentions and plans. This attempt at retrieval may be self-generated or set up by the instructions given to the subject.

The above hypothesis provides an adequate explanation of why lateral frontal lesions do not cause a generalized memory disorder. Performance on several standard memory tests can be normal after such lesions because it can be the automatic result of processing in the posterior temporal and parietal perceptual systems. For instance, when a stimulus that was seen before is again experienced through the visual modality the novel processing matches (i.e. triggers) pre-existing representations in posterior association cortex; this reactivation is sufficient to carry knowledge that the stimulus had been experienced before. Thus, performance on several basic recognition tasks that simply require awareness of familiarity of the stimulus can be normal after lateral frontal lesions. Similarly, when a subject reads or listens to a narrative story and that subject is subsequently asked to relate this story, the thematic relations between the various components of the story automatically trigger related pieces of information in posterior association cortex. Thus, the story is recalled even if the subject has suffered damage to the lateral frontal cortex. By contrast, when the subject is asked to recall specific pieces of information that are not automatically triggered by current sensory input or thematic and other strong relations, an active retrieval must be initiated to search for and retrieve the particular piece of information. According to the two-level hypothesis presented above, this type of search does require interactions between the ventrolateral frontal cortex and the posterior temporal and parietal association cortex.

In a recent series of studies with positron emission tomography, we attempted to test the prediction from the two-level hypothesis that the mid-ventrolateral frontal cortex (i.e. areas 45 and 47/12) is involved in the active explicit retrieval of specific information (Petrides *et al.* 1995; Doyon *et al.* 1996). In the first study, the aim was to establish whether the human mid-ventrolateral frontal cortex, in the left hemisphere, is involved in the strategic retrieval of verbal information from long-term memory (Petrides *et al.* 1995). To engage the subject in active retrieval of specific verbal information from long-term memory, the main experimental condition involved, during scanning, the free recall of a list of arbitrary words that had been studied before scanning. It is well known from experimental psychological studies that free recall under these conditions is the result of active strategic retrieval processes. Note that performance on such a free recall task cannot be simply the result of recognizing familiar words that are presented again, nor can it be the result of retrieving information by thematic relatedness, as in a logical story. The subject is now asked to recall a specific set of arbitrary words from his/her lexicon that were presented on a particular recent occasion under particular conditions, namely the specific set of words studied just before scanning.

As any recall task will require some degree of monitoring within working memory of the output from long-term memory, it was to be expected that during the performance of the above free recall task there should be significant activity in the mid-dorsolateral region of the frontal cortex, in addition to any ventrolateral activity that might be observed. Note that in our earlier work with PET (Petrides *et al.* 1993*b*), the mid-dorsolateral region of the frontal cortex, but not the ventrolateral, was shown to be specifically activated in relation to the monitoring, within working memory, of self-generated and externally generated verbal responses. Two control conditions were therefore employed to reveal any specific contribution of the left mid-ventrolateral frontal cortex to the active retrieval of verbal information. One of these scanning conditions required the simple repetition of auditorily presented words and was designed to control for processes involved in the listening, understanding and production of words. The other control condition was designed to involve easy verbal retrieval (i.e. at a level that would be significantly easier than that of the free recall task) but monitoring, within working memory, of the retrieved verbal output at about the same level as that in the free recall task. For this purpose, a verbal paired-associate task was used in which the pairs were very well learned before scanning and were therefore very easy to retrieve in comparison with the free recall task (Petrides *et al.* 1995).

In relation to the repetition control task, both the free recall task resulted in greater activation within both the mid-ventrolateral and mid-dorsolateral frontal cortex. The comparison between the free recall (i.e. difficult retrieval) and the highly learned paired-associate recall (i.e. easy retrieval) revealed significantly greater activity in the left mid-ventrolateral frontal cortex in the free recall task, but no difference between the tasks in the mid-dorsolateral frontal cortex (Petrides *et al.* 1995).

Significant activity in the dorsolateral frontal cortex had been previously observed in a number of other PET studies that examined retrieval from verbal episodic memory (Grasby *et al.* 1993; Shallice *et al.* 1994; Tulving *et al.* 1994; Buckner *et al.* 1995). In these studies, with the exception of Buckner *et al.* (1995), no activation of the ventrolateral frontal cortex was observed. The present results suggest that the earlier failure to observe activation in ventrolateral frontal cortex from retrieval of verbal episodic memory was due to the fact that the control tasks used also activated, to the same extent, ventrolateral frontal cortex. The results presented above indicate that the mid-dorsolateral and the mid-ventrolateral frontal cortex are involved in the performance of tasks requiring retrieval from verbal episodic long-term memory, but their contributions differ. The mid-dorsolateral frontal region participates in free recall by virtue of its role in the on-line monitoring, within working memory, of the output from long-term memory, whereas the mid-ventrolateral frontal cortex is more directly involved in active retrieval mechanisms (Petrides *et al.* 1995).

In another PET study, we tested the prediction that the right mid-ventrolateral frontal cortex would be involved in the active explicit retrieval of specific information in a visuospatial task (Doyon *et al.* 1996). The aim of this study was to compare neuronal activation between a condition in which the subjects performed a highly automatized visuospatial sequence under implicit control with a condition in which the subjects performed the same sequence but now with explicit knowledge and thus explicit retrieval of each move in the sequence. The prediction from the two-level hypothesis was that, in comparison with the automatic performance of the visuospatial sequence, explicit performance of the sequence should involve activity in the ventrolateral frontal cortex.

In this task, the subjects were faced with a touch-sensitive screen on which four blue response boxes were displayed. During testing, a red circle would appear above one of the response boxes and the subject was simply required to touch that box as quickly as possible (figure 8.3). As soon as the subject had touched the appropriate box, the red circle disappeared and, after a fixed interval (800 ms), the red circle would again appear above one of the boxes, thus initiating the next trial. As before, the subject's task was merely to touch the box that lay under the red circle as fast as possible. In every block of ten trials, the red circle moved in a predetermined fixed sequence, but the subject was not informed of this. The subjects were extensively trained on this task just before scanning. As expected, the result of this training was to reduce significantly the subject's reaction time on each trial, indicating learning of the repeating sequence (figure 8.3). The subjects were then scanned with PET as they performed this highly automatized visuospatial sequence of movements.

After the above training and scanning, the subjects were asked whether they had noticed that there was a sequence in the task and whether they knew the sequence. Although all subjects were aware that there was a repeating sequence of moves, none of them was able to generate the repeating sequence from memory. The subjects were then given explicit training on the sequence in the following manner. Instead of simply being required to press the box below which the red circle appeared, as in the implicit training, they were now asked to press the box where they thought the next stimulus in the visuospatial sequence would appear. This training procedure was continued until the subjects reached the learning criterion. The subjects were then scanned with PET under testing conditions that were identical to those of the implicit sequence performance.

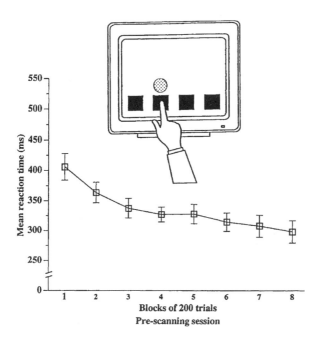

Fig. 8.3 Schematic diagram of the experimental arrangement in the visuospatial sequence task. On each trial, a red circle appeared above one of four blue response boxes. The subject's task was to touch that box as quickly as possible. The graph shows the mean reaction time data of the subjects tested in the visuospatial sequence task. Note the gradual reduction in reaction time implying implicit learning of the sequence as a result of the pre-scanning training session. Each data point in the training session corresponds to the reaction time averaged over two blocks of 100 trials (i.e. 200 trials). At the end of this training session, the subjects were scanned while they performed this task. Although behaviourally the subjects demonstrated learning of the sequence, they did not have explicit knowledge of the sequence when tested after scanning.

Note that in both the implicit and the explicit conditions, the subjects performed the same visuospatial sequence and made the same number of movements, as each response was guided by the appearance of the red circle every 800 ms. Thus, there was only one difference between the two conditions: In the explicit condition, the subject had explicit knowledge of the sequence and, after each response, would actively retrieve the next location where the red circle would appear; by contrast, in the implicit condition, although there was implicit anticipation of the next response (as indicated by the reaction times), the subject was not able to retrieve explicitly specific information about the next move. When activity in the two conditions was compared, there was greater activity within the right ventrolateral frontal cortex during the performance of the explicit sequence, in accordance with the predictions of the two-level hypothesis. Note that no other part of the frontal cortex exhibited increases in blood flow in the explicit condition in comparison with the implicit condition. It is also interesting to note that the increase was observed only in the right ventrolateral frontal cortex, as would be expected from the fact that the stimulus material was visuospatial.

In conclusion, the data reviewed above show that within the mid-lateral part of the frontal cortex, two systems can be distinguished: one centered on the mid-dorsolateral frontal cortex and the other on the mid-ventrolateral frontal cortex. The fundamental distinction between these two regions of the frontal lobe appears to be in terms of the nature of the executive processing that is being carried out, although within the dorsolateral and ventrolateral frontal regions there may be further specialization according to the sensory modality of the information processed.

Acknowledgements

This work was supported by grants from the National Sciences and Engineering Research Council of Canada, the Medical Research Council of Canada and the McDonnell-Pew Program in Cognitive Neuroscience.

References

Bachevalier, J. & Mishkin, M. 1986 Visual recognition impairment follows ventromedial but not dorsolateral prefrontal lesions in monkeys. *Behav. Brain Res.* **20**, 249–61.
Buckner, R. L., Petersen, S. E., Ojemann, J. G., Miezin, F. M., Squire, L. R. & Raichle, M. E. 1995 Functional anatomical studies of implicit and explicit memory retrieval tasks. *J. Neurosci.* **15**, 12–29.
Butters, N. & Pandya, D. 1969 Retention of delayed-alternation: effect of selective lesions of sulcus principalis. *Science* **165**, 1271–73.
Doyon, J., Owen, A. M., Petrides, M., Sziklas, V. & Evans, A. C. 1996 Functional anatomy of visuomotor skill learning in human subjects examined with positron emission tomography. *Eur. J. Neurosci.* **8**, 637–48.

Funahashi, S., Bruce, C. J. & Goldman-Rakic, P. S. 1993 Dorsolateral prefrontal lesions and oculomotor delayed-response performance: evidence for mnemonic 'scotomas'. *J. Neurosci.* **13**, 1479–97.

Goldman, P. S. & Rosvold, H. E. 1970 Localization of function within the dorsolateral prefrontal cortex of the rhesus monkey. *Exp. Neurol.* **27**, 291–304.

Goldman, P. S., Rosvold, H. E., Vest, B. & Galkin, T. W. 1971 Analysis of the delayed-alternation deficit produced by dorsolateral prefrontal lesions in the rhesus monkey. *J. Comp. Physiol. Psychol.* **77**, 212–20.

Goldman-Rakic, P. S. 1995 Architecture of the prefrontal cortex and the central executive. *Ann. N. Y. Acad. Sci.* **769**, 71–83.

Grasby, P. M., Frith, C. D., Frackowiak, R. S. J. & Dolan, R. J. 1993 Functional mapping of brain areas implicated in auditory-verbal memory function. *Brain* **116**, 1–20.

Gross, C. G. & Weiskrantz, L. 1962 Evidence for dissociation of impairment on auditory discrimination and delayed response following lateral frontal lesions in monkeys. *Exp. Neurol.* **5**, 453–76.

Jacobsen, C. F. 1936 Studies of cerebral function in primates. I. The functions of the frontal association areas in monkeys. *Comp. Psychol. Monogr.* **13**, 1–60.

Jonides, J., Smith, E. E., Koeppe, R. A., Awh, E., Minoshima, S. & Mintun, M. A. 1993 Spatial working memory in humans as revealed by PET. *Nature Lond.* **363**, 623–25.

McCarthy, G., Blamire, A. M., Puce, A. *et al.* 1994 Functional magnetic resonance imaging of human prefrontal cortex activation during a spatial working memory task. *Proc. Natl. Acad. Sci. U.S.A.* **91**, 8690–94.

Mishkin, M. 1957 Effects of small frontal lesions on delayed alternation in monkeys. *J. Neurophysiol.* **20**, 615–22.

Mishkin, M. & Manning, F. J. 1978 Non-spatial memory after selective prefrontal lesions in monkeys. *Brain Res.* **143**, 313–23.

Mishkin, M., Vest, B., Waxler, M. & Rosvold, H. E. 1969 A re-examination of the effects of frontal lesions on object alternation. *Neuropsychologia* **7**, 357–63.

Owen, A. M., Evans, A. C. & Petrides, M. 1996 Evidence for a two-stage model of spatial working memory processing within the lateral frontal cortex: a positron emission tomography study. *Cereb. Cortex* **6**, 31–38.

Passingham, R. E. 1975 Delayed matching after selective prefrontal lesions in monkeys (Macaca mulatta). *Brain Res.* **92**, 89–102.

Petrides, M. 1989 Frontal lobes and memory. In *Handbook of neuropsychology*, vol. 3 (ed. F. Boller & J. Grafman), pp. 75–90. Amsterdam: Elsevier.

Petrides, M. 1991 Monitoring of selections of visual stimuli and the primate frontal cortex. *Proc. R. Soc. Lond.* B **246**, 293–98.

Petrides, M. 1994 Frontal lobes and working memory: evidence from investigations of the effects of cortical excisions in nonhuman primates. In *Handbook of neuropsychology*, vol. 9 (ed. F. Boller & J. Grafman), pp. 59–82. Amsterdam: Elsevier.

Petrides, M. 1995*a* Functional organization of the human frontal cortex for mnemonic processing: evidence from neuroimaging studies. *Ann. N.Y. Acad. Sci.* **769**, 85–96.

Petrides, M. 1995*b* Impairments on nonspatial self-ordered and externally ordered working memory tasks after lesions of the mid-dorsal part of the lateral frontal cortex in the monkey. *J. Neurosci.* **15**, 359–75.

Petrides, M., Alivisatos, B., Evans, A. C. & Meyer, E. 1993*a* Dissociation of human mid-dorsolateral frontal cortex in memory processing. *Proc. Natl. Acad. Sci. U.S.A.* **90**, 873–77.

Petrides, M., Alivisatos, B., Meyer, E. & Evans, A. C. 1993*b* Functional activation of the human frontal cortex during the performance of verbal working memory tasks. *Proc. Natl. Acad. Sci. U.S.A.* **90**, 878–82.

Petrides, M., Alivisatos, B. & Evans, A. C. 1995 Functional activation of the human ventrolateral frontal cortex during mnemonic retrieval of verbal information. *Proc. Natl. Acad. Sci. U.S.A.* **92**, 5803–07.

Petrides, M. & Milner, B. 1982 Deficits on subject-ordered tasks after frontal-and temporal-lobe lesions in man. *Neuropsychologia* **20**, 249–62.

Petrides, M. & Pandya, D. N. 1994 Comparative architectonic analysis of the human and the macaque frontal cortex. In *Handbook of neuropsychology*, vol. 9 (ed. F. Boller & J. Grafman), pp. 17–58. Amsterdam: Elsevier.

Shallice, T., Fletcher, P., Frith, C. D., Grasby, P., Frackowiak, R. S. J. & Dolan, R. J. 1994 Brain regions associated with acquisition and retrieval of verbal episodic memory. *Nature Lond.* **368**, 633–35.

Tulving, E., Kapur, S., Markowitsch, H. J., Craik, F. I. M., Habib, R. & Houle, S. 1994 Hemispheric encoding/retrieval asymmetry in episodic memory: positron emission tomography findings. *Proc. Natl. Acad. Sci. U.S.A.* **91**, 2012–15.

9

Dissociating executive functions of the prefrontal cortex

T. W. Robbins

9.1 Introduction

The term 'executive functioning' generally refers to those mechanisms by which performance is optimized in situations requiring the operation of a number of cognitive processes (Baddeley 1986). Executive functioning is required when effective new plans of action have to be formulated, and appropriate sequences of responses must be selected and scheduled. Components may include the enhancement of information held temporarily or 'on line' (cf. Goldman-Rakic's 1987 concept of 'working memory'), the marshalling of attentional resources (Shallice 1982), the inhibition of inappropriate responses in certain circumstances (Shallice & Burgess 1993) and the 'monitoring' of behaviour with respect to affective or motivational state (Damasio 1994; Petrides 1996). Some insight into the nature and organization of executive functions can be gleaned from a psychometric approach (e.g. Duncan *et al.* 1995), but it is still not established to what extent they represent emergent properties of interactions between specialized cognitive subsystems or the operation of a single central executive (Baddeley 1986), possibly with dissociable components (Shallice & Burgess 1993).

As many of the deficits shown by patients with frontal lobe dysfunction are of an executive nature, a neural perspective may be useful. Equivalence between the prefrontal cortex and executive functioning cannot of course be assumed, especially in view of the occurrence of the 'dysexecutive syndrome' in patients with damage to other brain regions. However, it may be profitable to consider possibly distinct forms of executive dysfunction in the context of the considerable anatomical connectivity existing between the prefrontal cortex and other regions of the cerebral cortex, as well as the subcortical brain. Four particularly important forms of neural interaction involving the prefrontal cortex are with: (1) dedicated processing modules of the posterior cortex such as the parietal and temporal lobes; (2) limbic structures such as the amygdala and hippocampus; (3) the output of the striatum, which targets the frontal lobe; and (4) the ascending monoaminergic and cholinergic systems of subcortical origin, which exert potentially diverse effects on forebrain functioning. The fact that the prefrontal cortex itself is not a homogeneous structure, having several distinct cytoarchitectonic regions, also has implications for the nature and organization of executive functions (Pandya & Yeterian 1995).

9.2 Validation and standardization of tests sensitive to frontal lobe dysfunction

Our overall aim is to seek illuminating functional dissociations of executive and non-executive mechanisms, via comparative studies of brain-damaged humans and monkeys, psychometric analyses and studies of functional neuroimaging in intact human subjects. To this end, we have devised tests with executive as well as non-executive components for testing patients with frontal lobe damage.

For these studies, groups of patients with frontal lobe excisions, together with age-and IQ-matched controls, have been used (for full clinical details see Owen *et al.* 1990, 1993, 1996*a*). These patients ($n = 40$) include cases resulting from neurosurgery undertaken generally for the relief of epilepsy or the removal of tumours. The majority of cases are unilateral with a rough equivalence of numbers according to the side of the lesions. The group of frontal lobe lesioned patients is heterogeneous with respect to the exact location and extent of the lesion (confirmed on the basis of magnetic resonance imaging (MRI) or computerized tomographic (CT) scans and the notes of the neurosurgeon C. E. Polkey). Groups of patients with other cortical lesions or neurodegenerative diseases have been studied as positive controls, including temporal lobe excisions, amygdalo-hippocampectomy and basal ganglia disorders. Such controls may help to identify the nature of possible interactions with other components of the distributed neural networks in control of performance (see above), as well as helping to define the precise contribution of the prefrontal cortex itself.

The three main types of test probe aspects of executive functioning involving planning, working memory, response control and attentional shifting, and have been found to be sensitive to damage of the prefrontal cortex. The test of planning is based on the Tower of London task (Shallice 1982) but modified in several ways to obtain several independent measures of performance (Owen *et al.* 1990) and to maximize its 'look ahead' requirements (Owen *et al.* 1995*b*). The attentional set-shifting paradigm (Roberts *et al.* 1988; Owen *et al.* 1991) represents the decomposition of a test much used in clinical assessments of frontal lobe damage (the Wisconsin Card Sort Test or WCST), according to the principles of learning theory. The third test, of working memory (Morris *et al.* 1988; Owen *et al.* 1990), is based loosely on Passingham's (1985) adaptation of a food searching test for monkeys with dorsolateral prefrontal lesions, and on the 'self-ordered' memory tasks of Petrides & Milner (1982). The latter test not only measures memory performance, but is also amenable to analyses of the strategies adopted by subjects performing the task.

Data have been obtained from a large group of normal volunteers using these tests, as well as others from the Cambridge Neuropsychological Test Automated Battery (CANTAB) and subjected to factor analysis (Robbins *et al.* 1994, 1996). This analysis indicates that measures from some of the three main tests load on common factors (e.g. spatial working memory and planning), but some do not (attentional set-shifting). Further analyses show that tests of visual recognition memory or learning, or other tests of frontal lobe function such as verbal fluency, load on an independent factor. Moreover, a test of non-verbal 'fluid intelligence' (see Duncan *et al.* 1995), AH 4–2, loads across virtually all factors, including those that capture tests sensitive to frontal lobe dysfunction and those that do not (see Robbins *et al.* 1996).

This analysis indicates that these tests measure dissociable aspects of executive functioning which contribute to task performance over and above more basic cognitive functions, such as visual perception and short term storage. Moreover, the analysis indicates possible dissociations between basic memorial requirements of tasks and their executive components which control response selection, such as the adoption of an overall strategy or plan, or the utilization of specific attentional inhibitory mechanisms. This general hypothesis can be tested further by dissecting performance on these tasks at a neural level, for example by studies of humans and animals with defined lesions, or using functional neuroimaging.

9.3 Strategic versus memorial factors in performance

(a) Self-ordered working memory

Successful performance in control subjects on the self-ordered spatial working memory task often exemplifies a searching strategy which essentially retraces the 'route' previously employed by the subject in searching through the spatial array of boxes, but 'monitors' or 'edits' it to avoid previously reinforced locations. This strategy can be captured by an index which is demonstrably uncontaminated by overall mnemonic performance (Owen *et al.* 1990, 1996*a*) and yet which correlates highly with such performance (Owen *et al.* 1990; table 9.1). Use of this strategy can thus markedly reduce the load on memory caused by interference from previous unreinforced choices.

About 70% of frontal patients we have tested are markedly impaired (> 1 standard deviation from the control mean) on the self-ordered spatial working memory task, as shown by large increases in responses to locations that were previously reinforced ('between-search errors'). However, this apparent deficit in 'working memory' is accompanied by impairment in the use of an effective strategy (Owen *et al.* 1990, 1996*a*), suggesting that at least part of their deficit on the task arises from executive failure. Several other patient groups have equivalent deficits in overall performance on the spatial working memory tests,

Table 9.1 Inter-correlation matrix for task performance; normal subjects ($n = 200$) (The tasks and associated measures are described in detail in references cited in the text.)

	Extra-dimensional shift	Span	Spatial working memory Errors	Spatial working memory Strategy	Tower of London
Extra-dimensional shift (errors)	–	–0.227**	0.160	0.141	0.160
Spatial span		–	–0.435**	–0.230**	0.199*
Spatial working memory (errors)			–	0.518**	–0.379**
Spatial working memory (strategy score)				–	–0.326**
Tower of London (perfect solutions)					–

* $P < 0.01$; ** $P < 0.001$.

as measured by the between-search error score, but no significant deficits in the use of strategy. These groups include patients with early-in-the-course Alzheimer's disease (Sahgal et al. 1992), Parkinson's disease (Owen et al. 1992) and temporal lobe excisions or amygdalo-hippocampectomy (Owen et al. 1995a, 1996a). While patients with Huntington's disease (Lawrence et al. 1996) and Korsakoff's syndrome (Joyce & Robbins 1991) also exhibit marked impairments in strategy, as well as memory performance, these deficits might be expected to arise from the disruption of neural circuitry intimately associated with the prefrontal cortex, namely the striatum and mediodorsal thalamus, respectively. It would seem most unlikely that the deficit in strategy formulation is secondary to an impairment in the ability to remember the previous sequence of choices, as (1) a measure of a computerized form of the Corsi spatial span task showed no significant differences between frontal lesioned patients and controls; and (2) correlations between this span measure and the adoption of strategy are generally low and non-significant in frontal patients (table 9.2; Owen et al. 1996a), as well as in the normal population, especially when the stronger correlations between span and spatial working memory performance, and spatial working memory and strategy scores are partialled out (see table 9.1). This pattern of correlations remains robust when the effects of age, verbal and 'fluid' IQ (as measured by AH4–2) are partialled out, and suggests that performance on the spatial working memory task is governed by two major factors, one related to short-term spatial memory and the other to strategic factors.

Our data provide empirical support for suggestions made from previous studies (Passingham 1985; Petrides & Milner 1982) of an executive contribution to the 'frontal' deficits on such self-ordered tasks over and above their memorial requirements. If this is true there should be a smaller deficit in frontal

Table 9.2 Inter-correlation matrix for task performance; frontal patients ($n = 19$) (The tasks and associated measures are described in detail in references cited in the text. NART IQ and age partialled out.)

	Fluency	Extra-dimensional shift	Span	Spatial working memory Errors	Spatial working memory Strategy	Tower of London
Verbal fluency (FAS)	–	0.252	−0.492*	−0.557*	0.193	−0.040
Extra-dimensional shift (errors)		–	−0.299	0.284	0.310	−0.483*
Spatial span			–	−0.435*	−0.120	0.098
Spatial working memory (errors)				–	0.446*	−0.336
Spatial working memory (strategy score)					–	−0.406*
Tower of London (perfect solutions)						–

*$P < 0.05$.

patients on similar tasks where the strategic component is less prominent. This prediction has been confirmed using two tasks designed by A. M. Owen. They are direct verbal and visual analogues of the spatial working memory task described above. However, instead of searching spatial locations, subjects are required to search through changing arrays of abstract visual patterns or words without semantic content (based on surnames taken from the London telephone directory) (Owen *et al.* 1996*a*). For controls, there is considerably less evidence of an effective strategy based on the 'updating' of a repetitive sequence in either case. And there is no significant deficit on either task in the frontal group, although both tasks are considerably more difficult than the spatial working memory analogue. There is no obvious explanation of this difference in terms of the exact sites of the patients' lesions in the prefrontal cortex. However, performance is significantly impaired in the visual working memory task for a group of temporal lobe lesioned patients (Owen *et al.* 1996*a*), and for both tasks in a group of patients with Parkinson's disease (Owen *et al.* 1997).

  Therefore, it appears that the executive deficit in the spatial working memory task in frontal patients has a considerable degree of selectivity, but is not simply produced by damage to a short-term memory storage system. It also seems likely that performance on the task is a product of interactions between posterior cortical structures (including the hippocampus). Moreover, it is evident that frontal patients are not invariably impaired on difficult tasks that might be expected to depend on high levels of general intelligence. Rather, it appears that deficits are more evident when there are important strategic components to the task that might reflect the operation of an executive or 'supervisory attentional' system.

(b) Planning

The finding of impaired use of strategy in frontal patients is consistent with the clinical impression of their inability to plan in everyday life. However, there has been only limited empirical evidence for this view (Shallice & Burgess 1993). Our modifications of the Tower of London (or Stockings of Cambridge) test, in two separate formats, emphasize different aspects of planning, namely the reproduction of the appropriate motor sequence and the manipulation of appropriate mental imagery. In the first format the subjects solve problems by rearranging a configuration of stimuli in the bottom half of the screen to resemble a 'goal' configuration in the top half. A 'yoked motor control' condition enables thinking time to be estimated by subtracting motor latencies to make each move of the sequence. Using this test format, we have shown that frontal patients (irrespective of lesioned side) were less efficient in generating accurate solutions than controls. They also had longer 'thinking times' after the first move, suggesting that they had initiated solutions without fully 'thinking them through' (Owen et al. 1990). By contrast, patients with temporal lobectomies were not significantly impaired in any aspect of performance (Owen et al. 1995a).

It is important to distinguishing the three disc Tower of London puzzles from the four disc Tower of Hanoi tasks which depend on trial and error learning. Goel & Grafman (1995) criticize these latter tests for assessing planning functions because of the contaminating requirements to inhibit prepotent responses. As they concede, these difficulties are mainly avoided in the Tower of London problems. The difficulties are avoided to an even greater extent by our second version of the Tower of London problems, which can be solved by only a single overt response. For these problems, the subject inspects an array with two different arrangements of coloured balls. He or she is required to indicate the number of 'moves' it would take to transform the bottom arrangement into the top by touching an appropriate response panel labelled from 1 to 5. Both the accuracy and latency of responding can be measured. Frontal patients are again less accurate than controls, but do not take significantly longer to arrive at their correct choices, unlike patients with Parkinson's disease (Owen et al. 1995b). Therefore, it is difficult to argue that the effects arise merely from non-specific deficits in response control that produce impulsive forms of responding.

(c) Functional neuroimaging in normal volunteers

The design of both forms of the Tower of London test makes them suitable for studies of functional neuroimaging in normal subjects. When the 'mental' format was used changes in regional cerebral blood flow (rCBF) in both 'easy' (2–3 move) and 'difficult' (4–5 move) problems were compared using positron emission tomography (PET) with $H_2^{15}O$. A further comparison condition was with an array which required the subject to sustain attention to i before making a similar motor response (Baker et al. 1996). Both types o comparison indicated that the 'mental' task produced increases in rCBF in a distributed cortical network that included the superior occipito-parietal cortex and three main zones in the frontal cortex: the premotor area, a band of activation including the dorsolateral prefrontal cortex (Brodmann's areas 9/46) bilaterally and the frontopolar (Brodmann's area 10) cortex on the right. Similar areas were activated in a parallel study performed with the 'motor' format of the task, except that activations were greater on the left side (Owen *et al.* 1996*b*). This was conceivably because of the different requirements of the two tasks on spatial working memory and action production, although the differences might have arisen in part from a different type of comparison condition, in the latter case involving a memory sequencing task.

An important conclusion is that a complex planning task in humans activates discrete regions of the prefrontal cortex, predominantly in the dorsolateral and polar regions, in conjunction with posterior cortical systems implicated by other studies in the manipulation of mental imagery. The activation of the prefrontal cortical sites presumably reflects a functional interaction with this posterior system that leads to the generation and monitoring of candidate sequences of moves to solve the problems. There are striking parallels with the self-ordered memory task described above, where the goal is less clearly specified, but there is a more obvious memory load. This is seen not only from the correlations between performance on the memory and planning tasks shown in table 1, but also from recent functional imaging studies of a close analogue of our self-ordered task (Owen *et al.* 1996*c*). These studies indicated two major sites of activation in the dorsolateral and ventrolateral prefrontal cortex. Further data suggest that the ventrolateral area (Brodmann's area 47) may play a role in the 'passive' receipt of items for memory (as in spatial span performance), whereas the dorsolateral prefrontal cortex is important for the 'monitoring' role by which candidate sequences are compared with the goal sequence. This dissociation of two distinct factors contributing to the self-ordered spatial working memory task thus accords with the psychometric evidence shown in table 9.1. Further studies are required to elucidate the role of the right frontopolar area (Brodmann's area 10) in the planning task.

9.4 Attentional set shifting versus memorial factors in performance

Novel circumstances often dictate that the processes governing response selection in predictable situations must be countermanded to allow the expression of new intentions. A classical example is the fixation with particular ways of solving problems (or 'Einstellung' of the Gestalt psychologists) which interferes with the production of flexible strategies for problem solving. In the clinical context, perseveration on the WCST has often been used as an indication of frontal lobe dysfunction (Milner 1963), although there has been considerable disagreement about the psychological and neural specificity of this test in recent years. Some authors have argued that it provides yet another test of 'working memory' in which the subject has to keep the currently valid sorting principle constantly in mind. There has also been considerable disagreement over the extent to which it represents a 'pure' frontal test (Anderson *et al.* 1991), although the notion of a 'pure' test in itself is misleading, as it is apparent that neuropsychological tests consist of many interactive components that depend on the outputs of different neural systems. The obvious possibility that the test depends on discrete regions within the prefrontal cortex has never been resolved; there is no agreement concerning either the possible laterality of the effects, or their critical zone. An informative recent functional imaging study employing PET identified several neocortical regions that were activated by the WCST task, including both dorsolateral and orbitofrontal regions, as well as both temporal and parietal lobe structures (Berman *et al.* 1995).

We have also undertaken a functional analysis of the WCST, which recognizes that it has several cognitive components, at the core of which is the extra-dimensional shift test, derived from human and animal learning theory (Downes *et al.*, 1989; Roberts *et al.* 1988). In an extradimensional shift, attention to compound stimuli is transferred from one perceptual dimension (e.g. colour) to another (e.g. form), on the basis of changing reinforcement or feedback. Control tests include the ability to shift performance on the basis of altered feedback within a dimension (reversal learning) and the ability to shift performance to novel exemplars of the same dimension (intra-dimensional shift) (see Roberts *et al.* 1988; Owen *et al.* 1991).

About 50% of patients with frontal lobe damage have been shown to exhibit selective difficulties in reaching a learning criterion at the extra-dimensional shift, whereas patients with temporal lobectomies or amygdala-hippocampectomies were unimpaired (Owen *et al.* 1991). However, both of these temporal lobe lesions had some impact on performance at the extra-dimensional shifting stage, where the latencies to respond were significantly lengthened (Owen *et al.* 1991). Thus, this is the third of our tasks that requires processing in the posterior (in this case, temporal) cortex, presumably in conjunction with prefrontal mechanisms.

Patients with basal ganglia disorders also exhibit major deficits on the attentional set-shifting task, although these may differ qualitatively from those seen after frontal damage, in two main ways. There is a greater incidence of failures in patients with striatal dysfunction at those stages when the set is being acquired (Owen *et al.* 1992). They may also fail the extra-dimensional shift in a different way than frontal patients. This can be shown by changing one of the perceptual dimensions at the extra-dimensional stages with a novel dimension that replaces either the previously reinforced or non-reinforced dimension. Subjects are required either to shift responding to the novel dimension, ignoring the previously reinforced dimension, or to shift to the previously non-reinforced dimension, ignoring the novel one. These two conditions can be termed 'perseveration' and 'learned irrelevance', respectively. In simple terms the subject has to inhibit responding to the previously reinforced dimension in the perservation condition and to overcome inhibition to respond to the previously non-reinforced dimension in the learned irrelevance condition. The frontal patients have a selective deficit in the perservation condition, whereas patients with basal ganglia disorders make more errors in both conditions (Owen *et al.* 1993; see figure 9.1*a*).

These results identify the exact nature of the extra-dimensional deficit in frontal patients as a specific failure of response inhibition leading to perservation. The results also show that it is difficult to explain these patients' shifting impairment simply in terms of 'holding stimuli on-line in memory'. There was no deficit in the learned irrelevance condition which would appear to provide a similar load for memory as the perseveration condition. This argument also holds for the intra-dimensional stages of the task, where similar compound stimuli were employed and no deficits observed in the frontal group for these forms of associative learning. Thus, it can be argued from these data that frontal patients have major deficits in response inhibition that are not secondary to problems in short-term memory. These conclusions are substantiated by findings of intact extra-dimensional shift performance in the face of major short-term memory deficits in patients early in the course of Alzheimer's disease (Sahakian *et al.* 1990).

The failure of attentional shifting is probably importantly determined by the novelty, and hence learning requirements, of the test situation. Some evidence for this is provided from a recent study by R. D. Rogers in this laboratory in which subjects have been trained to shift continuously from one dimension ('letters of the alphabet') to another (digits), on the basis of learned cues. A group of patients with frontal excisions showing deficits on the perseveration component of the attentional set-shifting task failed to show any impairments on this pretrained shifting task, although considerable and equivalent costs of shifting were entailed in both the frontal lesioned and normal subjects.

9.5 Anatomical and pharmacological dissociations of executive dysfunction

The pattern of deficits shown by individual frontal patients in our sample (see also table 9.2) suggests the possibility of functional dissociations with anatomical correlates. However, interpretation of such data is compromised by the inconsistency and transient nature of frontal deficits, as well as the variability in the size and extent of the damage within the prefrontal cortex, which often fails to respect anatomical boundaries. Such considerations justify the use of tasks that can be used in experimental animals, as well as in humans, to study the effects of well-defined experimental lesions (cf. Goldman-Rakic 1987; Petrides 1996).

Our attentional set-shifting paradigm is one such task which can be used to study the neural basis of different aspects of response inhibition in monkeys. Thus, Dias *et al.* (1996) have studied the effects of excitotoxically-induced,

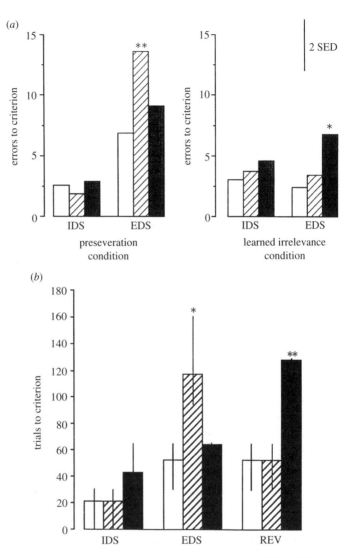

Fig. 9.1 (*a*) Errors to criterion for the intradimensional shift (IDS) and extradimensional shift (EDS) stages of the attentional set-shifting paradigm for the perseveration and learned irrelevance conditions by groups of patients with frontal excisions (hatched) or Parkinson's disease (PD) (medicated and unmedicated groups combined) (shaded bars), as well as age-and IQ-matched control subjects (open bars). Replotted from Owen *et al.* 1993. ** $P < 0.01$;* $P < 0.05$, compared with controls. 2 SED = 2 standard errors of the differences between means. (*b*) Trials to criterion for intradimensional shift (IDS) extradimensional shift (EDS) and reversal (REV) stages of the attentional set-shifting paradigm for marmosets with lesions of the lateral (hatched bars) or orbital prefrontal cortex (solid bars), or with sham surgery (open bars) (data replotted from Dias *et al.* 1996). Vertical lines refer to the range of scores. ** $P < 0.01$;* $P < 0.05$ compared with the other groups.

localized lesions of the prefrontal cortex of marmosets on performance of the intra-dimensional and extra-dimensional shifts, as well as on the reversal of associations for the compound stimuli following the extra-dimensional stage. A double dissociation of effects was found for lesions to the lateral prefrontal cortex (designated as area 9 by Brodmann) and to the orbitofrontal cortex (Brodmann's areas 11, 12 & 13). Specifically, the lateral lesion selectively impaired extra-dimensional shifting, whereas the orbitofrontal lesion selectively impaired reversal learning (see figure 9.1*b*). Neither lesion affected learning at the intradimensional stage.

These results suggest that distinct processes of response inhibition are recruited to control extra-dimensional shifting and associative reversal learning, represented in separable processing domains within the prefrontal cortex. Other evidence for the dissociation is provided by a demonstration of opposite patterns of effects of cortical cholinergic depletion, following lesions of the basal forebrain and of prefrontal dopamine depletion, produced by 6-hydroxydopamine, in marmosets (Roberts *et al.* 1992, 1994). Cholinergic depletion selectively impaired serial reversal learning, whereas prefrontal dopamine loss actually selectively enhanced extra-dimensional shifting. Furthermore, it is important to emphasize that these effects in monkeys, like those in humans, cannot be reduced to deficits in 'holding stimuli on line', as shown by the fact that marmosets with prefrontal dopamine loss that exhibited enhanced attentional shift performance were significantly impaired in the classic delayed response task (Roberts *et al.* 1994). Analogous dissociations between the test of spatial working memory described above, and other 'executive' functions have recently been reported following treatment of patients with dementia of the frontal lobe type with the alpha-2 adrenoceptor receptor antagonist idazoxan (Coull *et al.* 1996). The involvement of these subcortical systems may represent ways in which arousing or rewarding signals influence prefrontal function; these signals may potentially disrupt, as well as enhance processing in their terminal domains, depending on the test situation.

At a theoretical level the results show that these identical compound stimuli can be processed at more than one site in the prefrontal cortex, perhaps simultaneously. At one of these sites, processing allows a 'reward' tag to be shifted from one stimulus to another ('affective shifting'). At the other site, shifts are effected between responding to different dimensions (e.g. shapes rather than colours) of complex stimuli, rather than to particular exemplars, a seemingly higher-order cognitive process. On the basis of previous experience a 'set' is established for the control of responding, perhaps on the basis of processing in the posterior (e.g. inferotemporal) cortex. However, in novel situations, it is adaptive to relax that control, in order to allow the development of an alternative 'response set'. These data are not necessarily incompatible with hierarchical models of prefrontal cortex that emphasize the serial flow of information from sectors of the prefrontal cortex in receipt of basic perceptual and associative information to other, possibly superordinate regions (such as the dorsolateral prefrontal cortex) (Petrides 1996). However, the present double dissociation is more consistent with the parallel processing of information by relatively independent sectors of the prefrontal cortex (Pandya & Yeterian 1995).

9.6 Conclusions

Neuropsychological evidence obtained from subjects with frontal lobe lesions, as well as psychometric and functional neuroimaging data obtained from normal volunteers, have been presented that are consistent with the hypothesis that the prefrontal cortex plays a major and specific role in response selection processes, particularly when these have a possible function in the strategic control of responding. These response selection processes are sensitive to inhibitory influences at several functional levels, including mechanisms by which the effects of particular associations of stimuli with reward, and the superordinate effects of stimulus categories or dimensions, are attenuated hence facilitating the expression of voluntary behaviour in novel circumstances These dissociable aspects of executive function appear to be mediated by distinct neural systems that engage different regions of the prefrontal cortex.

Acknowledgements

I thank B. J. Everitt, A. M. Owen, A. C. Roberts, R. D. Rogers and B. J Sahakian for discussion, as well as other colleagues for their collaboration and assistance, in particular, North East Age Research (P. Rabbitt and L. McInnes and the Wellcome Dept. of Cognitive Neurology. The work was supported by the Wellcome Trust.

References

Anderson, S. W., Damasio, H., Dallas Jones, R. & Tranel, D. 1991 Wisconsin Card Sorting Test performance as a measure of frontal lobe damage. *J. Clin. Expt. Neu ropsych.* **13**, 909–22.
Baddeley, A. D. 1986 *Working memory*. Oxford: Clarendon Press.
Baker, S. C., Rogers, R. D., Owen, A. M. *et al.* 1996 Neural systems engaged by planning: A PET study of the Tower of London task. *Neuropsychologia* **34**, 515–26
Berman, K. F., Ostrem, J. L., Randolph, C. *et al.* 1995 Physiological activation of a cortical network during performance of the Wisconsin Card Sorting Test: a positron emission tomography study. *Neuropsychologia* **33**, 1027–46.
Coull, J. T., Sahakian, B. J. & Hodges, J. R. 1996 The alpha-2 antagonist idazoxan remediates certain attentional and executive forms of dysfunction in dementia of the frontal type. *Psychopharmacology* **123**, 239–49.
Damasio, A. 1994 *Descartes' error*. New York: Putnam Press.

Dias, R., Robbins, T. W. & Roberts, A. C. 1996 Dissociation in prefrontal cortex of attentional and affective shifts. *Nature* **380**, 69–72.

Downes, J. J., Roberts, A. C., Sahakian, B. J., Evenden, J. L. & Robbins, T. W. 1989 Impaired extra-dimensional shift performance in medicated and unmedicated Parkinson's disease: evidence for a specific attentional dysfunction. *Neuropsychologia* **27**, 1329–44.

Duncan, J., Burgess, P, & Emslie, H. 1995 Fluid intelligence after frontal lobe lesions. *Neuropsychologia* **33**, 261–68.

Goel, V. & Grafman, J. 1995 Are the frontal lobes implicated in 'planning' functions? Interpreting data from the Tower of Hanoi. *Neuropsychologia* **33**, 623–42.

Goldman-Rakic, P. S. 1987 Circuitry of primate prefrontal cortex and regulation of behavior by representational memory. In *Handbook of physiology. The nervous system* (ed. F. Plum), pp. 373–417. Bethesda, MD: American Physiological Society.

Joyce, E. M. & Robbins, T. W. 1991 Frontal lobe function in Korsakoff and non Korsakoff alcoholics: planning and spatial working memory. *Neuropsychologia* **29**, 709–23.

Lawrence, A. D., Sahakian, B. J., Hodges, J. R., Rosser, A. E., Lange, K. W. & Robbins, T. W. 1996 Executive and mnemonic functions in early Huntington's disease. *Brain*. (In the press.)

Milner, B. 1963 Effects of different lesions on card sorting. *Archives of Neurology* **9**, 100–10.

Morris, R. G., Downes, J. J., Sahakian, B. J., Evenden, J., Heald, A. & Robbins, T. W. 1988 Planning and spatial working memory in Parkinson's disease. *J. Neurol. Neurosurg. Psychiat.* **51**, 757–66.

Owen, A. M., Downes, J. J., Sahakian, B. J., Polkey, C. E. & Robbins, T. W. 1990 Planning and spatial working memory following frontal lobe lesions in man. *Neuropsychologia* **28**, 1021–34.

Owen, A. M., Roberts, A. C., Polkey, C. E., Sahakian, B. J. & Robbins, T. W. 1991 Extra-dimensional versus intradimensional set shifting performance following frontal lobe excision, temporal lobe excision or amygdalo-hippocampectomy in man. *Neuropsychologia* **29**, 993–1006.

Owen, A. M., James, M., Leigh, P. N. *et al.* 1992. Frontostriatal cognitive deficits at different stages of Parkinson's disease. *Brain* **115**, 1727–51.

Owen, A. M., Roberts, A. C., Hodges, J. R., Summers, B. A., Polkey, C. E. & Robbins, T. W. 1993 Contrasting mechanisms of impaired attentional set-shifting in patients with frontal lobe damage or Parkinson's disease. *Brain* **116**, 1159–79.

Owen, A. M., Sahakian, B. J., Semple, J., Polkey, C. E. & Robbins, T. W. 1995*a* Visuospatial short term recognition memory and learning after temporal lobe excisions, frontal lobe excisions or amygdala hippocampectomy in man. *Neuropsychologia* **33**, 1–24.

Owen, A. M., Sahakian, B. J, Hodges, J. R., Summers, B. A., Polkey, C. E. & Robbins, T. W. 1995*b* Dopamine-dependent fronto-striatal planning deficits in early Parkinson's disease. *Neuropsychology* **9**, 126–40.

Owen, A. M., Morris, R. G., Sahakian, B. J., Polkey, C. E. & Robbins, T. W. 1996*a* Double dissociations of memory and executive functions in self-ordered working memory tasks following frontal lobe excision, temporal lobe excisions or amygdala-hippocampectomy in man. *Brain* **119**, 1597–615.

Owen, A. M., Doyon, J., Petrides, M. & Evans, A. C. 1996*b* Planning and spatial working memory examined with positron emission tomography. *European J. Neurosci.* **8**, 353–64.

Owen, A. M., Evans, A. C. & Petrides, M. P. 1996c Evidence for a two-stage model of spatial working memory processing within the lateral frontal cortex: a positron emission tomography study. *Cerebral Cortex* **6**, 31–38.

Owen, A. M., Iddan, J. L., Hodges, J. R., Summers, B. A. E. & Robbins, T. W. 1997 Spatial and non-spatial working memory at different stages of Parkinson's disease. *Neuropsychologia* **35**, 519–32.

Pandya, D. P. & Yeterian, E. H. 1995 Morphological correlations of human and monkey frontal lobe. In *Neurobiology of human decision-making* (ed. A. E. Damasio, H. Damasio, & Y. Christen), pp. 13–46. New York: Springer.

Passingham, R. E. 1985 Memory of monkeys (Macaca mulatta) with lesions in pre-frontal cortex. *Behavioral Neuroscience* **9**, 3–21.

Petrides, M. P. 1996 Lateral frontal cortical contribution to memory. *Seminars in the Neurosciences* **8**, 57–63.

Petrides, M. P. & Milner, B. 1982 Deficits on subject-ordered tasks after frontal-and temporal lobe lesions in man. *Neuropsychologia* **20**, 249–62.

Robbins, T. W., James, M., Owen, A., Sahakian, B. J., McInnes, L. & Rabbitt, P. M. 1994 Cambridge Neuropsychological Test Automated Battery (CANTAB): a factor analytic study of a large sample of normal elderly volunteers. *Dementia* **5**, 266–81.

Robbins, T. W., James, M., Owen, A. M., Sahakian, B. J., McInnes, L. & Rabbitt, P. 1996 A neural systems approach to the cognitive psychology of ageing: using the CANTAB battery. In *Methodology of frontal and executive function* (ed. P. Rabbitt), pp. 215–38. Hove, East Sussex: Psychology Press.

Roberts, A. C., Everitt, B. J. & Robbins, T. W. 1988 Extra and intra-dimensional shifts in man and marmoset. *Q. J. Exp. Psychol.* **40B**, 321–42.

Roberts, A. C., Robbins, T. W., Everitt, B. J. & Muir, J. L. 1992 A specific form of cognitive rigidity following excitotoxic lesions of the basal forebrain in monkeys. *Neuroscience* **47**, 251–64.

Roberts, A. C., De Salvia, M. A., Wilkinson, L. S. *et al.* 1994 6-Hydroxydopamine lesions of the prefrontal cortex in monkeys enhance performance on an analogue of the Wisconsin Card Sorting test: Possible interactions with subcortical dopamine. *J. Neurosci.* **14**, 2531–44.

Sahakian, B. J., Downes, J. J., Roberts, A. C., Philpot, M., Levy, R. & Robbins, T. W. 1990 Preserved attentional function and impaired mnemonic function in dementia of the Alzheimer type. *Neuropsychologia* **28**, 1197–213.

Sahgal, A., Lloyd, S., Wray, C. J. *et al.* 1992 Does visuospatial memory in Alzheimer's disease depend on the severity of the disorder? *Int. J. Geriatric Psychiatry* **7**, 427–36.

Shallice, T. 1982 Specific impairments of planning. *Phil. Trans. R. Soc. Lond.* B **298**, 199–209.

Shallice, T. & Burgess P. 1993 Supervisory control of action and thought selection. In *Attention: selection, awareness and control* (ed. A. Baddeley, & L. Weiskrantz), pp. 171–87. Oxford: Clarendon Press.

10

Attention to action

R. E. Passingham

10.1 Introduction

We distinguish between those actions to which we attend and those to which we do not. For example, we do not attend to our breathing because we did not learn to breathe and it comes 'naturally'. We do not attend to riding a bicycle because, though we learnt to ride, it has become 'second nature'.

10.2 New learning and automatic performance

This paper reports studies in which Positron Emission Tomography (PET) has been used to study the changes that occur in the brain when a motor task is learned and then practiced until it has become automatic. The task was to learn a sequence of finger movements, eight moves long. The task is described by Jenkins *et al.* (1994). The subjects learned by trial and error. An example of a sequence is fingers 1, 3, 4, 3, 1, 4, 2, 3. A pacing tone sounded every 3 seconds and when the subjects heard the tone they pressed one of four keys. If they correctly identified the first keypress in the sequence, they were rewarded by a high-pitched tone; on the next trial they tried to identify the next press in the sequence. If they were wrong they heard a low-pitched tone, and at the next pacing tone they tried another key by pressing with a different finger. The end of the sequence was identified by three short high-pitched tones. The subjects then returned to the beginning, and continued to perform the task in the same fashion.

Regional cerebral blood flow (rCBF) was measured using $H_2^{15}O$. The subjects were scanned while they learned new sequences (NEW) and while they performed a prelearned sequence (PRE) which they had learned before scanning and had practised for one hour. They were also scanned during a baseline condition (BASE) in which they heard the pacing tones and the auditory feedback but made no movements.

We have carried out two studies using this task, one by Jenkins *et al.* (1994) and a more recent one by Jueptner *et al.* (1996) using a more sensitive scanner. In both studies the dorsal prefrontal cortex (areas 9, 46, 10) was extensively activated during new learning (NEW vs PRE, figure 10.1), but was not significantly activated above baseline levels when the subjects performed the

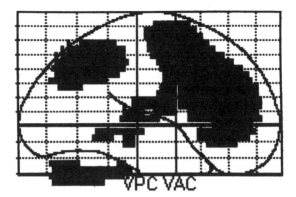

Fig. 10.1 Sagittal view of the brain showing activation in black for new motor learning compared with performance of the prelearned task (NEW vs PRE). In this and the other figures the brain is shown as if it were transparent, showing activation on the lateral surface of both hemispheres as well as in subcortical nuclei. Data from Jueptner *et al.*1996.

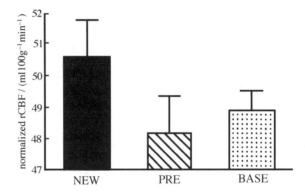

Fig. 10.2 Histograms showing regional cerebral blood flow in right dorsal prefrontal cortex (area 9/46) for new learning (NEW), performance of the prelearned task (PRE) and the baseline condition (BASE). Regional cerebral blood flow for the peak coordinate ($x = 38$, $y = 24$, $z = 28$). Data from Jueptner *et al.* (1996a).

prelearned task (PRE vs BASE, figure 10.2). The same pattern was found for the anterior cingulate, Brodmann's area 32.

We have also scanned subjects while they learned a verbal version of this task (Jenkins *et al.*, in preparation). As for the finger sequence, there were four elements. The difference was that these were the words 'the', 'with', 'how' and 'of'. Again, the subjects learned by trial and error. However, instead of moving one of four fingers on each trial, the subjects said one of the four words. As before, auditory cues told the subject whether the response was correct at that point in the sequence. The subjects were scanned while they learned new sequences (NEW) and also while they performed a sequence that they had learned and practised for one hour before scanning (PRE).

Again there was extensive activation of the prefrontal cortex (areas 9, 46, 10, 45, 47) during new learning (NEW vs PRE, figure 10.3). As for the finger sequence, the prefrontal cortex was no longer activated above resting levels when the subjects performed the overlearned verbal sequence (PRE vs BASE, figure 10.4). The pattern for the anterior cingulate area 32 was the same: it was activated during new learning (NEW vs BASE) but not during automatic performance (PRE vs BASE).

Raichle *et al.* (1994) have studied the learning of another verbal task. The task was verb generation: for each noun that was presented, the subject was required to produce a verb that was semantically related. The subjects were

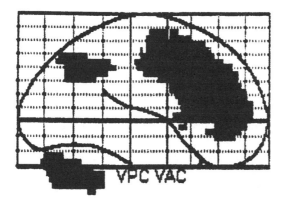

Fig. 10.3 Sagittal view of the brain showing activation in black for new verbal learning compared with performance of the prelearned task (NEW vs PRE). Data from Jenkins *et al.* (1996).

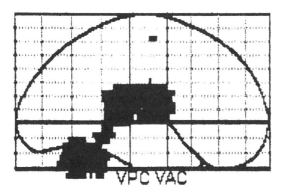

Fig. 10.4 Sagittal view of the brain showing activation in black for performance of the prelearned verbal sequence (PRE vs BASE). Data from Jenkins *et al.* 1996.

scanned while they produced verbs to a series of nouns. They were also scanned later after they had been repeatedly presented with the same nouns and their responses had become stereotyped. On the first trial of the task there was extensive activation of the left prefrontal cortex and the anterior cingulate cortex. However, these areas were no longer activated when the subjects had practised the task.

These studies of verbal and motor learning suggest that the prefrontal and anterior cingulate area 32 are engaged when subjects must concentrate on solving new problems but not when attention is no longer required because the task has become automatic. Frith *et al.* (1991) also distinguish between routine and non-routine performance. They showed that the prefrontal and anterior cingulate cortex were activated when the subjects had to perform non-routine tasks in which they generated either words or movements at will, but that the same areas were not activated when subjects said the same words on every trial or moved their fingers as indicated by the experimenter.

10.3 Dual task performance

The standard method for demonstrating that a task is automatic is to investigate whether it can be performed with minimal interference at the same time as another task. We therefore tested other subjects using a dual task paradigm. We taught 20 subjects a finger sequence outside the scanner; as before the sequence was 8 moves long (Watkins *et al.* unpublished data). They were trained in the same way as for the prelearned task in the imaging studies, except that they were required to make a movement every 2.5 seconds instead of every 3 seconds. On the first trial they learned the sequence by trial and error until they could perform the sequence in one run without error. They were then tested for a further 12 trials, each trial lasting for 90 seconds.

On trial 3 and trial 12 the subjects were required to perform a verbal task at the same time as the motor sequence. Every 2.5 seconds a word was presented on a computer monitor at the same time as the pacing tone. Ten subjects were required to repeat the word (noun repetition). The other ten subjects were required to produce a verb that was semantically appropriate for the noun (verb generation). These two tasks were chosen deliberately because it is known that the prefrontal cortex is activated in one (verb generation) but not in the other (noun repetition) (Petersen *et al.* 1988; Raichle *et al.* 1994).

Figure 10.5 shows the response times and the errors on the motor learning task for trials 3 (early stage) and 12 (late stage). For comparison, the times and errors are shown for the neighbouring trials in which the subjects only performed the motor task, that is for trials 2 + 4 (early stage), and for trials 11 + 13 (late stage). There was more interference when the subjects generated verbs than when they repeated nouns. Furthermore, there was a significant interaction between type of performance (dual task or not) and trial (early v late): for response times [$F(1,9) = 8.04$, $p = 0.02$] and for errors

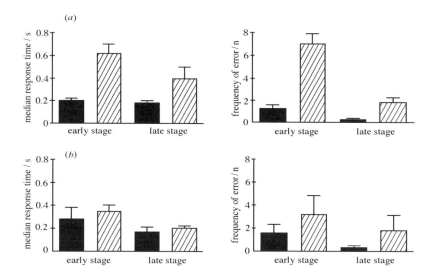

Fig. 10.5 Response times and errors on the motor sequence task. The data are shown during (*a*) performance of verb generation, and (*b*) performance of noun repetition. Single task denoted by solid bars; dual task denoted by hatched bars.

$[F(1,9) = 9.01, p = 0.015]$. The decline in interference between trials 3 and 12 was greater when subjects performed the verb generation task than it was when they performed the noun repetition task.

10.4 Central interference

These results prompt the question as to the stage in processing at which the interference occurs in the brain. Interference could occur if both tasks engaged the same perceptual or motor systems, or if they engaged common associative areas. Each possibility will be discussed in turn.

On the perceptual side, motor sequence learning engages the sensory and associative areas of the parietal lobe (Jenkins *et al.* 1994), whereas viewing words and generating words engage the striate and ventral prestriate areas and the ventral temporal lobe (Petersen *et al.* 1988; Raichle *et al.* 1994). On the motor side, the learning of finger sequences engages the lateral premotor cortex and the hand area of motor cortex (Jenkins *et al.* 1994), whereas producing words engages the frontal operculum and the face area of motor cortex (Petersen *et al.* 1988; Raichle *et al.* 1994).

We also found much less interference when subjects learned the motor sequence at the same time as repeating nouns. Yet the same perceptual and motor areas are engaged when subjects repeat nouns they read as when they generate verbs in response to nouns that they read. The supplementary motor area is also activated both in noun repetition (Petersen *et al.* 1988) and verb generation (Wise *et al.* 1991).

It appears, therefore, that there is interference centrally. The data for verb generation and noun repetition suggest that it occurs in the frontal lobe. The term 'frontal' is used rather than the more restrictive term 'prefrontal' because the frontal lobe includes the anterior cingulate cortex. When verb generation is compared with noun repetition, there is additional activation in the prefrontal and anterior cingulate cortex (Petersen *et al.* 1988; Raichle *et al.* 1994). The hypothesis is that when subjects are learning the motor sequence task on trial 3, there is still some activation of the frontal areas, and that interference occurs because the verb generation task also makes demands on these frontal areas. On trial 12 these areas are no longer activated during the motor sequence task, and thus they can be fully engaged by the task of generating verbs.

On this hypothesis, the reason why there is less interference with noun repetition is that this task does not engage the prefrontal and anterior cingulate cortex. Noun repetition is an overlearned skill which can be performed without attention. As mentioned earlier, we have taught subjects a verbal sequence and compared new learning (NEW) with performance of an overlearned sequence (PRE) (Jenkins *et al.* 1996). During new learning both Broca's area and the supplementary speech area were strongly activated, but neither area was engaged when the sequence had become automatic. When the sequence had been overlearned, there was extensive activation in the cerebellum and basal ganglia, but the motor output was limited to the insula and operculum at the base of the motor cortex (figure 10.4). Raichle *et al.* (1994) also found that when subjects generated verbs to a list they had practiced, there was activation in the sylvian-insular cortex. This area was similarly activated in noun repetition.

10.5 Attention to action

There is a relation between these findings concerning the brain and the subjective report that early in learning subjects must pay attention to the motor sequences but need not do so when the task has been practised for many trials. Shallice (1982) has previously argued that the prefrontal cortex acts as a 'supervisory attentional system' that influences the selection of action when subjects perform tasks that are non-routine. It should therefore be possible to show that the prefrontal and anterior cingulate cortex are activated when the subjects must pay attention to the task in hand.

In a recent study we have compared performance of a prelearned motor sequence with and without attention (Jueptner *et al.* 1996). In one condition the subject performed a prelearned motor sequence (PRE) which has been practiced for one hour before scanning. In the other condition the subjects performed the same sequence, but they were asked to attend to what they were doing (ATT). Specifically they were asked to think about the next movement. When these conditions were compared (ATT vs PRE) the only areas that were activated were the left dorsal prefrontal cortex (9, 46, figure 10.6a) and the right anterior cingulate cortex (areas 32, 24, figure 10.6b).

A distinction should be drawn between attention to action and attention to locations in the external world. There is activation in the parietal lobe when subjects are required to attend to spatial locations (Posner & Petersen 1990; Corbetta et al. 1993) or to aspects of complex stimuli (Haxby et al. 1994). However, in the present study, while the dorsal prefrontal cortex was activated when subjects were required to attend to their actions (ATT vs PRE), the parietal cortex was not.

The term 'attention to action' is not precise. There are many operations which may require attention. In new learning of motor sequences the subjects must generate new moves, monitor the outcomes and mentally rehearse the sequence. The dorsal prefrontal cortex is engaged when subjects must generate numbers, and monitor their responses, while remembering the ones that they have produced (Petrides et al. 1993). The sequence is also 'supraspan' and Grasby et al. (1993, 1994) have shown that the prefrontal cortex is activated when subjects must remember lists that are supraspan.

During performance of the prelearned task with attention (ATT) the subjects did not have to make new decisions, monitor the outcomes or mentally rehearse the sequence. When a comparison was made of new learning with the attention condition (NEW vs ATT), there was more activation of the dorsal prefrontal and anterior cingulate cortex (32) during new learning than in performance of the prelearned task with attention (Jueptner et al. 1996, figure 10.2). Any one or all of these processes may account for the extensive activation of the prefrontal cortex in new learning. The results do not indicate which of these processes cannot be performed without interference in the dual task paradigm.

During new learning of the motor sequences one of the operations that the subjects must perform is the generation of new responses. It has been shown in other studies that the dorsal prefrontal cortex is activated when subjects must decide of their own accord which movements to make (Deiber et al. 1991; Frith

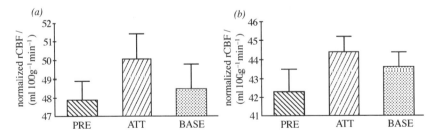

Fig. 10.6 Histograms showing regional cerebral blood flow in new learning of the motor task (NEW), performance of the prelearned task (PRE) and performance of the prelearned sequence with attention (ATT). Data from Jueptner et al. (1996a). (a) Left dorsal prefrontal cortex (area 9/46) ($x = -34, y = 20, z = 32$) (b) Right anterior cingulate cortex (area 32/24) ($x = 18, y = 10, z = 28$)

et al. 1991). We have also scanned subjects while they made decisions as to when to move their forefinger (Jahanshahi *et al.* 1995). In one condition the subjects themselves decided when to move the finger (SELF) and in the comparison condition they moved their finger when they heard a tone that functioned as an external trigger stimulus (EXT). The anterior cingulate cortex (areas 32, 24) was activated in both conditions (SELF VS BASE, EXT VS BASE) but the dorsal prefrontal cortex was only activated in the self-paced task (SELF VS BASE). Furthermore, the dorsal prefrontal cortex was the only area that was differentially activated when the two conditions were directly compared (SELF VS EXT, figure 10.7). This result implicates the dorsal prefrontal cortex in the process of making decisions concerning action.

Verb generation also requires subjects to make decisions. The subjects must produce a verb that is appropriate, but they themselves decide which of many possible verbs to produce. Frith *et al.* (1991) have also studied verbal fluency tasks in which the subjects are required to produce words that begin with particular letters. Again the subjects have a choice of which words to produce. Frith *et al.* (1991) showed that the prefrontal cortex and anterior cingulate cortex were activated when subjects performed the verbal fluency task.

Motor sequence learning and verb generation are alike in that before the subject responds there are no external prompts to specify which responses should be selected. In this sense they involve 'willed action' (Frith *et al.* 1991). They are also alike in that the subjects must reflect on and manipulate possible responses in the head (Frith & Grasby 1995).

Baddeley (1996) has also shown that there is considerable interference if subjects are required to generate a random sequence of key responses at the same time as producing a novel sequence of number and letters such as K-5-L-6-M-7. Interference on the motor task was measured by the decrease in randomness in the sequence of key responses. The subjects were also slow to

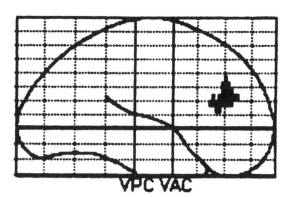

Fig. 10.7 Sagittal view of the brain showing activation in black for performance of the self-paced task (SELF) compared with performance of the externally paced task (EXT). Data from Jahanshahi *et al.* (1995).

produce the verbal sequence when required to perform both tasks at the same time. Baddeley argues that both tasks place a heavy load on the 'central executive' of working memory.

10.6 Prefrontal cortex and anterior cingulate

It is not clear whether interference occurs in prefrontal cortex, the anterior cingulate cortex or both.

(a) Prefrontal cortex

When subjects learn a finger sequence, there is activation in the dorsal prefrontal cortex (areas 9 and 46). However, Petersen *et al.* (1998) and Raichle *et al.* (1994) report that when subjects generate verbs there is a peak of activation in the ventral prefrontal cortex (area 45). Frith & Grasby (1995) have compared the peaks for activation reported in the literature for verbal and motor tasks, and they conclude that for verbal tasks there are peaks of activation in ventral prefrontal cortex whereas for motor tasks the peaks lie in the dorsal prefrontal cortex.

There are also differences in the laterality of the activation for verb generation and motor sequence learning. When subjects generate verbs the activation is restricted to the left prefrontal cortex (Petersen *et al.* 1988; Raichle *et al.* 1994). When subjects learn the finger sequence, there is activation in both the left and right prefrontal cortex, but the activation is more extensive on the right (Jenkins *et al.* 1994; Jueptner *et al.* 1996).

It could therefore be argued that verbal and motor tasks are processed in parallel systems within the prefrontal cortex. However, there is clear overlap between the systems.

First, Petersen *et al.* (1988) report that, as well as a peak in the ventral prefrontal cortex for verb generation, there is also a peak more dorsally. It lies within the conservative coordinates given by Rajkowksa & Goldman-Rakic (1995) for area 46. Furthermore, Raichle *et al.* (1994) present a figure (figure 10.4) showing the extent of the activation in lateral prefrontal cortex during verb generation, and it is clear that the activation overlaps with that found for motor-sequence learning (see Jenkins *et al.* 1994, figure 10.5). Second, Buckner *et al.* (1995) report that there is activation of the left frontal pole (area 10) during verb generation. Again, this activation overlaps with the activation seen during motor sequence learning (see Jenkins *et al.* 1994, figure 5).

(b) Anterior cingulate cortex

There is also extensive activation in the anterior cingulate cortex (area 32) when subjects generate verbs (Petersen *et al.* 1988; Raichle *et al.* 1994) or learn motor sequences (Jenkins *et al.* 1994; Jueptner *et al.* 1996). Frith & Grasby (1995) review the evidence that this area is activated when subjects must select between responses whether the tasks are verbal or motor.

Posner & Petersen (1990) have argued that the anterior cingulate cortex is especially activated when subjects must attend to the selection of responses. They base their argument on the claim that the activation of the anterior cingulate cortex increases as the number of targets to be detected increases. Frith & Grasby (1995) have reviewed attempts to distinguish between the functions of the anterior cingulate and prefrontal cortex. There is, as yet, no clear demonstration of a task that activates the anterior cingulate cortex without also activating the prefrontal cortex. For example, Pardo *et al.* (1990) claimed that only the anterior cingulate cortex was activated when subjects performed the Stroop task, but it has been shown more recently that the frontal polar cortex is also activated during this task (Carter *et al.* 1995).

(c) Scanning during dual task performance

One way to resolve the issue would be to scan subjects while they try to perform verb generation and learn motor sequences at the same time. We have not done this. However, Shallice *et al.* (1994) and Fletcher *et al.* (1995) have scanned subjects while they encoded verbal information at the same time as performing a motor task. When the motor task was easy, there was activation in the left prefrontal cortex during encoding of words. When the motor task was difficult, the prefrontal cortex was no longer significantly activated. However, there was an increase in the activation of the anterior cingulate cortex.

Unfortunately, this study does not decide the issue. The design of the experiment did not permit an assessment of the activation induced by the distractor task alone. It is true that Fletcher *et al.* (1995) report a comparison between the activation induced by the difficult compared with the easy motor task. However, this comparison does not show which areas were activated during performance of the more difficult motor task compared with a rest condition.

There is another issue that would be clarified by scanning subjects while they performed verb generation and motor sequences at the same time. figure 10.5 shows that even on trial 12 there was some interference as measured by the effect of verb generation on the response times for the motor task. One explanation would be that during dual task performance either the dorsal prefrontal or the anterior cingulate cortex were to some extent reactivated during performance of the motor sequence because the subjects were not confident of performing the motor sequence task without attention. D'Esposito *et al.* (1995) reported activation of these areas when subjects were faced with a dual task paradigm, even though these areas were not activated when the subjects performed either task alone. By scanning verb generation and the performance of the motor sequence on trial 12 it would be possible to see if there was more activation of the dorsal prefrontal or anterior cingulate cortex when the motor sequence was performed with verb generation than occurred without. The prediction would be that this would no longer happen if the motor sequence was overtrained for many more trials.

10.7 Conclusions

It has been claimed that interference may occur between two tasks if both tasks engage the prefrontal and anterior cingulate cortex. The advantage of this claim is that, if it is correct, there is an objective way of deciding whether a motor task is 'routine' or not. Shaffer (1975) has argued that the notion of automated performance begs the question of what is attention. It is proposed here that the more routine a task, the less the prefrontal and anterior cingulate cortex will be activated.

It is important to note that this is not a claim that this is the only stage of processing at which interference can occur. For example, it is known that there is interference with verbal memory if subjects are required to say 'la la la' either aloud or in their head at the same time as remembering the words (Baddeley 1986). Paulesu et al. (1993) have shown that when subjects remember letters, there is activation in left perisylvian areas: these include the superior temporal cortex, the inferior parietal cortex, Broca's area and the neighbouring ventral premotor cortex. In a recent experiment Paulesu et al. (1996) have found that one of these areas, the ventral premotor cortex, is activated when subjects repeat 'la la la' aloud or in their head. This result is consistent with the claim that interference can occur if two tasks engage a common area.

The claim made in the present paper concerns the interference that occurs when subjects must attend to the selection of more than one action at the same time. The claim is a version of the hypothesis that attentional selection occurs 'late' rather than 'early' (Allport 1991). The assumption is that the system is built to produce coherent action, and that it is adaptive to concentrate on one task at a time. Just as the animal scans the visual environment in a serial fashion, so it may pay to deal with problems concerning action in series. Serial processing at a late stage may be a design advantage, not a limitation.

Acknowledgements

I am grateful to the radiographers, Andreanna Williams, Andrew Blythe and Graham Lewington, for help with scanning. I am also grateful to Matthew Rushworth and Chris Frith for helpful discussions on this paper. The work is supported by the Wellcome Trust.

References

Allport, A. 1991 Visual attention. In: *Foundations of cognitive science* (ed. M. I. Posner), pp. 631–82. Cambridge: MIT Press.

Baddeley, A. 1986 *Working memory*. Oxford University Press

Baddeley, A. 1996 Exploring the central executive. *Q. J. Exp. Psychol.* **49a**, 5–28.

Buckner, R. L., Raichle, M. E. & Petersen, S. E. 1995 Dissociation of human prefrontal cortical areas across different speech production tasks and gender group. *J. Neurosci.* **74**, 2163–73.

Carter, C. S., Mintun, M. & Cohen, J. D. 1995 Interference and facilitation effects during selective attention. An H215O PET study of Stroop task performance. *Neuroimage* **2**, 264–72

Corbetta, M., Miezin, F. M., Shulman, G. L. & Petersen, S. E. 1993 A PET study of visuospatial attention. *J. Neurosci.* **13**, 1202–26.

Deiber, M.-P., Passingham, R. E., Colebatch, J. G., Friston, K. J., Nixon, P. D. & Frackowiak, R. S. J. 1991 Cortical areas and the selection of movement: a study with positron emission tomography. *Expl. Brain Res.* **84**, 393–402.

D'Esposito, M., Dejre, J. A., Alsop, D. C., Shin, R. K., Atlas, S. & Grossman, M. 1995 The neural basis of the central executive system of working memory. *Nature, Lond.* **378**, 279–81.

Fletcher, P. C., Frith, C. D., Grasby, P. M., Shallice, T., Frackowiak, R. S. J. & Dolan, R. J. 1995 Brain systems for encoding and retrieval of auditory-verbal memory. *Brain* **118**, 401–16.

Frith, C. D., Friston, K., Liddle, P. F. & Frackowiak, R. S. J. 1991 Willed action and the prefrontal cortex in man: a study with PET. *Proc. R. Soc. Lond.* B. **244**, 241–46.

Haxby, J. V., Horwitz, B., Ungerleider, L. G., Maisog, J. Ma., Pietrini, P. & Grady, C. L. 1994 The functional organization of human extrastriate cortex: a PET-rCBF study of selective attention to faces and locations. *J. Neurosci.* **14**, 6336–53.

Jahanshahi, M., Jenkins, I. H., Brown, R. G., Marsden, C. D., Passingham, R. E. & Brooks, D. J. 1995 Self-initiated versus externally triggered movements. I. An investigation using measurement of regional cerebral blood flow with PET and movement-related potentials in normal and Parkinson's disease subjects. *Brain* **118**, 913–33.

Jenkins, I. H., Brooks, D. J., Nixon, P. D., Frackowiak, R. S. J. & Passingham, R. E. 1994 Motor sequence learning: a study with positron emission tomography. *J. Neurosci.* **14**, 3775–90.

Jueptner, M., Stephan, K. M., Frith, C. D., Brooks, D. J., Frackowiak, R. S. J. & Passingham, R. E. 1996 The anatomy of motor learning. I. The frontal cortex and attention to action. *J. Neurophysiol* **77**, 1313–24.

Pardo, J. V., Pardo, P. J., Janer, K. W. & Raichle, M. E. 1990 The anterior cingulate cortex mediates processing selection in the Stroop attentional conflict paradigm. *Proc. Nat. Acad. Sci. U.S.A.* **87**, 256–59.

Paulesu, E., Frith, C. D. & Frackowiak, R. S. J. 1993 The neural correlates of the verbal component of working memory. *Nature, Lond.* **362**, 342–45.

Paulesu E., Passingham, R. E., Frackowiak, R. S. J. & Frith, C. D. 1996 Exploring the articulatory representations of verbal working memory with PET. *Neuroimage* **3**, 5555.

Petersen, S. E., Fox, P. T., Posner, M. I., Mintun, M. & Raichle, M. E. 1988 Positron emission tomographic studies of the cortical anatomy of single word processing. *Nature, Lond.* **331**, 585–89.

Petrides, M., Alivisatos, B., Meyer, E. & Evans, A. C. 1993 Functional activation of the human frontal cortex during the performance of verbal working memory tasks. *Proc. natn. Acad. Sci. U.S.A.* **90**, 878–82.

Posner, M. I. & Petersen 1990 The attention system of the human brain. *Ann. Rev. Neurosci.* **13**, 25–42.

Raichle, M. E., Fiez, J. A., Videen, T. O. *et al.* 1994 Practice-related changes in human brain functional anatomy during non-motor learning. *Cerebral Cortex* **4**, 8–26.

Rajkowska, G. & Goldman-Rakic, P. S. 1995 Cytoarchitectonic definition of prefrontal areas in the normal human cortex: II. Variability in locations of areas 9 and 46 and relationship to the Talairach coordinate system. *Cerebral Cortex* **5**, 323–37.

Shaffer, L. H. Multiple attention in continuous verbal tasks. In *Attention and performance* (ed. P. M. A. Rabbitt & S. Dornic), pp. 157–67. New York: Academic Press.

Shallice, T., Fletcher, P., Frith, C. D., Grasby, P., Frackowiak, R. S. J. & Dolan, R. J. 1994 Brain regions associated with acquisition and retrieval of verbal episodic memory. *Nature, Lond.* **368**, 633–35.

Wise, R., Chollet, F., Hadar, U., Friston, K., Hoffner, E. & Frackowiak, R. S. J. 1991 Distribution of cortical neural networks involved in word comprehension and word retrieval. *Brain* **114**, 1803–17.

11

Evidence for the importance of dopamine for prefrontal cortex functions early in life

Adele Diamond

There is considerable evidence that dorsolateral prefrontal cortex subserves critical cognitive abilities even during early infancy and that improvement in these abilities is evident over roughly the next 10 years. We also know that (a) in adult monkeys these cognitive abilities depend critically on the dopaminergic projection to prefrontal cortex and (b) the distribution of dopamine axons within dorsolateral prefrontal cortex changes, and the level of dopamine increases, during the period that infant monkeys are improving on tasks that require the cognitive abilities dependent on prefrontal cortex. To begin to look at whether these cognitive abilities depend critically on the prefrontal dopamine projection in humans even during infancy and early childhood we have been studying children who we hypothesized might have a selective reduction in the dopaminergic innervation of prefrontal cortex and a selective impairment in the cognitive functions subserved by dorsolateral prefrontal cortex. These are children treated early and continuously for the genetic disorder, phenylketonuria (PKU). In PKU the ability to convert the amino acid, phenylalanine (Phe), into another amino acid, tyrosine (Tyr), is impaired. This causes Phe to accumulate in the bloodstream to dangerously high levels and the plasma level of Tyr to fall. Widespread brain damage and severe mental retardation result. When PKU is moderately well controlled by a diet low in Phe (thus keeping the imbalance between Phe and Tyr in plasma within moderate limits) severe mental retardation is averted, but deficits remain in higher cognitive functions. In a four-year longitudinal study we have found these deficits to be in the working memory and inhibitory control functions dependent upon dorso-lateral prefrontal cortex in PKU children with plasma Phe levels 3–5 times normal. Prefrontal cortex abilities even during the first year of life. To test the hypothesis about the underlying biological mechanism we have reated the first animal model of early and continuously treated PKU. As predicted, the experimental animals had reduced levels of dopamine and the dopamine metabolite, homovanillic acid (HVA), in prefrontal cortex and showed impaired performance on delayed alternation, a task dependent on prefrontal cortex. Noradrenaline levels were unaffected; however, some reduction in serotonin levels and in dopamine levels outside the prefrontal cortex were found.

If prefrontal cortex functions are vulnerable in children with a moderate plasma Phe:Tyr imbalance because of the special properties of the dopamine neurons that project to prefrontal cortex, then other dopamine neurons that share those same properties should also be vulnerable in these children. The dopamine neurons in the retina share these properties (i.e. unusually high firing and dopamine turnover rates), and we have found that PKU children with plasma Phe levels 3–5 times normal are impaired in their contrast sensitivity, a behavioural measure sensitive to the retinal dopamine levels.

11.1   Introduction

One of the first demonstrated, and still one of the strongest, links between cognitive development and brain function is the improvement in infants' performance on the A-not-B, delayed response, and object retrieval tasks between $7\frac{1}{2}$ and 12 months of age and the dependence of successful performance on these tasks on the proper functioning of dorsolateral prefrontal cortex (see table 11.1). Human infants of $7\frac{1}{2}$–9 months, infant macaques of $\frac{1}{2}$–$\frac{1}{2}$ months, and adult macaques with bilateral removals of dorsolateral prefrontal cortex fail all three tasks under the same conditions and in the same ways. For reviews of this work see Diamond (1990*a, b*, 1991*a, b*). If maturation of the prefrontal neural system helps make possible cognitive advances reflected in improved performance on these tasks, in what aspects of the prefrontal system might one expect these maturational changes to be occurring? One candidate is in the levels of dopamine in prefrontal cortex. After briefly considering the abilities required

Table 11.1

	A$\bar{\text{B}}$	Delayed response	Object retrieval
Human infants show a clear developmental progression from $7\frac{1}{2}$–12 months.	Diamond 1985	Diamond & Doar 1988	Diamond 1988
Infant monkeys show a clear developmental progression from $1\frac{1}{2}$–4 months.	Diamond & Goldman-Rakic 1986	Diamond & Goldman-Rakic 1986	Diamond & Goldman-Rakic 1986
Adult monkeys with lesions of prefrontal cortex fail.	Diamond & Goldman-Rakic 1989	Diamond & Goldman-Rakic 1989	Diamond & Goldman-Rakic 1985
5-month-old infant monkeys, who received lesions of prefrontal cortex at 4 months, fail.	Diamond & Goldman-Rakic 1986	Diamond & Goldman-Rakic 1986	
Adult monkeys with lesions of parietal cortex succeed.	Diamond & Goldman-Rakic 1989	Diamond & Goldman-Rakic 1989	Diamond & Goldman-Rakic 1985
Adult monkeys with lesions of the hippocampal formation succeed.	Diamond *et al.* 1989	Squire & Zola-Morgan 1983	Diamond *et al.* 1989

for success on the A-not-B, delayed response, and object retrieval tasks, this paper will focus on recent work with children treated early and continuously for phenylketonuria (PKU), and with a corresponding animal model. That work sheds light on the importance of dopamine for prefrontal cortex function during early human life.

11.2   The cognitive abilities required by the A-not-B, delayed response, and object retrieval tasks

A-not-B (Piaget 1954, original French edition 1937) and delayed response (Jacobsen 1935) are two-choice hiding tasks. The ability of the subject to keep his or her mind on where the reward was hidden (whether one calls this 'working memory' or 'sustained attention') during the delay until retrieval is permitted appears to be essential. Evidence for this is, for example, that human infants, infant macaques, and infant or adult macaques with lesions of dorso-lateral prefrontal cortex generally perform well on the A-not-B and delayed response tasks if there is no delay, if the delay is shortened by 2–3 s, if they can look at the correct well during the delay, or if allowed to reach or move toward the correct well during the delay (in monkeys with dorsolateral prefrontal cortex ablations see Harlow *et al.* 1952; Bättig *et al.* 1960; Miles & Blomquist 1960; Pinsker & French 1967; Goldman & Rosvold 1970; Fuster & Alexander 1971; Diamond & Goldman-Rakic 1989; in human infants $7\frac{1}{2}$–9 months of age see Gratch & Landers 1971; Evans 1973; Harris 1973; Gratch *et al.* 1974; Cornell 1979; Fox *et al.* 1979; Diamond 1985).

The role of working memory or sustained attention is less prominent in the object retrieval task (Diamond 1988, 1990*b*), where the subject must detour around a small transparent box open on one side to retrieve the reward inside. Yet even here the ability to hold information in mind appears to be important in attaining mastery of the task. Infants of 6–8 months reach only at the side of the clear box through which they are looking. Thus, to retrieve the reward they must look through the opening and continue to do so as they reach inside. However, by $8\frac{1}{2}$–9 months when the front of the box is open, and by $9\frac{1}{2}$–10 months when the left or right side of the box is open, infants can look through the opening, then sit up and reach in while looking through a closed side; that is, the memory of having looked through the opening is enough. Looking along the route the hand will reach appears to be critical; at these ages infants still fail if they have not looked through the opening on a given trial. However, it is a major achievement to be freed from having to continue to do so. Even so, being able to divide or switch one's attention between the box and the reward appears to be more critical on the object retrieval task than does sustained attention or working memory.

The most obvious requirement of the object retrieval task is the ability to resist the strong pull to reach straight to the visible reward. For example, human infants, and macaques with dorsolateral prefrontal cortex ablations, perform much better when the box is opaque than when it is transparent

(Diamond 1990*b*). Inhibitory control also seems to be required for success on the A-not-B and delayed response tasks. Infants, and macaques with dorsolateral prefrontal cortex ablations, perform fine at the first hiding place, although the delay is just as long there as it is on subsequent trials. It would appear that errors occur when the reward is hidden in the other hiding place because, having been positively reinforced for finding the reward at 'A' the tendency of subjects to reach to 'A' has been strengthened and that must now be inhibited or overridden if the subject is to reach to 'B'.

Some errors can be elicited simply by taxing working memory or sustained attention, for example by using a long delay at the first hiding location (e.g. Sophian & Wellman 1983). Similarly, some errors can be elicited simply by taxing inhibitory control, for example some infants err on the reversal trials to 'B' even when the covers are transparent (e.g. Butterworth 1977; Willatts 1985). However, the vast majority of errors occur when subjects must both hold information in mind and also exercise inhibitory control over their behaviour; that is on reversal trials to 'B' when the covers are transparent and a delay is imposed.

An analogue of this type of error in normal adults might be a scenario such as: 'On going to the telephone to call an old friend, I reminded myself of my friend's new phone number and was resolved not to make the mistake of dialling the old number. However, as the old and new phone numbers began with the same initial digits, as I began dialling the number I got into the routine of dialling the number I had dialled so many times in the past and dialled the old number though I knew full well my friend's new phone number'. In infants this type of error is often manifest in the A-not-B task by the infant reaching to 'A' when the infant had seen a toy being hidden in 'B' just before the delay, but not looking in the A well to see if the toy were there, and instead uncovering 'B' and looking in there for the toy. It is as if at some level the infant knew the toy was not in 'A' since the infant did not look in that well after uncovering it, but for some reason that knowledge did not direct where the infant first reached. A less common but more dramatic error is for the infant to look straight at the correct well ('B'), indicating with the eyes that he or she 'knows' where the toy is, while at the same time reaching to the previously correct well ('A') and uncovering it. The error can also happen earlier in the behaviour sequence as when you forget that your friend's phone number has changed and so go to the telephone with the intention of dialling the old phone number, or when an infant looks genuinely surprised not to find the toy in well 'A'.

With effort we can all dial our friends' changed numbers correctly, but it certainly requires less effort to remember and correctly dial other phone numbers (even if they are less well-practised) that do not require the inhibition of another number. Similarly, it requires less effort to dial a friend's new phone number if we are looking at the number written down as we dial it. It is when we must *both* hold the number in mind and resist or override a strong tendency to dial a different number that errors are most likely to occur, and for that, I would contend, dorsolateral prefrontal cortex is most clearly required. To repeat, it is when we must act *in a different way than our first inclination and when at least some of the information needed for action must be held in mind that dorsolateral prefrontal cortex is most clearly required.*

While the studies summarized in table 11.1 provide some evidence that important maturational changes may be occurring within the dorsolateral prefrontal cortex neural system during the first year of life, dorsolateral prefrontal cortex is probably not fully mature until at least 10 years of age. Not surprisingly, then, if one uses slightly more difficult tasks, one can elicit A-not-B-type errors beyond the infancy period. For example, 3-year-old children can sort cards correctly by the first criterion, whether that criterion is colour or shape (just as infants correctly retrieve the reward from wherever it is first hidden). However, when instructed to switch and sort by the other criterion, 3-year-olds persist in sorting by the first criterion (Zelazo *et al.* 1995, 1996; just as infants persist in reaching to the first hiding place when the reward is later hidden at the other hiding location), even though the experimenter reminds the child of the new sorting criterion at the outset of every trial. Children 4–5 years of age fail other tasks that require holding information in mind plus inhibitory control, such as the day-night Stroop-like task (Gerstadt *et al.* 1994). On that task, the subject must hold two rules in mind ('Say "Night" when you see a white card with a picture of the sun, and say "Day" when you see a black card with a picture of the moon and stars') and must resist or override the tendency to say what the images on the cards really represent. In Diamond & Taylor (1996), we present additional evidence that the working memory and inhibitory control abilities dependent on dorsolateral prefrontal cortex may reach a critical level of maturity by 6 years of age.

If it is true that maturational changes in prefrontal cortex underlie some of the cognitive advances during early childhood, as I have suggested, what exactly is changing in the prefrontal system during the early years of postnatal life? One candidate is increasing levels of the neurotransmitter, dopamine. For example, dopamine levels increase in the rhesus macaque brain during the period when infant rhesus macaques are improving on the A-not-B, delayed response, and object retrieval tasks (Brown & Goldman 1977; Lewis & Harris 1991). As an initial way of looking at the role of dopamine in prefrontal cortex function in humans early in development, we have been investigating children who, there was reason to believe, might have a selective reduction in dopamine in prefrontal cortex without other abnormalities in the brain—children treated early and continuously for phenylketonuria (PKU). We have also been investigating animal models of this condition.

11.3   Why the dopamine system in prefrontal cortex might be selectively affected in early and continuously treated PKU (ECT-PKU)

The core problem in PKU is an inability to convert the amino acid Phe, into another amino acid Tyr. This problem is caused by a mutation of the gene in chromosome 12 (12q22–12q24.1) which codes for the enzyme, phenyl alanine hydroxylase (Woo *et al.* 1983; Lidsky *et al.* 1985). Levels of Phe in the bloodstream rise to well over 10 times normal ($\geqslant 20\mathrm{mgdL}^{-1}(1200\mu\mathrm{molL}^{-1})$), levels of Tyr in the bloodstream drop, and severe mental retardation results (Krause *et al.* 1985). Treatment consists of a diet low in Phe. This results in lower plasma Phe levels than if the child ate normally, and it succeeds in averting severe mental retardation. However, the reduced-Phe diet does not result in completely normal plasma Phe levels (roughly $2\mathrm{mgdL}^{-1}$). That is because the low-Phe diet reflects a compromise between the need to minimize Phe intake and the need for protein. The advice of the U.S. National Collaborative Study of Treated PKU has been that plasma Phe levels should not exceed five times normal ($10\mathrm{mgdL}^{-1}$; Williamson *et al.* 1981; Koch & Wenz 1987). Thus, dietary treatment for PKU reduces the plasma Phe elevation, but does not erase it, and does nothing to ameliorate the plasma Tyr reduction. Because plasma levels of Phe and Tyr are not fully normal in children treated for PKU, the door is open for neurological and cognitive problems to still be present, at least in some children.

There have been reports of cognitive impairments in children treated early and continuously for PKU (i.e. children on the low-Phe diet since shortly after birth). For example, the IQs of these children are often significantly lower than the IQs of their siblings. Children with PKU, even when they have been on the special diet since shortly after birth, typically have IQs in the 80s or 90s; that is, IQs in the normal range, but just barely (e.g. Dobson *et al.* 1976; Berry *et al.* 1979; Williamson *et al.* 1981). More recently, studies have reported problems in attentional control, problem-solving, or 'executive functions'. For example, children with early and continuously treated PKU tend to be more distractible, to be more limited in the amount of information they can hold in mind at one time and manipulate, and to have more difficulty maintaining set until a problem is solved or a goal attained (e.g. Krause *et al.* 1985; Pennington *et al.* 1985; Faust *et al.* 1986; Brunner *et al.* 1987; Smith & Beasley 1989). These problems are reminiscent of the deficits seen after damage to prefrontal cortex. Indeed, damage to prefrontal cortex typically results in IQs lowered to the 80s or 90s (Stuss & Benson 1986, 1987); that is, the same range as one sees in children treated for PKU.

Why might the cognitive deficits be specific to the functions of prefrontal cortex? The mild imbalance in the plasma Phe·Tyr ratio results in mildly reduced levels of Tyr reaching the brain. Phe and Tyr compete for the same transporter proteins to cross the blood–brain barrier (Chirigos *et al.* 1960; Oldendorf, 1973; Pardridge 1977). Indeed, those proteins have a higher affinity for Phe than for Tyr (Pardridge & Oldendorf 1977; Miller *et al.* 1985). Hence, a modest imbalance between Phe and Tyr in the bloodstream results in mildly reduced CNS Tyr levels.

The dopamine system in prefrontal cortex is more sensitive to a mild reduction in Tyr than are the dopamine systems in most other brain regions. Tyr is the precursor of dopamine. Most brain regions receiving dopaminergic input are unaffected by modest changes in CNS Tyr levels. However, prefrontal cortex is acutely sensitive to even a small reduction in Tyr. That is because the dopamine neurons that project to prefrontal cortex fire so rapidly and turn over dopamine so quickly (Thierry *et al.* 1977; Bannon *et al.* 1981, 1983; Wurtman *et al.* 1981; Tam *et al.* 1990). Indeed, moderate reductions in CNS levels of Tyr, that have little effect on dopamine synthesis in other neural regions (such as the striatum), profoundly reduce dopamine synthesis in prefrontal cortex (Bradberry *et al.* 1989). Hence, we hypothesized that here was a mechanism by which the moderate Phe:Tyr imbalance in the bloodstream of children treated for PKU might selectively affect prefrontal cortex.

It has also been known for some time that reducing dopamine in prefrontal cortex produces deficits in the cognitive abilities dependent on prefrontal cortex. Selectively depleting dorsolateral prefrontal cortex of dopamine can produce deficits as severe as those found when dorsolateral prefrontal cortex is removed altogether (Brozoski *et al.* 1979). Indeed, local injection of dopamine antagonists into dorsolateral prefrontal cortex impairs performance in a precise, dose-dependent manner on tasks dependent on prefrontal cortex (Sawaguchi & Goldman-Rakic 1991). Similarly, destruction of the dopamine neurons in the ventral tegmental area (VTA) that project to prefrontal cortex impairs performance on these tasks (Simon *et al.*, 1980). Injections of MPTP (1-methyl-4-phenyl-1,2,3,6- tetrahydropyridine) result in reduced levels of dopamine in the prefrontal-striatal neural system. Cumulative doses of 15–75 mg of MPTP do not produce Parkinsonian-type motor deficits in rhesus macaques, although larger doses do. At the lower doses of MPTP, the monkeys are impaired on delayed response and object retrieval (Schneider & Kovelowski 1990; Taylor *et al.* 1990), although they perform normally on other tasks such as visual discrimination. Hence, we hypothesized, the moderate Phe:Tyr imbalance in the bloodstream of children treated for PKU might result in deficits in the cognitive abilities dependent upon prefrontal cortex because of the effect of the Phe:Tyr imbalance on prefrontal dopamine levels.

11.4   Evidence of prefrontal cortex cognitive deficits in ECT-PKU children

In a large, four-year longitudinal study (Diamond 1994; Diamond *et al.* 1996) we found that PKU children, who had been on a low-Phe diet since the first month of life, but who had moderately elevated plasma Phe levels (levels roughly 3–5 times normal (6–10 mgdL^{-1}; $360 - 600\mu$molL^{-1})), were impaired on all six tests that required both holding information in mind and resisting or overriding a dominant response, that is, tasks dependent on dorsolateral prefrontal cortex. The tests were the A-not-B and the object retrieval tasks for infants; A-not-B with invisible displacement for toddlers; the day–night Stroop-like test, the tapping test, and the three pegs test for young children; (see figure 11.1).

(a)

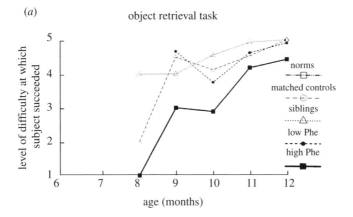

(b)

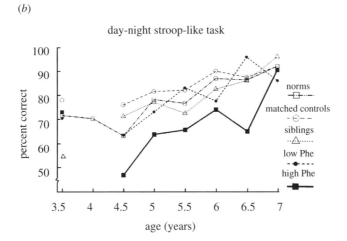

Fig. 11.1 ECT-PKU Children with 'higher' plasma Phe levels (Phe levels 3–5 times normal) performed significantly worse on tasks that required both working memory and inhibitory control than did other PKU and hyperPhe children with Phe levels closer to normal, their siblings, matched controls, and children from the general population. Examples of this can be seen in infants on (a) the object retrieval task (Diamond 1990, 1991) and (b) in young children on the day–night Stroop-like task (Gerstadt et al. 1994). The day–night Stroop-like task was not administered at 4 years of age to any of the groups followed longitudinally, because the control version of the task was administered instead. All groups performed normally on the control version, where they had to remember two rules, but did not have to resist the tendency to say what the scenes really represented (since the stimuli were abstract designs).

This is consistent with the results of other studies, the most relevant ones being those by Welsh et al. (1990) and Smith et al. (1996), as they too used cognitive tasks tailored to the functions of dorsolateral prefrontal cortex. The deficits we observed were evident in all age groups (infants, toddlers, and young children), and remained significant even after controlling for IQ, sex, health variables, and background characteristics. The deficits were clear whether the children were compared to (a) other ECT-PKU children with lower Phe levels, (b) their own siblings, (c) matched controls, or (d) children from the general population. Of the 24 comparisons between ECT-PKU children with Phe levels 3–5 times normal and the other groups of children on these six tasks (6 tasks × 4 comparisons per task), ECT-PKU children with higher Phe levels performed significantly worse on 21 of the 24 comparisons. The group differences obtained are robust because the children were tested repeatedly over time, which yielded several data points per subject and provided a more accurate and reliable indication of each child's ability and developmental trajectory than would have been possible had we tested each child only once. (Infants were tested every month from 6 to 12 months of age, toddlers every 3 months from 15 to 30 months, and young children every 6 months from $3\frac{1}{2}$ to 7 years of age.) In contrast to the marked differences between PKU children and other subjects on these tasks, of the 36 comparisons among the control groups (groups a-d above) on these six tasks (6 tasks × 6 comparisons per task), only six comparisons revealed a significant difference. That is, of the 60 pairwise group comparisons, 51 yielded results in the predicted direction. The cognitive deficits documented in several of the other studies of PKU children could be explained away by saying that (a) the plasma Phe levels of many of the children were outside the 'safe' range (i.e. > 5 times normal), (b) even if concurrent Phe levels were not excessively elevated earlier Phe levels had been (during the years the children had been off diet), and/or (c) the low-Phe diet had been started too late to avert early brain damage. None of those disclaimers is applicable here.

The higher a child's Phe level, the worse that child's performance tended to be on tasks that required acting counter to his or her initial tendency on the basis of information held in mind. Performance on these tasks was most strongly and consistently related to concurrent plasma Phe levels, rather than to mean Phe levels over a wide age range, during the first year of life, or during the first month. As current Phe levels varied so too, inversely, did behavioural performance.

Three tasks were administered that require memory of the choices one has already made or temporal order memory. The tasks were the three boxes test (boxes scrambled after each reach; Petrides 1988, 1989, 1991), the six boxes test (boxes scrambled after each reach), and the Corsi–Milner test of temporal order memory (Milner et al. 1991)). These tests tax working memory and require the functions of prefrontal cortex, but they do not tax inhibitory control and they do not require precisely the same region of prefrontal cortex as do tasks that tax both working memory + inhibitory control. Of the 12 comparisons between ECT-PKU children with Phe levels 3–5 times normal and the other groups of children on these three tasks (3 tasks × 4 comparisons per task), the children with higher Phe levels performed significantly worse than the comparison groups on only 0–2 of these 12 comparisons. Similarly, when plasma Phe level was treated as a continuous variable, no significant relationship between plasma Phe levels and any measure of performance on these three tasks was found. Perhaps the boxes and Corsi–Milner tasks failed to show an effect because of ceiling and floor effects, perhaps taxing both working memory and inhibitory control is critical, perhaps taxing inhibitory control is critical in and of itself, perhaps it has to do with regional differences within prefrontal cortex in the dopamine innervation, or perhaps the boxes and Corsi–Milner tasks did not lend themselves to the use of a strategy and so did not really require prefrontal cortex.

Dorsolateral prefrontal cortex consists primarily of Areas 9 and 46. In the rhesus macaque, Area 9 is much more densely innervated by dopamine than is Area 46 (Lewis *et al.* 1986; Lewis & Morrison 1989). The tasks on which we found no effect are more strongly linked to Area 9 than Area 46 (Petrides 1995). Perhaps the subregion of dorsolateral prefrontal cortex that enables us to hold information in mind and inhibit interfering actions or thoughts is more acutely sensitive to any small fluctuations in dopamine because it has so relatively little dopamine to start with, and hence might need all of its allotment all of the time.

Robbins and colleagues (Robbins, Chapter 9) and Mangels (1996) have found that prefrontal cortex is not required for memory of the choices one has already made or for temporal order memory when that information is processed incidentally, rather than intentionally, or when the task does not lend itself to use of a strategy (Owen *et al.* 1996). It is possible that the versions of self-ordered and temporal memory tasks we have used here might not require prefrontal cortex involvement. Certainly, on the Corsi–Milner test of memory for temporal order there was no meaningful order to the stimuli; the stimuli told no story, reflected no underlying organizing principles, and in general did not relate one to another. Perhaps if there had been some reason to remember the order in which the stimuli were being presented, other than because one would be tested on it, a group difference might have emerged.

Milner and her colleagues (Milner *et al.* 1991) found that patients with prefrontal cortex excisions were impaired on the temporal order test on which we found no impairment, but the excisions in their patients extended across subregions within prefrontal cortex and were not restricted to Areas 46 and 9. (Owen *et al.* 1996) found that prefrontal cortex was critically involved in remembering which stimuli one had already chosen when normal subjects were able to apply a strategy to the task. However, in a condition very much like our multiple boxes tasks, where the boxes were scrambled after each reach, Owen *et al.* found that subjects were not able to develop a strategy to solve the task, and prefrontal cortex did not appear to be required. However, Petrides (1995) found that monkeys were impaired on the three boxes tasks (boxes scrambled after each reach) after lesions of dorsolateral prefrontal cortex. The literature is contradictory on this point. Perhaps if we had included a test where temporal order memory, or memory of the reponses one has already made, was more amenable to the use of a strategy, we might have found an mpairment among subjects whose Phe levels were moderately elevated.

The same children who were impaired on all six working memory + inhibitory control tasks, performed normally on most of the ten control tasks, most of which required the functions of parietal cortex or the medial temporal lobe. The cognitive deficits, thus, appeared to be selective. The functions of parietal cortex and of the medial temporal lobe appeared to be spared. ECT-PKU children with higher Phe levels performed worse on only six out of the 40 comparisons on these tasks. The consistency of the deficits of the ECT-PKU children with Phe levels 3–5 times normal on the working memory + inhibitory control tasks and the paucity of deficits on all other tasks is unlikely to be a chance occurrence.

Visual paired comparison, delayed nonmatching to sample, and the Corsi–Milner test of recognition memory were the measures used of the recognition memory ability dependent on the medial temporal lobe. Of the 12 comparisons between children with Phe levels 3–5 times normal and the other groups of children on these three tasks (3 tasks × 4 comparisons per task), children with higher Phe levels performed significantly worse on only three of these 12 comparisons. However, at the longest delays on the visual paired comparison task (10 min), ECT-PKU infants, regardless of their plasma Phe level, performed significantly worse than infants from the general population and tended to perform worse than matched controls. Plasma Phe levels covaried inversely with performance on the task as well. Hence, on this condition of this one control task an impairment was found.

ECT-PKU children whose plasma Phe levels were closer to normal (< 3× normal) performed comparably to all control groups on our cognitive tests. This is consistent with another recent report that, when plasma Phe levels were kept below three times normal from birth to the present, ECT-PKU children showed no cognitive impairments (Stemerdink et al. 1995). This indicates that the cognitive deficits may well be preventable.

Are the cognitive deficits observed here indicative of a developmental delay or of absolute, lasting deficits? On the one hand, all children, even ECT-PKU children with higher Phe levels, improved over time on our tasks. On the other hand, the impression that ECT-PKU children may 'catch up' to other children is probably misleading. In almost all cases this 'catch up' was due to ceiling effects because the same tasks were administered over a wide age range, and these tasks tended to be too easy for children at the upper end of an age range. Many tests, such as IQ measures, increase the difficulty of the test as children get older, although the test may be called by the same name throughout. We found that when all groups of children appeared to be performing comparably, because all were near the ceiling, when we went to the next battery of tasks for the next age range, the differences between the groups reappeared. The impairment of the ECT-PKU children with higher Phe levels in working memory and inhibitory control was as evident in our oldest age range ($3\frac{1}{2}$–7-year-olds) as it was in our youngest age range (6–12-month-olds). There was little evidence of any narrowing of the gap between ECT-PKU children with Phe levels 3–5 times normal and their same-aged peers, at least from 6 months to 6 years of age. We stopped studying children at 7 years of age. One cannot tell from this study whether sometime after 7 years of age ECT-PKU children whose Phe levels remain only moderately elevated might no longer show the kinds of cognitive deficits we have documented. However, early cognitive deficits or developmental delays, especially when they extend over a long period (6 months–6 years) are likely to have profound and enduring effects, even if the cognitive deficits themselves are subsequently resolved. For example, children who have repeatedly seen themselves struggle with cognitive tasks which their peers find easy, come to believe themselves to be less able, and may continue to see themselves in this way long after the ability gap has been narrowed. Similarly, others around the child (parents, teachers, and peers) typically expect a child to perform as he or she always has, and people often perform as others expect them to perform. Because ECT-PKU children whose Phe concentrations are moderately elevated appear to have difficulty in getting their actions to reflect their intentions, because they sometimes get stuck in behavioural ruts from which they cannot easily extricate themselves, these children may be wrongly labelled as 'bad', 'intentionally difficult', or 'wilful'—and such labels can affect a child for life.

11.5   Is dorsolateral prefrontal cortex only required when the information to be held in mind concerns spatial location?

The tasks on which the infants and toddlers with plasma Phe levels 3–5 times normal failed (A-not-B, object retrieval, and A-not-B with invisible displacements), required holding information in mind about spatial location. One of the most influential and intriguing hypotheses about the functions of dorsolateral prefrontal cortex is that this region is required for holding spatial information in mind (Goldman-Rakic 1987). According to that hypothesis, information about object features is processed in ventrolateral prefrontal cortex, whereas dorsolateral prefrontal cortex is specialized to help us hold in mind information about spatial location. Also according to this hypothesis, a subject acts according to a prepotent response when the correct answer has been forgotten; the prepotent response is sort of a default when one does not know what to do. That is, subjects with dorsolateral prefrontal cortex damage do not err, even in part, because of a failure to exercise inhibitory control; they err because of a failure of working memory, specifically spatial working memory.

There were no spatial tasks on which ECT-PKU infants and toddlers with plasma Phe levels 3–5 times normal performed as well as controls, but there were also no spatial tasks that did not require both holding information in mind and inhibition of a strong response tendency. The prefrontal tasks on which we found no deficits (the multiple boxes and temporal order memory tasks) do not require memory of spatial information. That would be consistent with the spatial memory hypothesis. These tasks also required little or no inhibition, however the main findings that are inconsistent with the spatial memory hypothesis are that at least two of the tasks on which young children with moderate plasma Phe elevations failed (the day–night Stroop-like task and the tapping task) do not seem to require holding any spatial information in mind. (On the tapping task, as on the day-night task, the subject must hold two rules in mind and must resist making the response that would ordinarily be made (Diamond & Taylor 1996).)

In general, evidence is mixed concerning the possible specialized role of dorsolateral prefrontal cortex in handling spatial information in particular. Evidence in support of this role includes findings such as the following: rhesus monkeys with lesions of dorsolateral prefrontal cortex fail spatial alternation tasks but not object alternation tasks (Mishkin & Manning 1978; but see Bauer & Fuster 1976), and in rhesus monkeys neurons in dorsolateral prefrontal cortex have been found which are active during the delay period of the spatial delayed response task whereas neurons in the inferior convexity are active during the delay period of a conditional pattern discrimination task (Wilson *et al.* 1993). However, evidence contrary to the dorsolateral spatial memory hypothesis includes the following: in positron emission tomography (PET) studies with human subjects, Petrides and his colleagues report activation in ventrolateral prefrontal cortex, but not in dorsolateral prefrontal cortex, on a spatial memory span task (Petrides this volume), and activation in dorsolateral prefrontal cortex, but not in ventrolateral prefrontal cortex, on a non-spatial self-ordered memory task (Petrides *et al.* 1993 and this volume).

The tasks that most reliably and robustly elicit activation of dorsolateral prefrontal cortex in neuro-imaging studies, such as the two-back task (e.g. Cohen *et al.* 1993 and this volume), require both holding information in mind (whether spatial or non-spatial) and inhibiting a response tendency. For example, on the two-back test, the subject must remember the rule, 'Respond when, and only when, you see an "x" that follows two items after an "a",' and subjects must resist or override the propensity to respond when they see an "x" under all other circumstances. Some of the evidence on the centrality of inhibitory control problems in patients with damage to dorsolateral prefrontal cortex seems hard to reconcile with a model that proposes that this neural region is important only for working memory. For example, even when the current rule is displayed on all trials so one does not need to hold it in mind, patients with damage to dorsolateral prefrontal cortex have more difficulty switching from one rule to another (e.g. to switch between sorting by size to sorting by shape; Rubinstein *et al.* 1996) than do patients with more posterior damage. It has long been known that patients with damage to dorsolateral prefrontal cortex can sometimes tell you the correct criterion even as they continue to sort cards on the Wisconsin Card Sort Test incorrectly by the old criterion (e.g. Milner 1963; Luria & Homskaya 1964). In these instances, there is a failure of knowledge to result in the prepotent response being overridden. It is as if subjects get stuck in a behavioural rut from which they cannot readily extricate themselves despite their best intentions and despite knowing what correct performance entails.

11.6   An animal model of mild, chronic plasma Phe elevations

With children it was only possible to measure cognitive performance and plasma amino acid levels. To more directly investigate our hypothesis that the cognitive deficits associated with moderately elevated plasma Phe levels are produced by a selective reduction in dopamine metabolism in prefrontal cortex, we turned to an animal model. Building on work modelling the untreated PKU condition (Greengard *et al.* 1976; Brass & Greengard 1982), we developed and characterized the first animal model of ECT-PKU (Diamond *et al.* 1994). By administering a phenylalanine hydroxylase inhibitor (α methylphenylalanine) plus a small supplement of Phe we were able to mildly and chronically elevate the plasma Phe levels of rat pups.

The affected rats were impaired on a behavioural task dependent on prefrontal cortex (delayed alternation). On this task, the animal must remember which goal arm was last entered over the *delay* between trials and the animal is rewarded only if it *alternates* goal arms (i.e. if it selects the goal arm *not* selected on the previous trial). The hallmark of what one finds after ablation of prefrontal cortex is that subjects fail when a delay is imposed between trials, although they are unimpaired at learning the task or when no delay is used (in rats see for example Wikmark *et al.* 1973; Larsen & Divac 1978; Bubser & Schmidt 1990; in monkeys see for example Jacobsen & Nissen 1937; Bätting *et al.* 1960; Kubota & Niki 1971). Thus, they are impaired when they must hold in mind which arm of the maze they have just entered and when they have to inhibit repeating that response in order to alternate. We found that the rats with moderately elevated plasma Phe levels learned the delayed alternation task normally and performed well when there was no delay between trials, but failed when a delay was imposed between trials. That is, they showed the pattern of error associated with prefrontal cortex dysfunction.

As predicted, lower levels of dopamine and the dopamine metabolite, HVA, were found in prefrontal cortex in the PKU-model animals than in controls. (Medial prefrontal cortex in the rodent is considered the homologue of dorsolateral prefrontal cortex in the primate (Leonard 1969; Domesick, 1972 Kolb, 1984; Groenewegen 1988), although Preuss (1995) has recently called this homology into question. Medial prefrontal cortex is located immediately in front of the genu.) There was almost no overlap between HVA and dopamine levels in prefrontal cortex of controls and of either experimental group. In contrast, there was no effect of elevated plasma Phe levels on noradrenaline in any of the neural regions investigated (prefrontal cortex, anterior cingulate, caudate-putamen, and nucleus accumbens).

Our predictions were not perfectly confirmed, however. We found some effect on the serotoninergic system, and some effects on dopamine metabolism outside of prefrontal cortex. This could be because plasma Phe levels were raised a bit more than intended (6.5 times normal, rather than < 5 times normal) or because the neurochemical effects of moderately elevated plasma Phe levels are not as localized as we have hypothesized. Our lab is presently investigating this further with the genetic mouse model of PKU created by McDonald & Shedlovsky (McDonald *et al.* 1990; Shedlovsky *et al.* 1993). These mice have a mutation of the gene that causes PKU in humans; these mice have a mutation of the gene homologous to the one that causes PKU in humans; these mice, too, are severely impaired in converting Phe to Tyr.

11.7   Confirming evidence from research on vision

If we are correct that the special properties of the dopamine neurons that project to prefrontal cortex make the functions of that area particularly vulnerable to moderate increases in the ratio of Phe:Tyr in the bloodstream, then any other dopamine neurons that also have those properties should also be affected. It turns out that the dopamine neurons in the retina share those properties. They too have rapid firing and dopamine turnover rates (Iuvone *et al.* 1978, 1989; Fernstrom *et al.* 1986). Moreover, the competition at the blood–retinal barrier is comparable to that at the blood–brain barrier (Rapoport 1976; Hjelle *et al.* 1978; Fernstrom *et al.* 1986; Tornquist & Alm 1986). Therefore, we predicted that retinal functions dependent on dopamine should also be affected in PKU children with plasma Phe levels 3–5 times normal; that prediction has recently been confirmed.

If the retina is depleted of dopamine, one finds impaired sensitivity to contrast (Kupersmith *et al.* 1982; Regan & Neima 1984; Skrandies & Gottlob 1986; Bodis-Wollner *et al.* 1987; Bodis-Wollner 1990). (Contrast sensitivity refers to the threshold of how much contrast between black lines (sinusoid gratings) and a white background is required for a person to be able to detect the black lines.) Diamond and Herzberg (1996) found that children treated early and continuously for PKU were impaired in their sensitivity to contrast across all five spatial frequencies tested (1.5–18.0 cycles per degree). Indeed, at the next to highest spatial frequency (12 cycles per degree), the 'group' variable accounted for 70% of the variance, controlling for acuity, sex, age, and test site. At no spatial frequency was the contrast sensitivity performance of any child with PKU superior to the performance of his or her sibling. The poorer contrast sensitivity performance of subjects with PKU was found even when the analyses were repeated omitting the two subjects with mean plasma Phe levels above five times normal and omitting the two subjects with IQ scores less than 90. In short, we have found two superficially unrelated behavioural effects, a selective deficit in cognitive functions dependent on dorsolateral prefrontal cortex and a selective visual defect in contrast sensitivity, both of which had been predicted based on the same underlying hypothesis (that a moderate imbalance in the plasma Phe:Tyr ratio selectively affects those dopamine neurons that have the most rapid firing and dopamine turnover rates).

We knew, from work with rats, that the dopamine neurons that project to prefrontal cortex have unusual properties that set them apart from most other dopamine-containing neurons in the CNS. However, there was no evidence concerning this in humans. The results we have obtained with children treated early and continuously for PKU provide what is probably the first evidence suggesting that the prefrontally-projecting dopamine neurons may also have these special properties in humans. We knew from work with rhesus macaques, that during the period that infant monkeys are improving on the A-not-B, delayed response, and object retrieval tasks, striking changes in the distribution of tyrosine hydroxylase-immuno reactive fibres in prefrontal cortex (Area 9) are occuring (Lewis & Harris 1991), and the level of dopamine is increasing in the monkey brain (Brown & Goldman 1977). It is possible that one of the reasons that human infants are able to succeed on these tasks by 12 months of age, although they fail these tasks even under the simplest conditions below 8–9 months of age, has to do with developmental changes in the dopaminergic innervation of prefrontal cortex.

Acknowledgements

Support from NIH (R01 #MH41842, R01 #HD34346, BRSG S07 #RR07083–26 & MRRC P30 #HD26979) and from March of Dimes (#12–0718, #12–0554 & #12–253) is gratefully acknowledged.

References

Bannon, M. J., Bunney, E. B. & Roth, R. H. 1981 Mesocortical dopamine neurons: rapid transmitter turn-over compared to other brain catecholamine systems. *Brain Res.* **218**, 376–82.

Bannon, M. J., Wolf, M. E. & Roth, R. H. 1983 Pharmacology of dopamine neurons innervating the prefrontal, cingulate, and piriform cortices. *Eur. J. Pharmacol.* **92**, 119–25.

Bättig, K., Rosvold, H. E. & Mishkin, M. 1960 Comparison of the effects of frontal and caudate lesions on delayed response and alternation in monkeys. *J. Comp. Physiol.* **53**, 400–04.

Bauer, R. H. & Fuster, J. M. 1976 Delayed-matching and delayed- response deficit from cooling dorsolateral prefrontal cortex in monkeys. *J. Comp. Physiol. Psychol.* **90**, 293–302.

Berry, H. K., O'Grady, D. J., Perlmutter, L. J. & Bofinger, M. K. 1979 Intellectual development and achievement of children treated early for phenylketonuria. *Devl. Med. Child Neurol.* **21**, 311–20.

Bodis-Wollner, I. 1990 Visual deficits related to dopamine deficiency in experimental animals and Parkinson's disease patients. *TINS* **13**, 296–302.

Bodis-Wollner, I., Marx, M. S., Mitra, S., Bobak, P., Mylin, L. & Yahr, M. 1987 Visual dysfunction in Parkinson's disease. Loss in spatiotemporal contrast sensitivity. *Brain* **110**, 1675–98.

Bradberry, C. W., Karasic, D. H., Deutch, A. Y. & Roth, R. H. 1989 Regionally-specific alterations in mesotelencephalic dopamine synthesis in diabetic rats: association with precursor tyrosine. *J. Neural Transmission* **78**, 221–29.

Brass, C. A. & Greengard, O. 1982 Modulation of cerebral catecholamine concentrations during hyperphenylalaninaemia. *Biochem. J.* **208**, 765–71.

Brown, R. M. & Goldman, P. S. 1977 Catecholamines in neocortex of rhesus monkeys: regional distribution and ontogenetic development. *Brain Res.* **124**, 576–80.

Brozoski, T. J., Brown, R. M., Rosvold, H. E. & Goldman, P. S. 1979 Cognitive deficit caused by regional depletion of dopamine in prefrontal cortex of rhesus monkey. *Science* **205**, 929–32.

Brunner, R. L., Berch, D. B. & Berry, H. 1987 Phenylketonuria and complex spatial visualization; an analysis of information processing. *Devl. Med. Child Neurol.* **29**, 460–68.

Bubser, M. & Schmidt, W. J. 1990 6-hydroxydopamine lesion of the rat prefrontal cortex increases locomotor activity, impairs acquisition of delayed alternation tasks, but does not affect uninterrupted tasks in the radial maze. *Behav. Brain Res.* **37**, 157–68.

Butterworth, G. 1977 Object disappearance and error in Piaget's stage IV task. *J. Exptl. Child Psychol.* **23**, 391–401.

Chirigos, M., Greengard, P. & Udenfriend, S. 1960 Uptake of tyrosine by rat brain *in vivo*. *J. Biol. Chem.* **235**, 2075–79.

Cohen, J. D., Forman, S., Casey, B. J., Servan-Schreiber, D., Noll, D. C. & Lewis, D. A. 1993 Activation of dorsolateral prefrontal cortex in humans durng a working memory task using functional MRI. *Soc. Neurosci. Abstr.* **19**, 1285.

Cornell, E. H. 1979 The effects of cue reliability on infants' manual search. *J. Exptl. Child Psychol.* **28**, 81–91.

Diamond, A. 1985 Development of the ability to use recall to guide action, as indicated by infants' performance on AB̄. *Child Development* **56**, 868–83.

Diamond, A. 1988 Differences between adult and infant cognition: is the crucial variable presence or absence of language? In *Thought without language* (ed. L. Weiskrantz), pp. 337–70. Oxford University Press.

Diamond, A. 1990*a* The development and neural bases of memory functions, as indexed by the AB̄ and delayed response tasks, in human infants and infant monkeys. *Ann. N. Y. Acad. Sci.* **608**, 267–317.

Diamond, A. 1990*b* Rate of maturation of the hippocampus and the developmental progression of children's performance on the delayed non-matching to sample and visual paired comparison tasks. *Ann. N. Y. Acad. Sci.* **608**, 394–426.

Diamond, A. 1991*a* Frontal lobe involvement in cognitive changes during the first year of life. In *Brain maturation and cognitive development: comparative and cross-cultural perspectives* (ed. K. R. Gibson & A. C. Petersen), pp. 127–80. New York: Aldine de Gruyter.

Diamond, A. 1991*b* Neuropsychological insights into the meaning of object concept development. In *The epigenesis of mind: essays on biology and knowledge* (ed. S. Carey & R. Gelman), pp. 67–110. Hillsdale, New Jersey: Lawrence Erlbaum Associates.

Diamond, A. 1994 Phenylalanine levels of 6–10 mg/dl may not be as benign as once thought. *Acta Pædiatrica* **83** (Supplement 407), 89–91.

Diamond, A. 1995 Evidence of robust recognition memory early in live even when assessed by reaching behavior. *J. Exptl. Child Psychol.* **59**, 419–56.

Diamond, A., Ciaramitaro, V., Donner, E., Djali, S. & Robinson, M. 1994 An animal model of early-treated PKU. *J. Neurosci.* **14**, 3072–82.

Diamond, A. & Goldman-Rakic, P. S. 1989 Comparison of human infants and rhesus monkeys on Piaget's AB̄ task: evidence for dependence on dorsolateral prefrontal cortex. *Exptl. Brain Res.* **74**, 24–40.

Diamond, A. & Herzberg, C. 1996 Impaired sensitivity to visual contrast in children treated early and continuously for PKU. *Brain* **119**, 523–53.

Diamond, A., Prevor, M., Callender, G. & Druin, D. P. 1997 Prefrontal cortex cognitive deficits in children treated early and continuously for PKU *Monogr. Soc. Res. Child Devel.* **62**, 4, Serial 252.

Diamond, A. & Taylor, C. 1996 Development of an aspect of executive control: development of the abilities to remember what I said and to "Do as I say, not as I do". *Devtl. Psychobiol.* **29**, 315–33.

Dobson, J. C., Kushida, E., Williamson, M. L. & Friedman, E. G. 1976 Intellectual performance of 36 phenylketonuric patients and their non-affected siblings. *Pediatrics* **58**, 53–58.

Domesick, V. B. 1972 Thalamic relationships of the medial cortex in the rat. *Brain Behav. Evol.* **6**, 457–83.

Evans, W. F. 1973 The stage IV error in Piaget's theory of concept development: an investigation of the rise of activity. Doctoral dissertation, University of Houston.

Faust, D., Libon, D. & Pueschel, S. 1986 Neuro-psychological functioning in treated phenylketonuria. *International J. Psychiatry Med.* **16**, 169–77.

Fernstrom, M. H., Volk, E. A., Fernstrom, J. D. & Iuvone, P. M. 1986 Effect of tyrosine administration on dopa accumulation in light-and dark-adapted retinas from normal and diabetic rats. *Life Sciences* **39**, 2049–57.

Fox, N., Kagan, J. & Weiskopf, S. 1979 The growth of memory during infancy. *Genetic Psychology Monographs* **99**, 91–130.

Fuster, J. M. & Alexander, G. E. 1971 Neuron activity related to short-term memory. *Science* **173**, 652–54.

Gerstadt, C., Hong, Y. & Diamond, A. 1994 The relationship between cognition and action: Performance of $3\frac{1}{2}$–7 year old children on a Stroop-like day-night test. *Cognition* **53**, 129–53.

Goldman, P. S. & Rosvold, H. E. 1970 Localization of function within the dorsolateral prefrontal cortex of the rhesus monkey. *Exptl. Neurology* **27**, 291–304.

Goldman-Rakic, P. S. 1987 Circuitry of primate prefrontal cortex and regulation of behavior by representational knowledge. In *Handbook of physiology* (ed. F. Plum & V. Mountcastle), vol. 5, pp. 373–417. Bethesda MD: American Physiological Society.

Gratch, G., Appel, K. J., Evans, W. F., LeCompte, G. K. & Wright, N. A. 1974 Piaget's stage IV object concept error: evidence of forgetting or object conception? *Child Devl.* **45**, 71–77.

Gratch, G. & Landers, W. F. 1971 Stage IV of Piaget's theory of infant's object concepts: a longitudinal study. *Child Devl.* **42**, 359–72.

Greengard, O., Yoss, M. S. & DelValle, J. A. 1976 α-methylphenylalanine, a new inducer of chronic hyperphenylalaninemia in suckling rats. *Science* **192**, 1007–08.

Groenewegen, H. J. 1988 Organization of the afferent connections of the mediodorsal thalamic nucleus in the rat, related to the mediodorsal-prefrontal topography. *Brain Res.* **24**, 379–431.

Harlow, H. F., Davis, R. T., Settlage, P. H. & Meyer, D. R. 1952 Analysis of frontal and posterior association syndromes in brain- damaged monkeys. *J. Comp. Physiol. Psychol.* **54**, 419–29.

Harris, P. L. 1973 Perseverative errors in search by young infants. *Child Devl.* **44**, 28–33.

Hjelle, J. T., Baird-Lambert, J., Cardinale, G. Specor, S. & Udenfriend, S. 1978 Isolated microvessels: the blood-brain barrier *in vitro. Proc. Nat. Acad. Sci.* **75**, 4544–48.

Iuvone, P. M., Galli, C. L., Garrison-Gund, C. K. & Neff, N. H. 1978 Light stimulates tyrosine hydroxylase activity and dopamine synthesis in retinal amacrine neurons. *Science* **202**, 901–02.

Iuvone, P. M., Tigges, M., Fernandes, A. & Tigges, J. 1989 L Dopamine synthesis and metabolism in rhesus monkey retina: development, aging, and the effects of monocular visual deprivation. *Visual Neurosci.* **2**, 465–71.

Jacobsen, C. F. 1935 Functions of frontal association areas in primates. *Arch. Neurol. Psychiat.* **33**, 558–60.

Jacobsen, C. F. & Nissen, H. W. 1937 Studies of cerebral function in primates. The effects of frontal lobe lesions on the delayed alternation habit in monkeys. *J. Comp. Physiol. Psychol.* **23**, 101–12.

Koch, R. & Wenz, E. 1987 Phenylketonuria. *A. Rev. Nutr.* **7**, 117–35.

Kolb, B. 1984 Functions of the frontal cortex of the rat: a comparative review. *Brain Res. Rev.* **8**, 65–98.

Krause, W. L., Helminski, M., McDonald, L., Dembure, P., Salvo, R., Freides, D. & Elsas, L. J. 1985 Biochemical and neurophysiological effects of elevated plasma phenylalanine in patients with treated phenylketonuria, a model for the study of phenylalanine in brain function in man. *J. Clin. Invest.* **75**, 40–48.

Kubota, K. & Niki, H. 1971 Prefrontal cortical unit activity and delayed alternation performance in monkeys. *J. Neurophysiol.* **34**, 337–47.

Kupersmith, M. J., Shakin, E., Siegel, I. M. & Lieberman, A. 1982 Visual system abnormalities in patients with Parkinson's disease. *Arch. Neurol.* **39**, 284–86.

Larsen, J. K. & Divac, I. 1978 Selective ablations within the prefrontal cortex of the rat and performance on delayed alternation. *Physiological Psychol.* **6**, 15–17.

Leonard, C. M. 1969 The prefrontal cortex of the rat. I. Cortical projections of the mediodorsal nucleus. II. Efferent connections. *Brain Res.* **12**, 321–43.

Lewis, D. A., Campbell, M. J., Foote, S. L. & Morrison, J. H. 1986 The monoaminergic innervation of primate neocortex. *Hum. Neurobiol.* **5**, 181–88.

Lewis, D. & Harris, H. W. 1991 Differential laminar distribution of tyrosine hydroxylase-immunoreactive axons in infant and adult monkey prefrontal cortex. *Neurosci. Lett.* **125**, 151–54.

Lewis, D. A. & Morrison, J. H. 1989 The noradrenergic innervation of monkey prefrontal cortex: A dopamine-β-hydroxylase immunohistochemical study. *J. Comput. Neurosci.* **282**, 317–30.

Lidsky, A. S., Law, M. L., Morse, H. G., Kao, F. T. & Woo, S. L. C. 1985 Regional mapping of the human phenylalanine hydroxylase gene and the PKU locus on chromosome 12. *Proc. Nat. Acad. Sci.* **82**, 6221–25.

Luria, A. R. & Homskaya, E. D. 1964 Disturbance in the regulative role of speech with frontal lobe lesions. In *The frontal granular cortex and behavior* (ed. J. M. Warren & K. Akert), pp. 353–71. New York: McGraw-Hill.

Mangels, J. A. 1996 The relationship between strategic processing, interference and memory for temporal order in patients with frontal lobe lesions. *Neuropsychologia* **11**, 207–21.

McDonald, J. D., Bode, V. C., Dove, W. F. & Shedlovsky, A. 1990 Pah^{hph-5}: a mouse mutant deficient in phenylalanine hydroxylase. *Proc. Nat. Acad. Sci.* **87**, 1965–67.

Miles, R. C. & Blomquist, A. 1960 Frontal lesions and behavioral deficits in monkey. *J. Neurophsiol.* **23**, 471–84.

Miller, L., Braun, L. D., Pardridge, W. M. & Oldendorf, W. H. 1985 Kinetic constants for blood-brain barrier amino acid transport in conscious rats. *J. Neurochem.* **45**, 1427–32.

Milner, B. 1963 Effects of brain lesions on card sorting. *Arch. Neurol.* **9**, 90–100.

Milner, B., Corsi, P. & Leonard, G. 1991 Frontal-lobe contribution to recency judgements. *Neuropsychologia* **29**, 601–18.

Mishkin, M. & Manning, F. J. 1978 Nonspatial memory after selective prefrontal lesions in monkeys. *Brain Res.* **143**, 313–23.

Oldendorf, W. H. 1973 Stereospecificity of blood brain barrier permeability to amino acids. *Am. J. Physiol.* **224**, 967–69.

Owen, A. M., Morris, R. G., Sahakian, B. J., Polkey, C. E. & Robbins, T. W. 1996 Double dissociation of memory and executive functions in self-ordered working memory tasks following frontal lobe excisions, temporal lobe excisions or amygdala hippocampectomy in man. *Brain* **119**, 1597–615.

Pardridge, W. 1977 Regulation of amino acid availability to the brain. In *Nutrition and the brain* (ed. R. J. Wurtman & J. J. Wurtman), pp. 141–204. New York: Raven Press.

Pardridge, W. M. & Oldendorf, W. H. 1977 Transport of metabolic substrates through the blood-brain barrier. *J. Neurochem.* **28**, 5–12.

Pennington, B. F., VanDoornick, W. J., McCabe, L. L. & McCabe, E. R. B. 1985 Neuropsychological deficits in early treated phenylketonuric children. *Am. J. Deficiency* **89**, 467–74.

Petrides, M. 1988 Performance on a nonspatial self-ordered task after selective lesions of the primate frontal cortex. *Soc. Neurosci. Abstr.* **14**, 4–8.

Petrides, M. 1989 Frontal lobes and memory. In *Handbook of neuropsychology* (ed. F. Boller & J. Grafman), pp. 75–90. Amsterdam: Elsevier.

Petrides, M. 1991 Functional specialization within the dorsolateral frontal corex for serial order memory. *Proc. R. Soc. Lond.* B **246**, 299–306.

Petrides, M. 1995 Impairments on nonspatial self-ordered and externally ordered working memory tasks after lesions of the mid- dorsal part of the lateral frontal cortex in the monkey. *J. Neurosci* **15**, 359–75.

Petrides, M., Alvisatos, B., Evans, A. C. & Meyer, E. 1993 Dissociation of human mid-dorsalateral from posterior dorsolateral frontal cortex in memory processing. *Proc. Nat. Acad. Sci.* **90**, 873–77.

Piaget, J. 1954 *The construction of reality in the child.* New York: Basic Books. Original French edition, 1937.

Pinsker, H. M. & French, G. M. 1967 Indirect delayed reactions under various testing conditions in normal and midlateral frontal monkeys. *Neuropsychologia* **5**, 13–24.

Preuss, T. M. 1995 Do rats have prefrontal cortex? The Rose-Woolsey-Akert Program reconsidered. *J. Cog. Neurosci.* **7**, 1–24.

Rapoport, S. I. 1976 Sites and functions of the blood-aqueous and blood-vitreous barriers of the eye. In *Blood-brain barrier in physiology and medicine* (ed. S. I. Rapoport), pp. 207–32. New York: Raven Press.

Regan, D. & Neima, D. 1984 Low-contrast letter charts in early diabetic retinopathy, ocular hypertension, glaucoma, and Parkinson's disease. *Br. J. Opthalmol.* **68**, 885–89.

Rubinstein, J., Evans, J. E. & Meyer, D. E. 1996 Executive control of cognitive processes in task switching. (In preparation.)

Sawaguchi, T. & Goldman-Rakic, P. S. 1991 D1 dopamine receptors in prefrontal cortex: Involvement in working memory. *Science* **251**, 947–50.

Schneider, J. S. & Kovelowski, C. J., II. 1990 Chronic exposure to low doses of MPTP. I. Cognitive deficits in motor asymptomatic monkeys. *Brain Res.* **519**, 122–28.

Shedlovsky, A., McDonald, J. D., Symula, D. & Dove, W. F. 1993 Mouse models of human phenylketonuria. *Genetics* **134**, 1205–10.

Simon, H., Scatton, B. & LeMoal, M. 1980 Dopaminergic A10 neurones are involved in cognitive functions. *Nature, Lond.* **286**, 150–51.

Skrandies, W. & Gottlob, I. 1986 Alterations of visual contrast sensitivity in Parkinson's disease. *Hum. Neurobiol.* **5**, 255–59.

Smith, M. L., Klim, P., Mallozzi, E. & Hanley, W. B. 1996 A test of the frontal-specificity hypothesis in the cognitive performance of adults with phenylketonuria. *Devtl. Neuropsychol.* **12**, 327–41.

Smith, I. & Beasley, M. 1989 Intelligence and behaviour in children with early treated phenylketonuria. *Eur. J. Clin. Nutrition* **43**, 1–5.

Sophian, C. & Wellman, H. M. 1983 Selective information use and perseveration in the search behavior of infants and young children. *J. Exptl. Child Psychol.* **35**, 369–90.

Stemerdink, B. A., van der Meere, J. J., van der Molen, M. W., Kalverboer, A. F. *et al.* 1995 Information processing in patients with early and continuously-treated phenyl-ketonuria. *Eur. J. Pediatrics* **172**

Stuss, D. T. & Benson, D. F. 1986 *The frontal lobes.* New York: Raven Press.

Stuss, D. T. & Benson, D. F. 1987 The frontal lobes and control of cognition and memory. In *The frontal lobes revisited* (ed. E. Perecman), pp. 141–58. New York: IRBN Press.

Tam, S. Y., Elsworth, J. D., Bradberry, C. W. & Roth, R. H. 1990 Mesocortical dopamine neurons: high basal firing frequency predicts tyrosine dependence of dopa-mine synthesis. *J. Neural Transmission General Section* **81**, 97–110.

Taylor, J. R., Roth, R. H., Sladek, J. R., Jr. & Redmond, D. E., Jr. 1990 Cognitive and motor deficits in the performance of the object retrieval detour task in monkeys (*Cercopithecus aethiops sabaeus*) treated with MPTP: Long-term performance and effect of transparency of the barrier. *Behav. Neurosci.* **104**, 564–76.

Thierry, A. M., Tassin, J. P., Blanc, A., Stinus, L., Scatton, B. & Glowinski, J. 1977 Discovery of the mesocortical dopaminergic system: Some pharmacological and functional characteristics. *Adv. Biomed. Psychopharmacology* **16**, 5–12.

Tornquist, P. & Alm, A. 1986 Carrier-mediated transport of amino acids through the blood-retinal and blood-brain barriers. *Graefe's Archive for Clinical and Experimental Ophthalmology* **224**, 21–25.

Welsh, M. C., Pennington, B. F., Ozonoff, S., Rouse, B. & McCabe, E. R. B. 1990 Neuropsychology of early-treated phenylketonuria: specific executive function defi-cits. *Child Devl.* **61**, 1697–13.

Wikmark, R. G. E., Divac, I. & Weiss, R. 1973 Delayed alternation in rats with lesions in the frontal lobes: Implications for a comparative neuropsychology of the frontal system. *Brain Behav. Evol.* **8**, 329–39.

Willatts, P. 1985 Adjustment of means-ends coordination and the representation of spatial relations in the productions of search errors by infants. *Br. J. Devtl. Psychol.* **3**, 259–72.

Williamson, M. L., Koch, R., Azen, C. & Chang, C. 1981 Correlates of intelligence test results in treated phenyl-ketonuric children. *Pediatrics* **68**, 161–67.

Wilson, F. A., Scalaidhe, S. P. & Goldman-Rakic, P. S. 1993 Dissociation of object and spatial processing domains in primate prefrontal cortex. *Science* **260**, 1955–58.

Woo, S. L. C., Lidsky, A. S., Güttler, F., Chandra, T. & Robson, K. J. H. 1983 Cloned human phenylalanine hydroxylase gene allows prenatal diagnosis and carrier detec-tion of classical phenylketonuria. *Nature, Lond.* **306**, 151–55.

Wurtman, R. J., Hefti, F. & Melamed, E. 1981 Precursor control of neurotransmitter synthesis. *Pharmacological Rev.* **32**, 315–35.

Zelazo, P. D., Frye, D. & Rapus, T. 1996 An age-related dissociation between knowing rules and using them. *Cog. Devt.* **11**, 37–63.

Zelazo, P. D., Reznick, J. S. & Piñon, D. E. 1995 Response control and the execution of verbal rules. *Devetl. Psychol.* **31**, 508–17.

Prefrontal function in schizophrenia: confounds and controversies

Daniel R. Weinberger and Karen Faith Berman

12.1 Introduction

The possibility of prefrontal cortex pathology in schizophrenia has been of interest to researchers and clinicians throughout this century. Prior to the early 1970s, evidence of prefrontal involvement consisted primarily of unreliable reports of postmortem anatomical pathology and of interpretations of clinical phenomena and of neuropsychological test results (Zec & Weinberger 1986). The development in the 1960s of *in vivo* regional cerebral blood flow (rCBF) measurement; techniques offered a dramatic new approach to studying brain function in health and disease. In 1974 Ingvar & Franzen reported the first of their pioneering series of studies which found that chronic schizophrenic patients had less frontal relative to posterior rCBF when compared with controls, who tended to show the opposite pattern. This finding, which they referred to as 'hypofrontality,' correlated with the severity of symptoms, especially with so-called 'negative symptoms.' Their data presaged the results of a round of studies that were published over the subsequent fifteen years or so the majority of which reported similar findings (Berman & Weinberger 1991).

The relatively consistent results of this early period, however, have not been sustained in recent studies. With the widespread availability of modern tomographic neuroimaging techniques, the study of schizophrenic prefrontal physiology has emerged as a preoccupation of many research centres around the world. As more data have appeared, the literature has become increasingly confused and the consistency of the early results and the interpretation of their meaning have become uncertain. Several prominent emission tomography studies have failed to observe 'hypofrontality' (Ebmeier *et al.* 1993, 1995; Gur *et al.* 1992, 1995), and some studies of patients admitted with acute exacerbations of symptoms have reported 'hyperfrontality' instead (Ebmeier *et al.* 1993; Szechtman *et al.* 1988; Cleghorn *et al.* 1989). While functional neuroimaging studies of patients performing cognitive activation tasks have been more consistent in showing prefrontal hypofunction than have studies performed during the resting state, task associated rCBF data have been challenged as artefacts of performance differences between experimental groups (Ebmeier *et al*. 1995; Gur & Gur 1995; Frith *et al*. 1995). Such inconsistencies and uncertainties have prompted commentaries in the literature about the validity of prefrontal hypofunction in schizophrenia and about the relevance of prefrontal cortex in this illness. A number of important questions have been raised, such as: Is the finding of prefrontal hypofunction in some studies an artefact of chronicity, of drug treatment, or of other illness-related epiphenomena? Are the inconsistencies in the literature explained by differences in the behavioural characteristics of patients during the scans, especially with respect to resting versus cognitive activation? Are findings of prefrontal hypofunction during cognitive activation artefacts of differences between patients and controls in performance on the cognitive tasks? In this report, we will address these questions and the broad controversy about frontal, and in particular prefrontal, function in schizophrenia.

12.2 Clinical and basic research implicate prefrontal hypofunction in schizophrenia

The functional neuroimaging data about prefrontal function in schizophrenia do not exist in a research vacuum. Indeed, if there were no neuroimaging data, there would still be considerable indirect and some direct evidence for prefrontal cortical involvement. As Gur & Gur (1995) recently pointed out, the abundance of other data implicating prefrontal cortex in this illness probably contributed to the early enthusiasm for the neuroimaging results. The clearest indirect evidence comes from a wealth of neuropsychological studies showing deficits on tests of attention, of 'executive' functions, and of working memory that have been linked in human and nonhuman primate studies with prefrontal function (Goldman-Rakic 1991; Goldberg & Gold 1995). The neuropsychological deficits themselves have been shown to be independent of chronicity, of ongoing psychotic symptoms, and of treatment (Lawson *et al*. 1988; Liddle 1995; Goldberg *et al*. 1993*a*; Saykin *et al*. 1991). Moreover, the neuropsychological deficits are robust predictors of prognosis, much more so than are psychotic symptoms, and to some degree may be genetic markers of trait liability (Goldberg *et al*. 1993*b*).

Another robust clinical finding in patients with schizophrenia that is linked to abnormal frontal lobe function is a deficit in smooth pursuit eye movements (Holzman 1985). This deficit, which has been observed in almost every clinical study that has examined such eye movements, is modelled in the nonhuman primate by a lesion of the ventral aspect of the frontal eye fields (MacAvoy *et al*. 1991). It has also been shown to be independent of chronicity, of ongoing psychotic symptoms, and of treatment. Other clinical evidence that has been cited as likely to reflect frontal dysfunction includes so-called soft neurological signs on clinical examination, defect symptoms such as poor motivation, flat effect, and poor insight (Weinberger 1988), and findings from recent electro-physiological investigations (Liddle 1995).

Structural neuroimaging studies also have found evidence of pathology of prefrontal cortex. This includes dilated prefrontal sulci (Weinberger *et al.* 1979; Doran *et al.* 1987; Shelton *et al.* 1988) and diminished frontal lobe volume (Breier *et al.* 1992; Andreasen *et al.* 1994), though these anatomical findings have been less consistent than the neuropsychological and eye movement findings. Several postmortem investigations have reported reduced prefrontal cortical thickness (e.g. Benes *et al.* 1991; Selemon *et al.* 1995), though these results also are inconsistent (e.g. Akbarian *et al.* 1993). MRI spectroscopy studies have further implicated prefrontal cortex as a site of pathology, provid-ing evidence of reduced concentrations of N-acetyl aspartate, an intracellular marker of neuronal pathology (Bertolino *et al.* 1996). Numerous postmortem studies describing neurochemical changes in prefrontal cortex have also appeared. Taken together, results from a variety of clinical and basic studies indicate that the functional neuroimaging data about schizophrenia should be examined in a broader context. From the perspective of this broader database, the functional neuroimaging results might be questioned more for the studies that did not find hypofrontality than for the studies that did.

12.3 Hypofrontality is an inconsistent finding in resting studies

The conclusion that hypofrontality is an inconsistent finding in studies of patients with schizophrenia during the so-called resting state is inescapable. In our own series of rCBF studies of patients, whether medicated or medication-free, hypofrontality during rest has either not been observed (Berman *et al.* 1992) or has been seen only with normalized, not absolute, rCBF data and has been much less robust than during cognition (Weinberger *et al.* 1986, 1988*b*; Berman *et al.* 1986). In a recent review of functional neuroimaging studies of rCBF and of glucose utilization, we found that only around 60% of thirty-nine published reports could be interpreted as showing hypofrontality in patients with schizophrenia (Berman & Weinberger 1991). This percent is lower if cognitive activation studies are excluded. The addition of several recent negat-ive resting studies (e.g. Catafau *et al.* 1994; Ebmeier *et al.* 1995; Gur *et al.* 1995) probably further depresses the resting state hypofrontality hit rate, though positive resting studies also continue to be reported (e.g. Biver *et al.* 1995; Vita *et al.* 1995).

The reasons for the inconsistencies in studies of patients at rest are probably numerous, likely having to do with differences in patient populations, medica-tion status, and study procedures. While each of these confounds may con-tribute noise to the functional activity data, none of them seem by themselves to reliably explain the discrepancies. Chronic patients, especially those with pro-minent negative symptoms, are more likely to be 'hypofrontal' at rest (Ingvar & Franzen 1974; Volkow *et al.* 1987; Tamminga *et al.* 1992; Wolkin *et al.* 1992), but some resting studies even of chronic patients with prominent negative symptoms do not report hypofrontality (e.g. Weinberger *et al.* 1986; *Gur et al.* 1987; Ebmeier *et al.* 1995). Antipsychotic medications have been reported to reduce prefrontal rCBF and glucose metabolism in some studies (Bartlett *et al.* 1991; Holcomb *et al.* 1996; Wolkin *et al.* 1996), but the effects of medications also are inconsistent (e.g. Szechtman *et al.* 1988; Bartlett *et al.* 1991; Ebmeier *et al.* 1995) and hypofrontality at rest is not reliably observed even in studies of medicated patients (e.g. Berman *et al.* 1986; Szechtman *et al.* 1988; Kawasaki *et al.* 1993; Ebmeier *et al.* 1995; Gur *et al.* 1995).

The technical sophistication of data collection and analysis also varies widely across studies. For example, many of the early positive resting studies were nontomographic and had low spatial resolution (though it could be argued that because of partial volume effects, this limitation would diminish the likelihood of a finding). Some studies only found effects with normalized data (e.g. Buchsbaum *et al.* 1990, 1992; Biver *et al.* 1995), raising questions about whether the abnormality was in the numerator (i.e. prefrontal cortex) or the denominator (e.g. overactive posterior cortex) employed in the normalization procedure. Nevertheless, negative results have also been found with low resolution scanners and normalized rCBF data (e.g. the particular scanner used in the normalized rCBF study of Ebmeier *et al.* (1995) acquires much of the radioactivity counts in a given '15 mm thick' slice from outside that slice).

In our view, the inconsistencies and controversy surrounding the resting hypofrontality data are, to some degree, 'straw men'. They boil down mainly to two issues. The first is conceptual, that is, whether prefrontal function is impaired in schizophrenia. The functional imaging studies of the resting state have not been able to answer this question. The second is methodological, that is, whether the resting state is the appropriate condition under which the first question should be asked. If the clinical data cited above which independently implicate prefrontal dysfunction in schizophrenia are correct, then the resting state is clearly not the appropriate condition.

Why might the resting state be inappropriate to study prefrontal function in patients with schizophrenia? We believe the most likely explanation for this is that the resting state is uncontrollable and inherently variable at both experiential and physiological levels (Weinberger *et al.* 1986; Weinberger & Berman 1988; Andreasen *et al.* 199). There is abundant evidence that subtle changes in what a subject attends to, thinks about, or even imagines during the resting state will affect the rCBF data. For example, Corbetta *et al.* (1990) showed in normal subjects that posterior cortical rCBF changed significantly depending on which features of a constant visual scene occupied the subjects' attention. Incidental cognitive processing also has been shown to affect rCBF patterns (Frith *et al.* 1995). Kosslyn *et al.* (1995) reported that visual cortical activity changes significantly during eyes-closed visual imagery. Even activation of sensorimotor cortex by a simple somato-sensory stimulus can be significantly attenuated if subjects are distracted (Meyer *et al.* 1991). Individual differences in such psychological and cognitive factors that are not controlled during the resting state could obscure a signal that may be a feature of the pathophysiology of an illness. This seems especially likely if the pathophysiological signal is a subtle one and if data are averaged across subjects, as is standard procedure in most emission tomography studies. While this confound concerns any condition, not just the resting state, its potential impact on the group data would probably be greater during the resting state because there is no prescribed behaviour to focus brain activity and provide for a common physiological signal.

In defence of the resting state, the reliability of resting patterns across time has been noted (Gur & Gur 1995). It is unclear what such reliability reflects. Random noise, for example, would be especially reliable over time. Moreover, reliability may reflect insensitivity. This possibility, that some of the methods used in resting studies of patients with schizophrenia are not sensitive enough to detect the subtle differences that characterize such patients, may be particularly relevant for studies that have looked at glucose utilization with fluorodeoxyglucose (FDG) and at rCBF with static SPECT tracers. The FDG data reflect metabolic information averaged over a long time period (approximately 30 minutes), and thus subtle pathophysiological signals may be obscured by signals related to nonpathological processes that are averaged during the acquisition. This possible limitation of FDG data is illustrated in studies of patients undergoing hypnosis (Grond et al. 1995) and of patients with cortical blindness (Bosley et al. 1991). In each of these instances, remarkably little has been found in the FDG PET data, though the conditions all involve dramatic deviations from normal awareness. SPECT rCBF tracers have also been shown to be relatively insensitive to subtle changes in cortical activity, probably for different reasons (Crosson et al. 1994).

Regardless of whether resting studies are inconsistent because the state itself is, or whether some of the techniques are not sensitive enough to reliably detect subtle effects against a physiologically noisy background, the resting state has not produced clear data in assessing function of prefrontal cortex, or for that matter any brain region, in patients with schizophrenia. Studies of patients during cognitive activation paradigms have been much more consistent, but the results have been challenged as artefacts of poor performance.

12.4 Prefrontal hypofunction is reliably found during cognitive activation paradigms

We have explored prefrontal function during cognitive tasks in seven separate studies of independent samples of patients with schizophrenia. In all instances, we found that prefrontal function was reduced during cognitive states that enlisted prefrontal activation in normal subjects. Each of these studies involved paradigms that emphasized working memory. Five studies had patients and controls performing an automated version of the Wisconsin Card Sort Task (WCST) (Berman et al. 1986; Weinberger et al. 1986, 1988b; Berman et al. 1992, *vide infra*), one had subjects perform a delayed alternation learning task (Gold *et al.* 1996, data in schizophrenia not published), and one a 'two-back' working memory paradigm (Callicott *et al.* 1996). We demonstrated in these studies that the finding could not be attributed to medication status, as patients were just as likely to be hypofrontal during the tasks whether medicated or medication-free (Berman *et al.* 1986), and never medicated patients also appeared 'hypofrontal' during such conditions (Callicott *et al.* 1996). This conclusion is supported by other recent studies showing failure of prefrontal activation in medication-naïve patients performing analogous tasks (e.g. Rubin *et al.* 1991; Andreasen *et al.* 1992; Catafau *et al.* 1994).

In our earlier review of functional neuroimaging studies of patients with schizophrenia, we noted that approximately 90% of studies performed during a cognitive activation procedure have found 'hypofrontality' (Berman & Weinberger 1991). Over the past five years, the number of activation-type studies has more than doubled, with the percentage of positive results remaining at least as robust. Clearly, during cognitive activation, prefrontal hypofunction is a reliable finding in patients with schizophrenia. The controversy involves the interpretation of the results.

12.5 Poor task performance: does it explain hypofrontality?

A variety of factors might account for prefrontal hypofunction during cognitive activation in patients with schizophrenia other than pathophysiology of prefrontal cortex. The most problematic include attention, motivation and mental effort, and level of performance. We have addressed the issues of attention, motivation, and mental effort in previous studies and discussions (Berman *et al.* 1986, 1988*a*; Weinberger & Berman 1988; Berman & Weinberger 1991), and therefore, will concentrate herein on the matter of task performance. A prominent criticism of the cognitive activation literature concerns the fact that patients as a group perform poorer than controls on the tasks. Thus, it has been argued that the physiological data, rather than being responsible for the behavioural deficits, are an artefact of such deficits (Frith *et al.* 1995; Gur & Gur 1995; Liddle 1995). Ebmeier *et al.* (1995, p. 452) concluded that the 'poorer performance of "frontal" activation tasks by patients with schizophrenia is probably sufficient explanation for the difference from controls)'.

The performance issue is a conundrum; a reasonable theoretical case can be made for either the abnormal cognition or the abnormal physiology being the horse that leads the other variable as the cart. In at least three of our studies, we found in patients a significant relationship between prefrontal activity and task performance (Weinberger *et al.* 1986; Goldberg *et al.* 1995, *vide infra*), indicating, at least, that the cart and horse are paradigmatically connected. As emphasized by the critics of this literature, poor performance could conceivably be the horse. On the other hand, if prefrontal pathophysiology is a characteristic of schizophrenia, then prefrontal-type cognitive deficits would be expected to follow as the cart. What do the experimental data suggest is the correct interpretation?

There are several research approaches that have been taken to address the role of performance. One is to study patients with other disorders who perform poorly on the same task. In principal, if the prefrontal physiological deficit found in patients with schizophrenia is an epiphenomenon of poor performance *per se*, then other subjects who perform as poorly should have similar prefrontal function. We have explored this question in patients with Huntington's disease, who perform as poorly as patients with schizophrenia on the WCST (Weinberger *et al.* 1988*a*; Goldberg *et al.* 1990), in otherwise healthy elderly subjects matched for performance with schizophrenic patients (Esposito *et al.* 1995), and in patients with Down's syndrome (Berman *et al.* 1988*b*), who perform much more poorly. In none of these studies did the other groups appear hypofrontal. Thus, poor performance *per se* on the WCST does not by itself account for the finding in patients with schizophrenia.

A second approach has been to study patients during tasks that they also perform more poorly than normals, but that do not normally enlist as robust prefrontal activity. Again in principal, if poor performance *per se* explains the hypofrontality data, than patients should appear hypofrontal on any task that they cannot perform as well as normals. In two studies, one of an attention/ vigilance task, the continuous performance task (Berman *et al.* 1986), and one of an abstract reasoning intelligence task, Ravens Progressive Matrices (Berman *et al.* 1988*a*), patients who were hypofrontal during the WCS had relatively normal prefrontal function during both of these tasks, even though their performance was well below normal. We proposed that prefrontal function was relatively normal in patients with schizophrenia during these tasks because the tasks depended less on prefrontal activation than did the WCST. This suggested that task-associated hypofrontality related to the frontal demands of the task and presumably to selective neural systems.

A third approach is to match patients and normal controls for level of performance. There are two ways that this has been explored. The first is illustrated by a series of studies from the Hammersmith PET Group, using a cued and paced verbal production ('fluency') task. This group of investigators argues that this task matches performance of patients and controls and thus obviates this potential confound (Frith *et al.* 1995; Liddle 1995). In studies of patients performing this task, which requires them to utter a word of a certain semantic category every five seconds following a visual cue, they produce the same number of words as normals and they show significant prefrontal activation (Frith *et al.* 1995). Does this mean that they do not have a prefrontal functional deficit? Most likely, it means only that the prefrontal activation effect of this task is not different in normals and in patients. The interpretation of these data are confounded by their own set of problems. When patients perform normally on a task, it may mean that the task does not require function from the neural systems that are affected by the disease process. The prefrontal neural functions enlisted during the cued verbal production task may

not be the same as those enlisted by tasks such as the WCST. Cognitive activation rCBF studies have demonstrated that many different neuropsychological
tasks are associated with activation of prefrontal cortex (Weinberger 1993).
Patients with schizophrenia do many things normally, presumably because
many functional brain systems can perform within normal limits. Thus, tasks
that are associated with normal performance, which are generally simple tasks,
may not have the specificity (or power) to reveal pathophysiological aspects of
schizophrenic brain function. This issue is analogous to the controversy about
matching patients with schizophrenia and controls on IQ. Since schizophrenia
affects IQ (Goldberg & Gold 1995), selecting for patients with normal IQ, in
effect, selects out a potentially important aspect of the illness.

Another problem that can occur with the interpretation of results
from paradigms that involve ostensibly normal performance is that all aspects
of performance in patients may not be isomorphic with normals. For example,
with the cued verbal production task, patients appear to have a delayed reaction time in responding to the cue (R. Dolan, personal communication).
This may reflect that they do not occupy the five second intercue interval in
the same manner as the normals. The observation that unlike normals who
deactivate temporal neocortex, patients activate this region during this task,
while possibly reflecting abnormal intracortical function (Dolan *et al.* 1995;
Frith *et al.* 1995), might more critically be interpreted as an indication that
their minds tend to wander during the intercue interval. Instead of focusing
on or preparing for the next response, they are attending to extraneous, perhaps
internal, auditory stimuli. These considerations illustrate that the strategy
of employing simple tasks that result in some measures of performance being
normal in patients is not as straightforward an approach to the question
of prefrontal hypofunction in schizophrenia as it may appear. Normal prefrontal rCBF in patients during such a task does not mean that prefrontal
function is normal, nor does it mean that the task is performed the same as
in normals.

Another approach to matching performance in patients and normals is to
find normals who perform as poorly as patients. This approach at least has
the potential to answer the question of whether normals and patients fail by
the same mechanisms. We have managed to collect WCST rCBF data from
groups matched for percent correct on this test (61% for normals and 60%
for patients). Patients (mean age 37, range 26–56) and controls (28, range
26–60) underwent PET rCBF scanning during the WCS as previously described
(Berman *et al.* 1995). The data, displayed as SPM images in slices through
prefrontal cortex (significance threshold is $P < 0.005$), are shown in the
figure. This figure illustrates that the normals activate Brodmann areas 9 and
46 bilaterally at this level, as well as a part of cingulate cortex. In contrast, the
patients, who overall turn on less of prefrontal cortex than the normals,
actually activate a different area of prefrontal cortex (that includes area
10), an area that does not correspond to any of the areas activated in normals.
The other panels of the figure illustrate that the region of prefrontal cortex

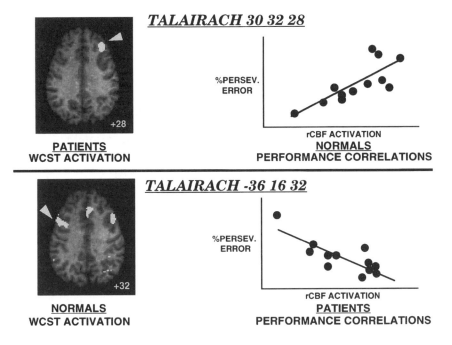

Fig. 12.1   Relationship of performance and prefrontal activation during the WCST in patients and controls. See text for explanation.

activated in the patients appears to be qualitatively the wrong region with respect to predicting better performance. The upper right panel shows that if we look in the normal subjects at the region that is activated in the patients, which normals do not significantly activate, the more normals tend to activate this region, the worse they perform. In the lower right panel we are looking in the patients at the region that is consistently activated in our studies of normals (i.e. areas 9 and 46), but that is not significantly activated in patients; the more patients tend to activate this region the better they do. This analysis illustrates that matching for poor performance has the potential to explore subtle distinctions in the physiological mechanisms that may differentiate the groups. The data suggest that poor performance is not the explanation for poor prefrontal function during the WCST in patients with schizophrenia but that a qualitatively abnormal regional physiological response to the task is. This conclusion is consistent with data from our study of monozygous twins discordant for schizophrenia in which we found that in addition to hypofunction of prefrontal cortex, the affected twin had hyperfunction of hippocampal formation during the WCST (Weinberger et al. 1993), a qualitatively abnormal pattern that represents a double dissociation with respect to the normals. Analogous results with the paced verbal production task have recently been described by Friston et al. (1996).

12.6 Comment

That the clinical syndrome of schizophrenia involves a deficit in functions of the prefrontal cortex seems highly probable. Prefrontal dysfunction, however, is a nonspecific characteristic of many brain conditions (Weinberger 1993), and precisely what mechanism is associated with schizophrenia and whether it is specific to this disorder are unclear. It is clear, however, that functional neuro-imaging studies can be constructed that either show evidence of prefrontal dysfunction or not, depending particularly on the experimental conditions. Studies performed during the resting state have a relatively low probability of revealing prefrontal hypofunction, unless, perhaps, patients are selected for prominent negative symptoms, especially poverty of speech (Liddle 1995). We have found that patients consistently are deficient in prefrontal activity, regard-less of their symptomatic profile, during tasks that require working memory and that appear to exceed their capacity for normal task performance. The data from studies of other neurological disorders and of normal subjects who have difficulty with such tasks suggest that the finding in patients with schizophrenia is not the result of their poor performance, but rather is the likely explanation for it. Nevertheless, the possibility that performance differences confound the physiological data cannot be definitively excluded. Comparing patients and controls on simple tasks involving no performance difference (at least on some measures) does not solve the problem, as other at least as problematic confounds are introduced. It is doubtful that any single functional neuro-imaging study performed during a cognitive task can by itself answer the 'carthorse' riddle. Multiple experiments with varied approaches are necessary to approximate the correct answer.

The contrasts between patients with schizophrenia and other groups of subjects who perform poorly on the WCST but activate prefrontal cortex illustrate that the relationships between prefrontal activation during a task and performance on the task are complex. This point is further underscored by a recent study which found that pharmacological ablation of gonadal steroid hormones in normal subjects significantly attenuated prefrontal activation during the WCST without affecting task performance (Berman *et al.* 1995a). Thus, activation or no activation (i.e. as defined in a statistical analysis of rCBF data) of the cortical region normally associated with performance of a parti-cular task does not guarantee good or poor performance, respectively. The complexity of the activation–performance relationship may involve multiple factors, including variations in temporal concordances between processing centres, changes in processing efficiency and thus signal-to-noise, the possible recruitment of alternative neural systems to subserve a particular task, and variations in functional connectivity of the region involved. The anatomical and functional connectivity of prefrontal cortex appears to be an especially important factor in accounting for variations of prefrontal activity in several neurological conditions (Weinberger 1993).

The mechanism of the deficit in prefrontal function in schizophrenia is obscure. Simple models of too little (or too much) activity do not adequately characterize prefrontal function in schizophrenia, any more than a single cognitive task accounts for all prefrontal functions. It has recently been proposed that a more informative perspective is to view prefrontal activity in schizophrenia in relation to activity in other regions (Weinberger & Lipska 1995; Friston *et al.* 1996). For example, as noted above, during the WCST, patients with schizophrenia are hypoactive in prefrontal cortex while they are hyperactive in hippocampus, suggesting an abnormal pattern of correlative intracortical activity. Analogous findings of mesial temporal cortical hyperactivity during the cued verbal production task have been interpreted as evidence that prefrontal cortex fails to inhibit temporolimbic cortex (or is inhibited by it), again implicating an abnormality of intracortical functional connectivity (Frith *et al.* 1995; Friston *et al.* 1996). The results of a study that found a strong correlation between hippocampal volume reduction and prefrontal rCBF during the WCST in patients with schizophrenia is further potential evidence of such an abnormality of cortical interactions (Weinberger *et al.* 1992). Nevertheless, as appealing as this interpretation may be, it is not clear how such a deficit translates into prefrontal hypoactivity during working memory tasks. It is conceivable that the overactivity in nonfrontal areas, rather than being a primary part of the problem in schizophrenic cortex, is an epiphenomenon of a primary deficit of prefrontal cortex. Perhaps, in an effort at a solution to the cognitive demands, patients are searching the nexus of neural circuitry to find a substitute for a prefrontal cortex that cannot fit the bill. Future studies will hopefully resolve these uncertainties.

References

Akbarian, S., Bunney Jr, W. E., Potkin, S. G., Wigal, S. B., Hagman, J. O., Sandman, C. A. & Jones, E. G. 1993 Altered distribution of nicotinamide-adenine dinucleotide phosphate-diaphorase cells in frontal lobe of schizophrenic implies disturbances of cortical development. *Arch Gen Psychiatry* **50**, 169–77.

Andreasen, N. C., Flashman, L., Flaum, M., Arndt, S., Swayze V, I. I., O'Leary, D. S., Ehrhardt, J. C. & Yuh, W. T. C. 1994 Regional brain abnormalities in schizophrenia measured with magnetic resonance imaging. *JAMA* **272**, 1763–69.

Andreasen, N. C., O'Leary, D. S., Cizadlo, T., Arndt, S., Rezai, K., Watkins, G. L., Ponto, L. L. B. & Hichwa, R. D. 1995 Remembering the past: Two facets of episodic memory explored with positron emission tomography. *Am J. Psychiatry* **152**, 1576–85.

Andreasen, N. C., Rezai, K., Alliger, R., Swayze, V. W., Flaum, M., Kirchner, P., Gohen, G. & O'Leary, D. S. 1992 Hypofrontality in neuroleptic-naive patients and in patients with chronic schizophrenia. *Arch Gen Psychiatry* **49**, 943–58.

Bartlett, E. J., Wolkin, A., Brodie, J. D., Laska, E. M., Wolf, A. P. & Sanfilipo, M. 1991 Importance of pharmacologic control in PET studies: Effects of thiothixene and haloperidol on cerebral glucose utilization in chronic schizophrenia. *Psychiatry Res: Neuroimaging* **40**, 115–24.

Benes, F. M., McSparren, J., Bird, E. D., SanGiovanni, J. P. & Vincent, S. L. 1991 Deficits in small interneurons in prefrontal and cingulate cortices of schizophrenic and schizoaffective patients. *Arch Gen Psychiatry* **48**, 996–1001.

Berman, K. F., Illowsky, B. & Weinberger, D. R. 1988a Physiological dysfunction of dorsolateral prefrontal cortex in schizophrenia. IV. Further evidence for regional and behavioral specificity. *Arch Gen Psychiatry* **45**, 616–22.

Berman, K. F., Randolph, C., Gold, J., Goldberg, T. E., Coppola, R., Ostrem, J. L., Garson, R. E., Herscovitch, P. & Weinberger, D. R. 1995b Physiological activation of a cortical network during performance of the Wisconsin Card Sorting Test: A Positron Emission Tomography study. *Neuropsychologia* **33**, 1027–46.

Berman, K. F., Schapiro, M. B., Friedland, R. P., Rappaport, S. I. & Weinberger, D. R. 1988b Regional cortical blood flow during cognitive activation in Down's Syndrome. *Soc Neurosci Abstracts* pp. 10–12.

Berman, K. F., Schmidt, P. J., Ostrem, J. L., Danaceau, M. A., Van Horn, J. D., Esposito, G., Rubinow, D. R. Weinberger, D. R. 1995a The effects of gonadal steroid hormones on cognitively-related regional cerebral blood flow: A positron emission tomography study. *J Cereb Blood Flow Metab* **15**, S133.

Berman, K. F., Torrey, E. F., Daniel, D. G. & Weinberger, D. R. 1992 Regional cerebral blood flow in monozygotic twins discordant and concordant for schizophrenia. *Arch Gen Psychiatry* **49**, 927–34.

Berman, K. F., Weinberger, D. R. 1991 Functional localization in the brain in schizophrenia. In *American Psychiatric Press Review of Psychiatry Volume* 10 (ed. A. Tasman & S. M. Goldfinger), pp. 24–59. Washington: American Psychiatric Press, Inc.

Berman, K. F., Zec, R. F. & Weinberger, D. R. 1986 Physiological dysfunction of dorsolateral prefrontal cortex in schizophrenia. II: Role of medication, attention, and mental effort. *Arch Gen Psychiatry* **43**, 126–35.

Bertolino, A., Nawroz, S., Mattay, V. S., Duyn, J. H., Moonen, C. T. W., Barnett, A. S., Frank, J. A., Tedeschi, G. & Weinberger, D. R. 1996 A specific pattern of impaired neuronal metabolism in schizophrenia as assessed by multislice proton magnetic resonance spectroscopic imaging. *Am, J, Psychiatry*. **153**, 1554–63.

Biver, F., Goldman, S., Luxen, A., Delvenne, V., Maertelaer, V. D., Fuente, J. D. L., Mendlewicz, J. & Lotstra, F. 1995 Altered frontostriatal relationship in unmedicated schizophrenic patients. *Psychiatry Res* **61**, 161–71.

Bosley, T. M., Kiyosawa, M., Harbour, R., Zimmerman, R., Savino, P. J., Sergott, R. C., Alavi, A., Reivich, M. 1991 Neuroimaging and positron emission tomography of congenital homonymous hemianopsia. *Am J Ophthalmol* **111**, 413–18.

Breier, A., Buchanan, R. W., Elkashef, A., Munson, R. C., Kirkpatrick, B. & Gellad, F. 1992 Brain morphology and schizophrenia: A magnetic resonance imaging study of limbic, prefrontal cortex, and caudate structures. *Arch Gen Psychiatry* **49**, 921–26.

Buchsbaum, M. S., Haier R. J., Potkin, S. G., Nuechterlein, K., Bracha, H. S., Katz, M., Lohr, J., Wu, J., Lottenberg, S., Jerabek, P. A., Trenary, M., Tafalla, R., Reynolds, C. & Bunney Jr, W. E. 1992 Frontostriatal disorder of cerebral metabolism in never-medicated schizophrenics. *Arch Gen Psychiatry* **49**, 935–42.

Buchsbaum, M. S., Nuechterlein, K. H., Haier, R. J., Wu, J., Sicotte, N., Hazlett, E., Asarnow, R., Potkin, S. & Guich, S. 1990 Glucose metabolic rate in normals and schizophrenics during the continuous performance test assessed by positron emission tomography. *Br J Psychiatry* **156**, 216–27.

Callicott, J. H., Ramsey, N., Tallent, K., Bertolino, A., Knable, M. B., Coppola, R., Goldberg, T., van Gelderen, P., Mattay, V. K., Frank, J., Moonen, T. W. & Weinberger, D. R. 1998 3-D PRESTO fMRI of a working memory task in schizophrenia. *Arch Gen Psychiatry* **18**, 186–96.

Catafau, A. M., Parellada E., Lomeña, F. J., Bernardo, M., Pavía, J., Ros, D., Setoaìn, J. & Gonzalez-Monclús, E. 1994 Prefrontal and temporal blood flow in schizophrenia: Resting and activation technetium-99m-HMPAO SPECT patterns in young neuro-leptic-naive patients with acute disease. *J Nucl Med* **35**, 935–41.

Cleghorn, J. M., Garnett, E. S., Nahmias, C., Firnau, G., Brown, G. M., Kaplan, R., Szechtman H. & Szechtman, B. 1989 Increased frontal and reduced parietal glucose metabolism in acute untreated schizophrenia. *Psychiatry Res* **28**, 119–33.

Corbetta, M., Miezin, F. M., Dobmeyer, S., Shulman, G. L. & Petersen, S. E. 1990 Attentional modulation of neural processing of shape, color, and velocity in humans. *Science* **248**, 1556–59.

Crosson, B., Williamson, D. J. G., Shukla, S. S., Honeyman, J. C. & Nadeau, S. E. 1994 A technique to localize activation in the human brain with technetium-99m-HMPAO SPECT: A validation study using visual stimulation. *J Nucl Med* **35**, 755–63.

Dolan, R. J., Fletcher, P., Frith, C. D., Friston, K. J., Frackowiak, R. S. J. & Grasby, P. M. 1995 Dopaminergic modulation of impaired cognitive activation in the anterior cingulate cortex in schizophrenia. *Nature* **378**, 180–82.

Doran, A. R., Boronow, J., Weinberger, D. R., Wolkowitz, O. M., Breier, A. & Pickar, D. 1987 Structural brain pathology in schizophrenia revisited: Prefrontal cortex pathology is inversely correlated with CSF levels of homovanillic acid. *Neuropsychopharmacology* **1**, 25–32.

Ebmeier, K. P., Blackwood, D. H. R., Murray, C., Souza, V., Walker, M., Dougall, N., Moffoot, A. P. R., O'Carroll, R. E. & Goodwin, G. M. 1993 Single-photon emission computed tomography with 99m Tc-exametazime in unmedicated schizophrenic patients. *Biol Psychiatry* **33**, 487–95.

Ebmeier, K. P., Lawrie, S. M., Blackwood, D. H. R., Johnstone, E. C. & Goodwin, G. M. 1995 Hypofrontality revisited: A high resolution single photon emission computed tomography study in schizophrenia. *J Neurol Neurosurg Psychiatry* **58**, 452–56.

Esposito, G., Kirkby, B. S., Van Horn, J. D., Weinberger, D. R. & Berman, K. F. 1995 Different pathophysiological mechanisms of altered Wisconsin Card Sort performance in schizophrenics and elderly normal subjects. *Soc Neurosci Abstracts* **21**, 747.

Friston, K. J., Herold, S., Fletcher, P., Silbersweig, D., Cahill, C., Dolan, R. J., Liddle, P. F., Frackowiak, R. S. J. & Frith, C. D. 1996 Abnormal frontotemporal interactions in patients with schizophrenia. In *Biology of schizophrenia and affective disease* (ed. S. J. Watson), pp. 421–49. London: American Psychiatric Press, Inc.

Frith, C. D., Friston, K. J., Herold, S., Silbersweig, D., Fletcher, P., Cahill, C., Dolan, R. J., Frackowiak, R. S. J. & Liddle, P. F. 1995 Regional brain activity in chronic schizophrenic patients during the performance of a verbal fluency task: Evidence for a failure of inhibition in left superior temporal cortex. *Br J Psychiatry* **167**, 343–49.

Frith, C. D., Kapur, N., Friston, K. J., Liddle, P. F. & Frackowiak, R. S. J. 1995 Regional cerebral activity associated with the incidental processing of pseudo-words. *Hum Br Map* **3**, 153–60.

Gold, J. M., Berman, K. F., Randolph, C., Goldberg, T. E. & Weinberger, D. R. 1996 PET validation and clinical application of a novel prefrontal task. *Neuropsychology* **10**, 3–10.

Goldberg, T. E., Berman, K. F., Moore, E. & Weinberger, D. R. 1990 rCBF and cognition in Huntington's disease and schizophrenia: A comparison of patients matched for performance on a prefrontal-type task. *Arch Neurol* **47**, 418–22.

Goldberg, T. E. & Gold, J. M. 1995 Neurocognitive deficits in schizophrenia. In *Schizophrenia* (ed. S. R. Hirsch & D. R. Weinberger), pp. 146–62. London: Blackwell.

Goldberg, T. E., Gold, J. M., Greenberg, R., Griffin, S., Schulz, S. C., Pickar, D., Kleinman, J. E. & Weinberger, D. R. 1993*a* Contrasts between patients with affective disorder and patients with schizophrenia on a neuro-psychological screening battery. *Am J Psychiatry* **150**, 1355–62.

Goldberg, T. E., Torrey, E. F., Gold, J., Ragland, D., Bigelow, L. B. & Weinberger, D. R. 1993*b* Learning and memory in monozygotic twins discordant for schizophrenia. *Psychol Med* **23**, 71–85.

Goldberg, T. E., Torrey, E. F., Gold, J. M., Bigelow, L. B., Ragland, R. D., Taylor, E. & Weinberger, D. R. 1995 Genetic risk of neuropsychological impairment in schizophrenia: A study of monozygotic twins discordant and concordant for the disorder. *Schizophr Res* **17**, 77–84.

Goldman-Rakic, P. S. 1991 Prefrontal cortical dysfunction in schizophrenia: The relevance of working memory. In *Psychopathology and the brain* (ed. B. J. Carroll & J. E. Barrett), pp. 1–23.

Grond, M., Pawlik, G., Walter, H., Lesch, O. M. & Heiss, W.-D. 1995 Hypnotic catalepsy-induced changes of regional cerebral glucose metabolism. *Psychiatry Res: Neuroimaging* **61**, 173–79.

Gur, R. C. & Gur, R. E. 1995 Hypofrontality in schizophrenia: RIP. *Lancet* **345**, 1383–84.

Gur, R. E., Mozley P. D., Resnick, S. M., Mozley, L. H., Shtasel, D. L., Gallacher, F., Arnold, S. E., Karp, J. S., Alavi, A., Reivich, M. & Gur, R. C. 1995 Resting cerebral glucose metabolism in first-episode and previously treated patients with schizophrenia relates to clinical features. *Arch Gen Psychiatry* **52**, 657–67.

Gur R. E., Resnick S. M., Alavi, A., Gur, R. C., Caroff, S., Dann R., Silver F. L., Saykin, A. J., Chawluk, J. B., Kushner, M. & Reivich, M. 1989 Regional brain function in schizophrenia. I. A positron emission tomography study. *Arch Gen Psychiatry* **44**, 119–25.

Holcomb, H. H., Cascella, N. G., Thaker, G. K., Medoff, D. R., Dannals, R. F. and Tamminga, C. A. 1996 Functional sites of neuroleptic drug action in the human brain: PET/FDG studies with and without haloperidol. *Am J Psychiatry* **153**, 41–49.

Holzman, P. S. 1985 Eye movement dysfunctions and psychosis. *Int Rev Neurobiol* **77**, 179–205.

Ingvar, D. H. & Franzen, G. 1974 Distribution of cerebral activity in chronic schizophrenia. *Lancet* **2**, 1484–86.

Kawasaki, Y., Maeda, Y., Suzuki, M., Urata, K., Higashima, M., Kiba, K., Yamaguchi, N., Matsuda, H. & Hisada, K. 1993 SPECT analysis of regional cerebral blood flow changes in patients with schizophrenia during the Wisconsin Card Sorting test. *Schizophr Res* **10**, 109–16.

Kosslyn, S. M., Thompson, W. L., Kim, I. J. and Alpert, N. M. 1995 Topographical representation of mental images in primary visual cortex. *Nature* **378**, 496–98.

Lawson, W. B., Waldman, I. N. & Weinberger, D. R. 1988 Schizophrenic dementia: Clinical and CT correlates. *J Nerv Ment Dis* **176**, 207–12.

Liddle, P. F. 1995 Brain imaging. In *Schizophrenia* (ed. S. R. Hirsch & D. R. Weinberger), pp. 425–39. London: Blackwell.

MacAvoy, M. G., Bruce, C. J. and Gottlieb, J. P. 1991 Smooth pursuit eye movement representation in the primate frontal eyefield. *Cereb Cortex* **1**, 95–102.

Meyer, E., Ferguson, S. S. G., Zatorre, R. J., Alivisatos, B., Marrett, S., Evans, A. C. & Hakim, A. M. 1991 Attention modulates somatosensory cerebral blood flow response to vibrotactile stimulation as measured by positron emission tomography. *Ann Neurol* **29**, 440–43.

Rubin, P., Holm, S., Friberg, L., Videbeck, P., Andersen, H. S., Bendsen, B. B., Stromso, N., Larsen, J. K., Lassen, N. A. & Hemmingsen, R. 1991 Altered modulation of prefrontal and subcortical brain activity in newly diagnosed schizophrenia and schizophreniform disorder: A regional cerebral blood flow study. *Arch Gen Psychiatry* **48**, 987–95.

Saykin, J. A., Gur, R. C., Gur, R. E., Mozley, D., Mozley, L. G., Resnick, S. M., Kester, B. & Stafiniak, P. 1991 Neuropsychological function in schizophrenia: Selective impairment in memory and learning. *Arch Gen Psychiatry* **48**, 618–24.

Selemon, L. D., Rajkowska, G. & Goldman-Rakic, P. S. 1995 Abnormally high neuronal density in the schizophrenic cortex: A morphometric analysis of prefrontal area 9 and occipital area 17. *Arch Gen Psychiatry* **52**, 805–18.

Shelton, R. C., Doran, A. R., Pickar, D. & Weinberger, D. R. 1988 Cerebral structural pathology in schizophrenia. Evidence for a selective prefrontal cortical deficit. *Am J Psychiatry* **145**, 154–63.

Szechtman, H., Nahmias, C., Garnett, S., Firnau, G., Brown, G. M., Kaplan, R. D. & Cleghorn, J. M. 1988 Effect of neuroleptics on altered cerebral glucose metabolism in schizophrenia. *Arch Gen Psychiatry* **45**, 523–32.

Tamminga, C. A., Thaker, G. K., Buchanan, R., Kirkpatrick, B., Alphs, L. D., Chase, T. N. & Carpenter, W. T. 1992 Limbic system abnormalities identified in schizophrenia using positron emission tomography with fluorodeoxyglucose and neocortical alterations with deficit syndrome. *Arch Gen Psychiatry* **49**, 522–30.

Vita, A., Bressi, S., Perani, D., Invernizzi, G., Giobbio, G. M., Dieci, M., Barbarini, M., Sole A. D. & Fazio, F. 1995 High-resolution SPECT study of regional cerebral blood flow in drug-free and drug-naive schizophrenic patients. *Am J Psychiatry* **152**, 876–82.

Volkow, N. D., Wolf, A. P., Gelder, P. V., Brodie, J. D., Overall, J. E., Cancro, R. & Gomez-Mont, F. 1987 Phenomenological correlates of metabolic activity in 18 patients with chronic schizophrenia. *Am J Psychiatry* **144**, 151–58.

Weinberger, D. R. 1988 Schizophrenia and the frontal lobes. *Trends Neurosci* **11**, 367–70.

Weinberger, D. R. 1993 A connectionist approach to the prefrontal cortex. *J Neuropsych Clin Neurosci* **5**, 241–53.

Weinberger, D. R. & Berman, K. F. 1988 Speculation on the meaning of cerebral metabolic 'hypofrontality' in schizophrenia. *Schizophr Bull* **14**, 157–68.

Weinberger, D. R., Berman, K. F., Iadarola, M., Driesen, N., & Zec, R. F. 1988*a* Prefrontal cortical blood flow and cognitive function in Huntington's Disease. *J Neurol Neurosurg Psychiatry* **51**, 94–104.

Weinberger, D. R., Berman, K. F. & Illowsky, B. 1988*b* Physiological dysfunction of dorsolateral prefrontal cortex in schizophrenia. III. A new cohort and evidence for a monoaminergic mechanism. *Arch Gen Psychiatry* **45**, 609–15.

Weinberger, D. R., Berman, K. F., Ostrem, J. L., Abi-Dargham, A. & Torrey, E. F. 1993 Disorganization of prefrontal-hippocampal connectivity in schizophrenia: A PET studies of discordant MZ twins. *Soc Neurosci Abstracts* **19**, 7.

Weinberger, D. R., Berman, K. F., Suddath, R. & Torrey, E. F. 1992 Evidence for dysfunction of a prefrontal-limbic network in schizophrenia: An MRi and rCBF study of discordant monozygotic twins. *Am J Psychiatry* **149**, 890–97.

Weinberger, D. R., Berman, K. F. & Zec, R. F. 1986 Physiological dysfunction of dorsolateral prefrontal cortex in schizophrenia. I: Regional cerebral blood flow (rCBF) evidence. *Arch Gen Psychiatry* **43**, 114–25.

Weinberger, D. R. Lipska, B. K. 1995 Cortical maldevelopment, anti-psychotic drugs, and schizophrenia: A search for common ground. *Schizophr Res* **16**, 87–110.

Weinberger, D. R., Torrey, E. F., Neophytides, A. & Wyatt, R. J. 1979 Structural abnormalities of the cerebral cortex in chronic schizophrenia. *Arch Gen Psychiatry* **36**, 935–39.

Wolkin, A., Sanfilipo, M., Duncan, E., Angrist, B., Wolf, A. P., Cooper, T. B., Brodie, J. D., Laska, E. & Rotrosen, J. P. 1996 Blunted change in cerebral glucose utilization after haloperidol treatment in schizophrenic patients with prominent negative symptoms. *Am J Psychiatry* **153**, 346–54.

Wolkin, A., Sanfilipo, M., Wolf, A. P., Angrist, B., Brodie, J. D. & Rotrosen, J. 1992 Negative symptoms and hypofrontality in chronic schizophrenia. *Arch Gen Psychiatry* **49**, 959–65.

Zec, R. F. & Weinberger D. R. 1986 Brain areas implicated in schizophrenia. In *The Neurology of Schizophrenia* (ed. H. A. Nasrallah & D. R. Weinberger), pp. 175–206. Amsterdam: Elsevier N Holland.

13

The role of the prefrontal cortex in self-consciousness: the case of auditory hallucinations

Chris Frith

13.1 The signs and symptoms of schizophrenia

The diagnosis of schizophrenia is based largely on the patient's behaviour (signs) and his self-report of his mental state (symptoms). As yet no marker has been found which can validate the diagnosis at the level of physiology. Many different patterns of signs and symptoms can lead to a diagnosis of schizophrenia, and so one patient can differ markedly from another. In addition, the severity of signs and symptoms can fluctuate and the pattern can change over time in the same patient. In these circumstances we would expect to see marked differences in the pattern of 'resting' neural activity across an unselected group of schizophrenic patients corresponding to their marked differences in mental state. This expectation has been confirmed in studies using regional cerebral blood flow (rCBF) as an index of neural activity (Liddle *et al.* 1992; Ebmeier *et al.* 1993) and there is some evidence that neural activity is more strongly related to current mental state than to diagnosis (Dolan *et al.* 1993). Given these results, I have chosen to explore the neural basis of particular symptoms rather than the patho-physiology of schizophrenia in general. An essential component of this exploration is an attempt to formulate cognitive mechanisms for the production of particular symptoms, rather than simply observing associations between symptoms and patterns of neural activity.

' For the purposes of this essay, my target symptom will be auditory hallucinations. However, I shall also consider other symptoms for which similar cognitive mechanisms may be involved. Hallucinations (experiencing a percept in the absence of any external stimulus) are a common feature of schizophrenia (Sartorius *et al.* 1974) although not unique to this disorder. These hallucinations usually take the form of hearing voices (Kendell 1985) and certain particular forms, such as when the patient hears people talking about him in the third person, are considered to be especially associated with schizophrenia (Schneider 1959). Example 1 is taken from an autobiographical account of a mental breakdown that occurred well before the diagnostic criteria for schizo-phrenia were first put forward by Kraepelin in 1896.

Example 1

Only a short time before I was confined to my bed I began to hear voices, at first only close to my ear, afterwards in my head, or as if one were whispering in my ear—or in various parts of the room... These voices commanded me to do, and made me believe a number of false and terrible things.

(From John Percival Esq., *A narrative of the treatment experienced by a gentleman, during a state of mental derangement*, London, 1840).

The description of the voices in the example are typical of the descriptions given by patients today (Chadwick & Birchwood 1994). There are three aspects of these abnormal experiences that I shall consider in this essay.

1. An auditory-verbal experience occurs in the absence of sensation.
2. 'Self-generated' activity is perceived to come from an external source.
3. The voice is perceived to come from an 'agent' intending to influence the patient.

My basic thesis is that these abnormal experiences occur because of dis-ordered interactions between prefrontal cortex and posterior brain regions.

13.2 What is the nature of auditory hallucinations?

Hallucinations are perceptions that occur in the absence of any sensory stimu-lation. Although auditory hallucinations are the most frequently reported schizophrenic patients can also experience visual, olfactory and tactile halluci-nations (see table 13.1). However, experimental studies of hallucinations are restricted almost entirely to auditory hallucinations. Patients report that the severity of auditory hallucinations (e.g. loudness and duration) fluctuates from moment to moment. Furthermore this severity is influenced by concurrent auditory input. Margo *et al.* (1981) have shown that unstructured auditory input (such as white noise) increases the severity of hallucinations, while severity is reduced by listening to speech or music and markedly reduced by reading aloud. These results show that auditory hallucinations share resources with systems concerned with the analysis of auditory sensations.

In some cases it has been shown that what the 'voices' say closely corres-ponds to the content of whispers or sub-vocal speech produced by the patient (Gould 1949; see example 2). This observation suggests that auditory hallucina-tions may be associated with inner speech. In line with this suggestion Bick & Kinsbourne (1987) have claimed that in some patients deliberate articulation reduces the severity of hallucinations. Also David (1994) has reported one case in which the occurrence of thought broadcasting (a particular form of auditory

Table 13.1   Types of hallucination

Types of hallucination	(Perception in the absence of sensation)
Visual	seeing frightening faces, dwarf figures
Tactile	feeling heat, being pricked, being strangled
Olfactory	food is tasteless or repulsive, room smells of gas
Auditory	hearing voices
	hearing one's thoughts spoken aloud (thought echo)
	voices speaking to the patient (second person hallucinations)
	voices speaking about the patient (third person hallucinations)

hallucination in which the patient hears his own thoughts spoken aloud) inter-fered with verbal short-term memory tasks in the same manner as articulatory suppression (saying 'blah blah blah blah') does in normal subjects (Baddeley 1986). All these behavioural observations suggest that auditory hallucinations arise in the same systems that are engaged when people listen to external speech or generate inner speech.

Example 2.   Hallucinations and subvocal speech

Whisper: She knows. She's the most wicked thing in the whole wide world. The only voice I hear is hers. She knows everything. She knows everything about aviation.
Patient: I heard them say I have a knowledge of aviation.
   (From Gould 1949).

Brain imaging studies confirm this conjecture at the physiological level. McGuire *et al.* (1996) have delineated the brain regions activated when normal volunteers are engaged with inner speech or imagining the sound of some one else speaking. Inner speech activates Broca's area (left inferior frontal gyrus), while imagining the sound of someone else speaking engages a number of additional areas including left premotor cortex, supplementary motor area (SMA) and left superior temporal gyrus (STG). Imaging the brain activity associated with hallucinations is difficult since the target event is involuntary and its timing cannot be predicted. Using single photon emission computerised tomography (SPECT) McGuire *et al.* (1993) observed activity in Broca's area during hallucinations and, to a lesser extent, in left STG. Cleghorn *et al.* (1992) also observed activity in left STG. Silbersweig *et al.* (1995) developed a much more sensitive technique for imaging hallucinations using positron emission tomography (PET) and observed activity in auditory association cortex. The precise location of this activity varied from patient to patient. In the extreme case of a patient who experienced visual hallucinations, the location of the activity clearly corresponded to the content of the hallucination.

All these results essentially confirm the reports of the patients. When the patients hear voices they show a similar pattern of behaviour and brain activity to those observed in normal people engaged in inner speech and/or auditory verbal imagery.

13.3 Self-monitoring

In the normal case people have no difficulty in recognizing that inner speech and auditory verbal imagery is self-generated. Thus, the first key question we have to answer about auditory hallucinations is why do the patients perceive their inner speech as coming from an external source. The ability to distinguish between self-generated images and externally caused sensations is a special case of the more general ability to attribute the source of knowledge. One example of this problem, the attribution of the source of memories, has been extensively studied in patients with various kinds of amnesia. The consensus view is that impaired source memory results from damage to the prefrontal cortex (Janowsky et al. 1989). The precise role of prefrontal cortex in source memory is not yet known. Recent brain imaging studies have shown that retrieval of items from episodic memory is associated with activity in right prefrontal cortex (Shallice et al. 1994). This activity seems to be associated with successful retrieval rather than the attempt to retrieve and lasts much longer (several seconds) than necessary for the successful recognition of an item presented previously. It is possible that this activity reflects the reconstruction and verification of an image of the past experience. Such reconstruction would include recovery of the source of the various components of the image.

Studies of source memory in neurological patients typically require the subject to distinguish between two external sources (list A vs list B; male voice vs female voice). In the case of hallucinations the distinction is between an external source and self-generated material. Johnson et al. (1993) have studied the ability of normal people to make this kind of distinction. Their results suggest that rather different processes are involved from traditional source memory. In particular such distinctions are very much easier to make.

A small number of studies of schizophrenic patients have been reported in which this kind of source memory has been studied. The results are somewhat equivocal. Bentall et al. (1991) asked patients either to generate category items (e.g. a fruit) or read out category items (plum). A week later they were asked to identify the source of these items (read or generated). Psychotic patients were worse than normal volunteers at this task whether or not they were hallucinating. Hallucinating patients were slightly more likely to attribute to the reading lists items they had generated themselves. Frith et al. (1991) asked patients to generate items in a category (e.g. animals) and then listen while the experimenter generated additional items from the same category. Ten minutes later the patient was asked to distinguish between the items he had generated and those produced by the experimenter. Once again schizophrenic patients were not good at this task, but the poor performance was related to incoherence of speech (thought disorder) rather than hallucinations.

In the experiment by Harvey (1985), patients were first asked to distinguish between words that had been read out by two different experimenters. The patients had no difficulty with this task. In the second experiment patients were shown words which they either read aloud or imagined reading aloud. Subsequently they had to distinguish between words they had read aloud and words they had imagined. Thought disordered patients were found to be bad at this task, but unfortunately the author does not report whether or not performance was related to hallucinations. Taken together these results suggest that some patients with schizophrenia do have difficulty with source memory tasks. However, the problem does not seem to relate closely to the presence of hallucinations.

There is one crucial aspect of self-monitoring in hallucinations that source memory experiments do not capture. In a source memory experiment the subject is required to make the distinction between sources sometime after the original experience. In contrast, the hallucinating patient has the immediate experience that what he is experiencing is coming from an external source when in fact it is not. This is clearly not a problem of memory.

Whenever we perform an action like speaking or moving a limb we receive sensory feedback about the consequences of this action. We can hear the sound of our own voice and we can feel the new position of our hand. In isolation this sensory information cannot indicate its own source. From the feel of my hand I cannot tell whether I moved it to its new position or it was moved passively by some outside force. However, studies of motor control and motor learning show that there are many other types of information from which knowledge of the source of sensation can be derived. In particular it is very likely that the brain uses 'forward modelling' to predict the consequences of action (Wolpert *et al.* 1995; see figure 13.1). In other words it is possible to calculate the sensory outcome of an action on the basis of the motor commands that were issued to generate that action. This information can tell us about the source of sensations. If the predicted sensory outcome does not match the observed sensory outcome then some external influence must have been at work. The information provided by forward modelling has a number of other important advantages for the performance and learning of motor skills. First, for example, errors can be detected before the arrival of the sensory feedback which indicates the consequences of the action. This is because the predictions from the forward model are available much sooner than the information from the feedback occurring after the action has been completed. The desired sensory outcome (e.g. the desired final position of the hand) can be compared with the position predicted by the forward model. If they do not match, it is likely that the wrong motor commands have been issued. These processes occur largely automatically and below the level of awareness.

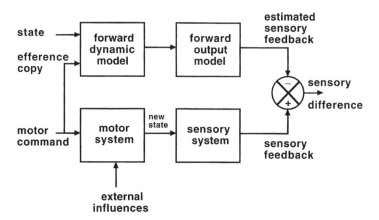

Fig. 13.1 How do we distinguish self-generated from external sensory events? This figure shows how a 'Forward model' can predict the sensory consequences of action (estimated sensory feedback). This feedback can be used to 'Cancel out' self-generated sensory events, thus distinguishing them from sensory events with an external cause.

I have already indicated how forward modelling allows the distinction to be made between external and internally generated influences. If the output from the forward model matches the intended outcome, but not the observed outcome then external influences must have occurred. If something went wrong with this mechanism, it might happen that mismatches between expected and observed sensory outcome would occur in the absence of external influences. In this case internally generated events could be misperceived as arising from external influences. Such misperceptions might underlie the 'Delusion of control', in which patients with schizophrenia describe feeling that their own actions are being controlled by alien forces. Forward modelling is a general strategy that can be applied to all kinds of actions and has been most extensively studied in relation to limb and eye movements. However, a failure in a forward modelling process applied to overt and covert speech could underlie auditory hallucinations. If we interpret auditory hallucinations in this way, then there are a number of other symptoms which fall into the same category (table 13.2). Among these are the so-called 'passivity' experiences or 'made' actions in which the patient feels that his own actions are being initiated by external forces. I have hypothesized that all these symptoms might be the result of something going wrong with the internal self-monitoring mechanism (maybe in the forward model) that normally permits the distinction between internally generated and external influences. As a result the patient perceives his own actions as being associated with external influences. If these patients have something wrong with the system that controls action then they should show specific types of action errors. For example, as indicated above rapid corrections of errors without feedback depends on the use of a forward model.

Table 13.2   Symptoms reflecting disorders in self-monitoring

Auditory hallucinations (thought broadcasting)	'It was like my ears being blocked up and my thoughts shouted out.'
Delusions of control (passivity of volition)	'My fingers pick up the pen, but I don't control them. What they do is nothing to do with me.'
Thought insertion (passivity of thought)	'the thoughts of Eamon Andrews come into my mind. He treats my mind like a screen and flashed his thoughts onto it.'

Two experiments suggest that schizophrenic patients do have difficulty with making rapid error corrections in the absence of visual feedback (Malenka *et al.* 1982; Frith & Done 1989). In the study by Frith & Done (1989) this difficulty was more marked in patients with passivity experiences. Mlakar *et al.* (1994) also found that such patients had difficulty subsequently recognizing designs that they had drawn in the absence of visual feedback. This would be consistent with the failure to use a forward model to construct the appearance of what had been drawn on the basis of the motor movements used. As yet there have been few investigations of this kind of control system in relation to speech. Leudar *et al.* (1992) observed the self corrections that schizophrenic patients made during the production of speech. They found that patients with hallucinations could detect their own errors as well as other patients, but found it much more difficult to self-repair them.

Clearly it will be possible to localize in the brain the various components of this model for control of action (Teuber 1964). But, as yet, we do not know where, for example, the forward model of action is computed or represented. Nor do we know in detail about the location of information about the desired or expected outcome of actions (but see Gray *et al.* 1992 for interesting speculations). Nevertheless, in broad terms the system must depend upon interactions between high level motor and sensory systems. This implies interactions between frontal/prefrontal cortex and posterior sensory association cortex. In a simple, but elegant brain imaging experiment, Paus *et al.* (1995) have shown that when subjects move their eyes in the dark at different rates, then rate related increases in activity can be seen in frontal eye fields, while rate related decreases are seen in visual areas. A similar result has been obtained by Wenzel *et al.* (1996) in relation to involuntary eye movements caused by vestibular stimulation. These results reflect a simple mechanism which permits a sensory system to discount changes in sensation due to eye movements and may correspond to the phenomenon of saccadic suppression. The same phenomenon has been observed in the somatosensory system. Elevated thresholds for perception of stimuli applied to the finger have been observed during movement of the finger (Rushton *et al.* 1981). Similar observations have also been made for the auditory system. Müller-Preuss & Ploog (1981) have found cells in the auditory cortex of the squirrel monkey which respond to the vocalizations of other monkeys, but not when the monkey itself vocalizes. Creutzfeldt *et al.* (1989) used implanted electrodes in the temporal lobes of patients undergoing neurosurgery and identified areas where the was a decrease in activity when the patient was vocalizing.

The abnormal experiences associated with schizophrenia might result from a failure of the modulation of sensory association cortex when prefrontal cortex is generating motor activity. This might be manifest as a functional disconnection between the appropriate areas, i.e. a lack of a (negative) correlation between activity in the two areas over time. Evidence for such a functional disconnection has been found in studies of schizophrenic patients performing word generation or word repetition tasks. When normal subjects perform the word generation task there is an increase in frontal and cingulate activity and a decrease in activity in the superior temporal gyrus (STG) relative to the word repetition task (Frith *et al.* 1991). This decrease was not observed in two studies of patients with schizophrenia (Frith *et al.* 1995; Dolan *et al.* 1995). Measures of functional connectivity suggest that there is a functional disconnection between frontal areas and left STG in these patients (Friston & Frith 1995).

13.4 The perception of agency

The typical hallucination described by a patient with schizophrenia is not merely a voice. It is a voice emanating from someone who is trying to influence the patient in some way (i.e. an agent). In many cases this agent is instructing the patient to perform some act which may cause violence either to the patient himself or to others. Patients expend much effort and experience much distress as they try to resist such instructions (Chadwick & Birchwood 1994). The involvement of external agents in hallucinations is a feature that puts this symptom in the same class as a large number of other symptoms common in schizophrenia (table 13.3). These are symptoms which involve false beliefs about agents, for instance that certain people are communicating with the patient (delusions of reference) or that people intend harm to the patient (delusions of persecution).

In a recent experiment we examined the effect of distorted feedback on the patient's perception of his own voice (Cahill & Frith 1996). Patients received

Table 13.3 Symptoms reflecting experience of agents

Auditory hallucinations (second person)	'We won't be so lenient next time. We're going to make your eyes roll up.'
Delusions of reference	'I saw someone scratching his chin which meant that I needed a shave.'
Delusions of persecution	'People at work are victimising me. A bloke at work is trying to kill me with some kind of hypnosis.'
	(From Chadwick & Birchwood 1994, and Frith 1992)

immediate feedback of their own voice distorted in pitch. In an acute phase of the illness, but not when well, they reported that they heard another person speaking when they spoke (example 3). This willingness to attribute their own voice to another person was significantly correlated with the severity of their current delusions, but not with hallucinations. It seems that deluded patients have a strong bias to attribute unusual experiences to the actions of other agents. This tendency is often associated with hallucinations, but need not be. It seems that the tendency to attribute events to external agents is to some extent independent of the tendency to perceive inner events as coming from an external source. Thus delusional beliefs about the actions of agents can occur in the absence of hallucinations. Furthermore, when recovering from an acute episode, patients may report that they still hear the voices, but that they know they are not 'real'.

Example 3.   Effects of distorted feedback

High pitch
'It only speaks when I speak. Sounds like the sound a deaf person might make'.
High pitch
'Any time I try to speak it speaks with me'.
Low pitch
'The voice has changed to a masculine voice. Same as a deaf masculine voice. I think it's an evil spirit speaking when I speak'.
(from Cahill & Frith 1996).

In this essay I use the word agent to refer to a being who acts on the basis of wishes and intentions. The recognition that other beings act on such a basis is often called 'Having a theory of mind' (Premack & Woodruff 1978). By assuming that other people have minds we are able to predict and control their behaviour on the basis of their knowledge and beliefs. Intensive research suggests that humans have a highly developed theory of mind, while other primates have this in a most rudimentary form, if at all (Cheney & Seyfarth 1990). Deluded patients seem to have an overactive theory of mind. They perceive intentions when none are present and sometimes attribute intentions to inanimate objects.

The acid test of having a theory of mind is the ability to handle false beliefs (Wimmer & Perner 1983). We can recognize that a person will act on the basis of a belief even when we know that this belief is incorrect. This is not possible for children under about four years of age or for most people with autism. A good example of their problem involves lying. Lying is a strategy for manipulating the behaviour of others by instilling in them a false belief. Young children and people with autism fail to use the strategy of lying (Sodian & Frith 1992). Preliminary results with schizophrenic patients suggest that they may also have difficulty with tasks which involve inferring the mental states of others (Corcoran et al. 1995; Frith & Corcoran 1996).

The observation that people with autism can be otherwise quite intelligent, but still not be able to handle false belief tasks suggests that there may be a fairly circumscribed neural system for having a theory of mind which can be damaged while the rest of the brain remains intact (U. Frith *et al.* 1991). We have explored this possibility by imaging brain activity while normal volunteers read stories in which the behaviour of the characters can only be understood on the basis of their intentions and beliefs about the situation described. When compared with control stories in which the mental states of the characters are irrelevant we observed an area of activation in the medial prefrontal cortex on the left (Brodmann area 8) which only appeared during the mental state stories (Fletcher *et al.* 1995). A similar result has been obtained in a French study where volunteers simply listened to stories (Mazoyer *et al.* 1993).

Since animals other than man do not seem to be able to perform false belief tasks we have little relevant information from lesion studies or single cell recordings. It is therefore hardly surprising that we know little about this medial frontal area in terms of its function or its connections with other areas. However, activity has been observed in this area in a number of relevant PET studies (table 13.4). Wise and his colleagues (personal communication) observed activity in this area during performance of a task in which normal subjects had to distinguish between speech sounds and similar computer generated sounds. Such a task can be interpreted as requiring the detection of agents (humans) from among non-agents (computers). This area was also implicated in two studies directly concerned with hallucinations. Silberswieg *et al.* (1995) observed the activity associated with hallucinations in an untreated schizophrenic patient. This patient experienced combined auditory and visual hallucinations in which rolling, disembodied heads spoke to him, giving instructions. Activity associated with these experiences was observed in a number of areas including a medial frontal area close to that observed In the 'Theory of mind' study (see table 13.4). McGuire *et al.* (1995) studied auditory-verbal imagery in schizophrenic patients who experience hallucinations when ill, but who were symptom free at the time of testing. These patients showed significantly less activity in this medial frontal area than control subjects when they were imagining the sound of someone speaking. Taken together, these results suggest that a) the medial prefrontal area has a role in tasks which involve detecting and dealing with agents and b) that this area is implicated in hallucinations. The precise interpretation of the results is not easy since we know so little about either the cognitive mechanisms underlying agency detection tasks or about the function and anatomy of this area of prefrontal cortex.

The problems associated with interacting with agents (i.e. predicting and influencing the behaviour of other people) are conceptually very similar to those associated with the control of our own actions. In the control of action forward modelling can be used to predict the new state (sensations and perceptions) that will result from an action. When interacting with an agent, forward modelling could be used in the same way to predict the effect of our action on the inner state of the other person rather than ourselves. Likewise, just as we

Table 13.4   Activity in medial frontal cortex (BA8)

Study	Condition	Coordinates		
		x	y	z
Fletcher *et al.* 1995	Theory of mind	-12	42	36
Wise et al. (see text)	Computer vs human speech	-6	40	36
McGuire *et al.* 1996	Alien vs distorted speech	-2	36	36
McGuire *et al.* 1995	Auditory imagery, low in hallucinators	-12	44	36
Silbersweig *et al.* 1995	During hallucinations	-2	35	39

can use an inverse model to compute the executive commands necessary to reach a desired state for ourselves, we could use an inverse model to work out what sort of behaviour on our part would produce the desired state in another.

At present we know rather little about how forward and inverse models are implemented in the brain during the control of action, and almost nothing about the mechanisms that allow us to interact with other people. There is clearly an important role for medial prefrontal areas in interactions with others, but these areas must be part of an extended system yet to be identified. The phenomenology of auditory hallucinations suggests that the two systems (controlling actions of the self and controlling interactions with others) are related although not identical. Hallucinations (perception in the absence of sensation) and delusions about influences from other people are usually, but not always associated. The observations that hallucinations and delusions fluctuate markedly over time and are influenced by drugs implies that the problem arises in the dynamics of interactions between brain regions rather than some more static structural abnormality. This dynamic interaction undoubtedly involves prefrontal cortex, but the details of the system are yet to be determined.

References

Baddeley, A. 1986 *Working memory*. Oxford: Oxford University Press.

Bentall, R. P., Baker, G. A. & Havers, S. 1991 Reality monitoring and psychotic hallucinations. *Br. J. Clin. Psychol.* **30**, 213–22.

Bick, P. A. & Kinsbourne, M. 1987 Auditory hallucinations and subvocal speech in schizophrenic patients. *Am. J. Psychiat.* **144**, 222–25.

Cahill, C. & Frith, C. D. 1996 False perceptions or false beliefs? Hallucinations and delusions in schizophrenia. In *Methods in madness* (ed. P. W. Halligan and J. C. Marshall), pp. 2677–91. Hove: Psychology Press.

Chadwick, P. & Birchwood, M. 1994 The omnipotence of voices. A cognitive approach to auditory hallucinations. *Br. J. Psychiat.* **164**, 190–201.

Cheney, D. L. & Seyfarth, R. M. 1990 *How monkeys see the world*. Chicago: Chicago University Press.

Cleghorn, J. M., Franco, S., Szetchtman, B., Kaplan, R. D., Szetchtman, H., Brown, G. M., Nahmias, C. & Garnett, E. S. 1992 Towards a brain map of auditory hallucinations. *Am. J. Psychiat.* **149**, 1062–69.

Corcoran, R., Mercer, G. & Frith, C. D. 1995 Schizophrenia, symptomatology and social inference: Investigating 'Theory of mind' in people with schizophrenia. *Schiz. Res.* **17**, 5–13.

Creutzfeldt, O., Ojeman, G. & Lettich, E. 1989 Neuronal activity in the human lateral temporal lobe II. Responses to the subject's own voice. *Exp. Brain. Res.* **77**, 476–89.

David, A. S. 1994 The neuropsychological origin of auditory hallucinations. In: *Neuropsychology of schizophrenia* (ed. A. S. David & J. Cutting), pp. 269–313. Hove: Lawrence Erlbaum Associates.

Dolan, R. J., Bench, C. J., Liddle, P. F., Friston, K. J., Frith, C. D., Grasby, P. M. & Frackowiak, R. S. J. 1993 Dorsolateral prefrontal cortex dysfunction in the major psychoses: symptom or disease specificity? *J. Neurol. Neursurg. Psychiat.* **56**, 1290–94.

Dolan, R. J., Fletcher, P., Frith, C. D., Friston, K. J., Frackowiak, R. S. J. & Grasby, P. M. 1995 Dopaminergic modulation of impaired cognitive activation in the anterior cingulate cortex in schizophrenia. *Nature, Lond.* **378**, 180–82.

Ebmeier, K. P., Blackwood, D. H., Murray, C., Souza, V., Walker, M., Dougall, N., Moffoot, A. P., O'Carroll, R. E. & Goodwin,-G. M. 1993 Single-photon emission computed tomography with 99mTc-exametazime in unmedicated schizophrenic patients. *Biol. Psychiat.* **33**, 487–95.

Fletcher, P., Happé, F., Frith, U., Baker, S. C., Dolan, D. J., Frackowiak, R. S. J. & Frith, C. D. 1995 Other minds in the brain: a functional imaging study of 'theory of mind' in story comprehension. *Cognition* **57**, 109–28.

Friston, K. J. & Frith, C. D. 1995 Schizophrenia: A Disconnection Syndrome? *Clin. Neurosci.* **3**, 89–97.

Frith, C. D. 1992 *The cognitive neuropsychology of schizophrenia.* Hove: Lawrence Erlbaum.

Frith, C. D. & Corcoran, R. 1996 Exploring 'theory of mind' in people with schizophrenia. 1996 *Psychol. Med.* **26**, 521–30.

Frith, C. D. and Done, D. J. 1989 Experiences of alien control in schizophrenia reflect a disorder in the central monitoring of action. *Psychol. Med.* **19**, 359–63.

Frith, C. D., Friston, K. J., Herold, S., Silbersweig, D., Fletcher, P., Cahill, C., Dolan, R. J., Frackowiak, R. S. J. & Liddle, P. F. 1995 Regional brain activity in chronic schizophrenic patients during the performance of a verbal fluency task. *Br. J. Psychiat.* **167**, 343y349.

Frith, C. D., Friston, K. J., Liddle, P. F. & Frackowiak, R. S. J. 1991 Willed action and the prefrontal cortex in man: a study with PET. *Proc. R. Soc. Lond.* B **244**, 241–46.

Frith, C. D., Leary, J., Cahill, C. & Johnstone, E. C. 1991 Disabilities and circumstances of schizophrenic patients – a follow-up study. IV. Performance on psychological tests: demographic and clinical correlates of the results of these tests. *Br. J. Psychiat.* **159**, (suppl. 13), 26–29.

Frith, U., Morton, J. & Leslie, A. M. 1991 The cognitive basis of a biological disorder: autism. *TINS* **38**.

Gould, L. N. 1949 Auditory hallucinations and subvocal speech. *J. Nerv. M. Dis.* **109**, 418–27.

Gray, J., Feldon, J., Rawlins, J., Hemsley, D. & Smith, A. 1991 The neuropsychology of schizophrenia. *Behav. Brain. Sci.* **14**, 1–84.

Harvey, P. D. 1985 Reality monitoring in mania and schizophrenia. *J. Nerv. Ment. Dis* **173**, 67–73.

Janowsky, J. S., Shimamura, A. P. & Squire, L. R. 1989 Source memory impairment in patients with frontal lobe lesions. *Neuropsychologia* **27**, 1043–56.

Johnson, M. K., Hashtroudi, S. & Lindsay, D. S. 1993 Source monitoring. *Psychol. Bull.* **114**, 3–28.

Kendell, R. E. 1985 Schizophrenia: clinical features. In *Psychiatry*, vol. 1 (ed. R. Michels & J. O. Cavenar), p. 8. Basic Books: London.

Leudar, I., Thomas, P. & Johnson, M. 1992 Self-repair in dialogue and schizophrenics: effects of hallucinations and negative symptoms. *Brain Lang.* **43**, 478–511.

Liddle, P. F., Friston, K. J., Frith, C. D., Hirsch, S. R., Jones, T. & Frackowiak, R. S. J. 1992 Patterns of cerebral blood flow in schizophrenia. *Br. J. Psychiat.* **160**, 179–86.

Malenka, R. C., Angel, R. W., Hampton, B. & Berger, P. A. 1982 Impaired central error correcting behaviour in schizophrenia. *Arch. Gen. Psychiat.* **39**, 101–07.

Margo, A., Hemsley, D. R. & Slade, P. D. 1981 The effects of varying auditory input on schizophrenic hallucinations. *Br. J. Psychiat* **139**, 122–27.

Mazoyer, B. M., Tzourio, N., Frak, V., Syrota, A., Murayama, N., Levrier, O., Salamon, G., Dehaene, S., Cohen, L. & Mehler, J. 1993 The cortical representation of speech. *J. Cog. Neurosci.* **5**, 467–79.

McGuire, P. K., Shah, P. and Murray, R. M. 1993s Increased blood flow in Broca's area during auditory hallucinations in schizophrenia. *Lancet* **342**, 703–06.

McGuire, P. K., Silbersweig, D. A., Wright, I., Murray, R. M., David, A. S., Frackowiak, R. S. J. & Frith, C. D. 1995 Abnormal inner speech: a physiological basis for auditory hallucinations. *Lancet* **346**, 596–600.

McGuire, P. K., Silbersweig, D. A., Murray, R. M., David, A. S., Frackowiak, R. S. J. & Frith, C. D. 1996 Functional anatomy of inner speech and auditory verbal imagery. *Psychol. Med.* **26**, 29–38.

Mellors, C. S. 1970 First-rank symptoms of schizophrenia. *Br. J. Psychiat.* **117**, 15–23.

Mlakar, J., Jensterle, J. & Frith, C. D. 1994 Central monitoring deficiency and schizophrenic symptoms. *Psychol. Med.* **24**, 557–64.

Müller-Preuss, P. & Ploog, D. 1981 Inhibition of auditory cortical neurones during phonation. *Brain Res.* **215**, 61–76.

Nathaniel-James, D. & Frith, C. D. 1996 Confabulation in schizophrenia: evidence of a new form? *Psychol. Med.* **26**, 391–99.

Paus, T., Marrett, S., Evans, A. C. & Worsley, K. 1995s Neurophysiology of saccadic suppression in the human brain. *4th IBRO World Congress of Neuroscience* **478**.

Premack, D. & Woodruff, G. 1978 Does the chimpanzee have a theory of mind? *Behav. Brain Sci.* **4**, 515–26.

Rushton, D. N., Rothwell, J. C. & Craggs, M. D. 1981 Gating of somatosensory evoked potentials during different kinds of movement in man. *Brain* **104**, 465–91.

Sartorius, N., Shapiro, R. & Jablensky, A. 1974 The international pilot study of schizophrenia. *Schiz. Bull.* **1**, 21–35.

Schneider, K. 1959 *Clinical psychopathology*. New York: Grune & Stratton.

Shallice, T., Fletcher, P., Frith, C. D., Grasby, P., Frackowiak, R. S. J. & Dolan, R. J. 1994 Brain regions associated with acquisition and retrieval of verbal episodic memory. *Nature, Lond.* **368**, 633–35.

Silbersweig, D. A., Stern, E., Frith, C. D., Cahill, C., Holmes, A., Grootoonk, S., Seaward, J., McKenna, P., Chua, S. E., Schnorr, L., Jones, T. & Frackowiak, R. S. J. 1995 A functional neuroanatomy of hallucinations in schizophrenia. *Nature, Lond.* **378**, 176–79.

Sodian, B. & Frith, U. 1992 Deception and sabotage in autistic and normal children. *J. Child Psychol. Psychiat.* **33**, 591–605.

Teuber, H-L. 1964 The riddle of frontal lobe function in man. In *The frontal granular cortex and behavior* (ed. J. M. Warren & K. Akert), pp. 410–44. New York: McGraw-Hill.

Wenzel, R., Bartenstein, P., Dieterich, M., Danek, A., Weindl, A., Minoshima, S., Ziegler, S., Schwaiger, M. & Brandt, Th. 1996 Deactivations of human visual cortex during involuntary ocular oscillations. *Brain* **119**, 101–10.

Wimmer, H. & Perner, J. 1983 Beliefs about beliefs: representation and constraining function of wrong beliefs in young children's understanding of deception. *Cognition* **21**, 103–28.

Wolpert, D. M., Ghahramani, Z. & Jordan, M. I. 1995 An internal model for sensory motor integration. *Science* **269**, 1880–82.

A computational approach to prefrontal cortex, cognitive control, and schizophrenia: recent developments and current challenges

Jonathan D. Cohen, Todd S. Braver and Randall C. O'Reilly

14.1 Introduction

(a) Prefrontal cortex and cognitive control

One of the central concepts within modern cognitive psychology is a distinction between controlled and automatic processing. Controlled processing is classically defined as relying on a limited capacity attentional system, while automatic processing is assumed to occur independently of attentional resources. Most contemporary theories posit that there is actually a continuum between controlled and automatic processing. Nevertheless, virtually all theorists acknowledge the need for some mechanism, or set of mechanisms responsible for the coordination of processing in a flexible fashion—particularly in novel tasks—and their relationship to attentional control. Perhaps the most explicit of these is Baddeley's theory of working memory (Baddeley 1986), which postulates a specific subcomponent responsible for executive control. The postulation of a cognitive system involved in executive control closely parallels theories concerning frontal lobe involvement in executive functions (Bianchi 1922; Damasio 1985; Luria 1969), and the long-standing clinical observation that patients with frontal lesions exhibit a 'dysexecutive syndrome.' However, traditional theories have not specified the mechanisms by which the executive operates, either at the psychological or neurobiological levels. Recent advances have begun to address this need for more explicit theorizing.

Shallice (1982) has proposed the 'Supervisory Attentional System' (SAS) as a mechanism by which PFC coordinates complex cognitive processes, and Gathercole (1994) has suggested that this may provide a mechanism by which the executive controller operates in Baddeley's theory of working memory. Shallice's theory is described in terms of a production system architecture. This has appeal, as it relates the executive functions of frontal cortex to the well characterized mechanisms of other production system theories, which include the active maintenance of goal states to coordinate the sequences of production firings involved in complex behaviours (Anderson 1983). One feature of goal representations is that they are actively maintained throughout the course of a sequence of behaviours, which coincides with the observation that PFC appears to be specialized for the active maintenance of task-relevant information (discussed below). Kimberg and Farah (1993) have also proposed a model of frontal function using a production system architecture, that they have used to simulate performance in a variety of tasks considered to rely on frontal lobe function. However, because both this and Shallice's SAS theory are cast in production system terms, they lack a transparent mapping onto specific neurobiological mechanisms. While neurobiological plausibility is not a requirement, *per se*, of a theory that seeks to explain the cognitive functions of PFC, this does become important if our goal is to understand the cognitive manifestations of a complex neuropsychiatric disorder, such as schizophrenia, in terms of its underlying pathophysiological processes. This goal has been one of the important motivations in our effort to understand how cognitive control may arise from the neurobiological mechanisms housed within PFC.

(b) A connectionist approach

Toward this goal, we have begun to develop a theory of PFC function using a computational architecture closer to the one used by the brain. We have done this within the connectionist, or parallel distributed processing framework (Rumelhart & McClelland 1986). The principles of this framework capture central features of computation as it is carried out in the brain (e.g. multiple simple processing units, graded flow of activation, modifiable connection weights, etc.), and allow us to explore their influence on behaviour by simulating performance in specific cognitive tasks (Cohen & Servan-Schreiber 1992). The central hypothesis that has emerged from this work is that PFC is used to represent context information, which we define as information necessary to mediate an appropriate behavioural response. This can be a set of task instructions, a specific prior stimulus, or the result of processing a sequence of prior stimuli (e.g. the interpretation resulting from processing a sequence of words in a sentence). We consider context representations to be closely related to goal representations within production system architectures. Thus, the actions associated with a particular goal may, in other contexts, be relatively infrequent or 'weak' behaviours. Such actions require the maintenance of an internal representation of the goal, or of goal-related knowledge to favour their execution, to suppress competing, possibly more compelling behaviours, and to coordinate their execution over temporally extended periods.

We have begun to implement this theory in models of performance in specific cognitive tasks that tap simple forms of cognitive control. Our initial work focused on performance in the Stroop task (Cohen *et al.* 1990), in which subjects must selectively attend to one dimension of information (e.g. the colour in which a word is displayed) and ignore information in a competing, but prepotent dimension (e.g. the word itself). Our model of this task illustrates the close relationship between goals, context representations, and attentional effects, all of which we argue reflect the functioning of PFC. In the model, a task (i.e. goal) is specified by the appropriate pattern of activation over a set of units (context layer) that represents each of the two dimensions over which stimuli can vary. Activation of the appropriate units modulates the flow of activity along the pathway from input to response (attention), favouring processing in the task-relevant pathway over the stronger competing one. What provides the context layer with the capacity for control of processing is that it has representations of the stimulus dimensions that are relevant to the task, and that activating these biases processing in favour of one pathway over the other. This observation is fundamental to our hypothesis of how PFC is involved in cognitive control: representations in PFC bias processing in posterior neocortex in favour of task-relevant pathways.

We have used these mechanisms to simulate detailed aspects of normal human performance in the Stroop task (Cohen *et al.* 1990), and a variety of other tasks involving attentional control (Cohen *et al.* 1994; Cohen & Servan-Schreiber 1992; Cohen *et al.* 1992). We have also used them to help understand the mechanisms underlying other cognitive functions that have typically been associated with frontal function, and that are of relevance to schizophrenia: active memory and behavioural inhibition. We have argued that both of these functions reflect the operation of the context layer under different task conditions. Under conditions of response competition, when a strong response tendency must be overcome for appropriate behaviour, the context module can be seen to play an inhibitory role, by supporting the processing of task relevant information, which can then compete more effectively with irrelevant information. This is exemplified by our model of the Stroop task (see figure 14.1). In contrast, when there is a delay between information relevant to a response and the execution of that response, then the context module can be seen to play a role in memory, by actively maintaining that information over time, so that it can be used later to mediate the appropriate response. This is exemplified by our model of the AX version of the continuous performance task, in which the correct response to one stimulus depends on the identity of a previous one (described in detail below; see figure 14.3). This theory has allowed us to account for a wide, and seemingly disparate array of cognitive deficits that arise in schizophrenia, in terms of a disturbance of frontal function. Frontal dysfunction has long been considered to be a central pathophysiological feature of schizophrenia (Kolb & Whishaw 1983; Kraeplin 1950; Levin 1984), and our simulation models of frontal function have begun to provide an integrated and explicit account of how frontal impairment could give rise to specific patterns of cognitive deficit observed in this illness.

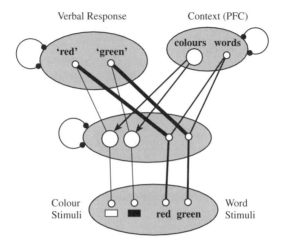

Fig. 14.1 Simulation model of the Stroop task. Heavier lines in the word reading pathway indicate stronger connections in this pathway. Larger circles indicate active (solid) or potentiated (open) units. Arrows indicate flow of activity. Loops with dots indicate lateral inhibitory connections among units within the module.

14.2 Applications to schizophrenia

(a) Simulation studies

One of the most overt features of schizophrenia is a failure of cognitive control. This is manifest in clinical symptoms such as distractibility, loosening of associations, and disorganized or socially inappropriate behaviour. In the laboratory, these disturbances have been observed as deficits of attention (Zubin 1975; Kornetsky & Orzack 1978; Wynne *et al.* 1978; Nuechterlein 1991; Cornblatt & Keilpk 1994;), working memory (Weinberger *et al.* 1986; Goldman-Rakic 1991; Park & Holzman 1992), and behavioural inhibition (Wapner & Krus 1960; Chapman *et al.* 1964; Storms & Broen 1969; Abramczyk *et al.* 1983; Wysocki & Sweet 1985; Manschreck *et al.* 1988; Carter *et al.* 1993; Cohen & Carter 1996). We have proposed that these deficits can be understood in terms of a disturbance in the processing of context, arising from a disturbance in frontal function. We have made this explicit, by committing performance in cognitive tasks that tap these cognitive functions to explicit simulation models, and showing that when damage is introduced to the context layer, the models are able to simulate schizophrenic performance in these tasks. For example, in Cohen & Servan-Schreiber (1992), we reported computer simulation models of three tasks that have commonly been considered to tap different cognitive processes: the Stroop task (selective attention and behavioural inhibition), the identical pairs version of the CPT (vigilance and signal detection ability), and a lexical disambiguation task (language processing). Models of all three tasks used a similar architecture. We showed that, in simulations of these tasks, a single disturbance to the layer used to represent context produced changes in performance that both quantitatively and qualitatively matched those observed for schizophrenics.

As noted above, our models suggest that both the active memory and behavioural inhibition functions commonly ascribed to PFC may reflect the operation of the context layer, under different behavioural conditions. This hypothesis has begun to receive empirical support in studies of normal cognitive function (Roberts *et al.* 1994), however it also has direct relevance to schizophrenic cognitive disturbances. Deficits of both active memory and inhibition have been reported in schizophrenia. However, to our knowledge, these have never been studied together under controlled task conditions. According to our theory, the ability to process context should be most important when there is both a need to maintain information over time and use that information after a delay to inhibit a habitual response. Below, we will discuss recent empirical results demonstrating that schizophrenics show selective and specific deficits under such conditions.

Our simulation studies also suggest that memory and inhibition effects are differentially sensitive to disturbances of the context layer. With mild to moderate disturbances, a deficit appears only when there is a delay between the context and a response. This is because, with partial degradation of context information, a suffiicient amount may remain at short or no delays to mediate a contextually appropriate response (i.e. inhibit the irrelevant response). At longer delays, however, degraded representations succumb to the cumulative effects of noise, and a failure to inhibit the habitual (but incorrect) response may be observed. Thus, the models predict that mild to moderate disturbances in patients with schizophrenia should manifest primarily at long delays, which might be viewed as a memory deficit. With sufficiently severe disturbances of the context mechanism, however, deficits should begin to emerge without any delay, which might be viewed as a deficit of inhibition. Assuming a Kraeplinian view of schizophrenia, this may map onto the course of the illness, with a 'memory' deficit early in the course and, as the illness progresses, a gradual reduction in the delay that can be tolerated. Eventually, late in the illness, a deficit would be observed even without a delay and may be perceived clinically as a 'failure of inhibition.' In both cases, the same mechanism is impaired, though to a different degree. Thus, our models make an interesting, and counterintuitive prediction: that 'memory' deficits should emerge earlier than 'inhibitory' deficits. This is counterintuitive insofar as inhibitory deficits require suppression of strong competing responses, something that might otherwise be considered to be more demanding and therefore subject to earlier failure, than simply maintaining information over a brief delay.

(b) Empirical studies

Recently, we have begun to use a variety of cognitive tasks to test predictions made by our models, and the theory upon which they are based. As an example of this work, we will focus on studies using the continuous performance test (CPT; Rosvold et al. 1956). This task was chosen to make contact between our computational models and an extensive literature concerning schizophrenic deficits (for reviews see Nuechterlein 1991; Cornblatt & Keilpk 1994). The task is simple enough to be able to simulate, yet generates a rich set of empirical findings that can be used to test detailed predictions made by the models. In this task, subjects observe sequences of letters presented one at a time, and must respond to a designated target. A version of this task in common use is the AX-CPT, which requires subjects to respond to a probe (e.g. the letter x), but only when it follows a designated cue (e.g. A). Performance in this task depends on the representation and maintenance of context information, insofar as the correct response to the probe depends on knowledge of the previous cue (A or not A). In standard versions of this task, target sequences (e.g. A-X) are typically low frequency (20%), and the delay between these is short (1 s). We modified this standard procedure, in order to probe both the inhibitory and memory functions associated with the processing of context. First, to assess 'inhibition,' we introduced a strong response bias by increasing the frequency of target sequences to 80%, with remaining trials evenly divided between two types of distractor sequences (B-X and A-Y, where 'b' corresponds to any non-A stimulus, and 'y' to any non-x). This required subjects to respond to x in 7 of every 8 trials that it appeared, thus producing a strong bias to respond to x. This, in turn, required the use of context (non-A cue) to override this response. A schizophrenic failure to process context would predict an increase in false alarms on BX trials. This runs counter to the usual finding for schizophrenics: an increase in misses, but no increase in false alarms. It also circumvents concerns about a general lack of motivation or tendency to respond as a basis for schizophrenic failures, since we predict that they will make a greater number of responses in this condition (i.e. BX false alarms) as compared to controls. Finally, we manipulated the delay between the cue and the probe (1 vs 5 s), predicting that schizophrenic failures to actively maintain context would produce a selective increase in BX errors at the long vs short delay condition. Conversely, we predicted that control subjects would perform equally or better at the long delay, given the slower pace of the task (Parasuraman 1979).

We have completed two studies using this paradigm. In the first study (Servan-Schreiber et al. 1996) we tested medicated and unmedicated schizo-phrenics and patient controls. Both overall performance, and sensitivity to context (D-prime computed for AX hits and BX false alarms) were measured for all three groups. Both groups of schizophrenics showed overall worse performance than control subjects. However, there was a significant interaction between group and delay, with unmedicated schizophrenics exhibiting a pre-dicted significant increase in AX misses and BX errors at the long delay, but not at the short delay (see figure 14.2). Groups did not differ in any other conditions of the task. Furthermore, the lack of a delay effect in either the control subjects, or the medicated schizophrenics who performed as poorly

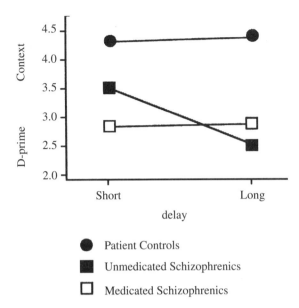

Fig. 14.2   Context sensitivity in the AX-CPT task. 'D-prime context' refers to D-prime calculated for AX hits vs. BX false alarms (see text for explanation).

overall as the unmedicated schizophrenics, satisfies the criteria proposed by Chapman & Chapman (1978) for establishing psychometric equivalence across task conditions, and demonstrating a true differential deficit. Thus, unmedicated schizophrenics exhibited a selective and specific deficit, as predicted by our model of PFC function, its role in the processing of context, and its disturbance in schizophrenia.

We have continued to study subjects in this task, including patients who present with a first episode of psychosis, prior to treatment with neuroleptic medication. Diagnosis is established at 6 month follow-up, which yields a population of subjects with a confirmed diagnosis of schizophrenia, and another with non-schizophrenia-spectrum diagnoses. The latter represent a valuable control population, as they are closely matched in demographic characteristics to the first-episode schizophrenics and, most importantly, present in a form clinically indistinguishable from the schizophrenics. Therefore, any laboratory measures that can distinguish between schizophrenics and these subjects are likely to reflect fundamental pathophysiological features of this illness, and hold promise as valuable clinical instruments. Analysis of the performance of these subjects in the AX-CPT indicate that the neuroleptic-naive first-episode schizophrenics display the predicted pattern of deficits in this task, whereas the non-schizophrenic subjects do not. This distinction in performance between schizophrenic and non-schizophrenic subjects, at a time when they are clinically indistinguishable, is potentially of great significance, strongly suggesting the specificity of our findings to schizophrenia, the sensitivity of our cognitive tasks, and the value of the theoretical approach that guided their design.

In another study (Cohen *et al.* 1996), we compared performance in the AX-CPT with two other cognitive tasks designed to probe processing of context, as a test of our hypothesis that a disturbance in the processing of context can provide a unified account of schizophrenic performance deficits across a variety of tasks. Performance in these tasks showed a modest but significant correlation in context-sensitive conditions (average $r = 0.38, P < 0.05$), but not control conditions (average $r = -0.02, P > 0.15$) matched for psychometric properties. These cross-task correlations are an important result, and contrast with historical failures to find such correlations among tasks that individually elicit schizophrenic performance deficits (Kopfstein & Neal 1972; Asarnow & MacCrimmon 1978). In previous studies, the detection of schizophrenic deficits, but failure to observe correlations, may have resulted from the use of tasks that included context-sensitive conditions (thus eliciting schizophrenic deficits), but measures of performance that were not sufficiently specific to these conditions. Aided by our computational models, our theory allowed us to decompose a set of disparate tasks, identify the conditions maximally sensitive to the processing of context, and demonstrate a predicted pattern of schizophrenic deficits across these tasks.

(c) Recent advances in simulation models

Our initial efforts involved models designed independently to address performance in a variety of different tasks. Recently, we have begun to adapt these models to conform to a more tightly constrained, and biologically plausible set of processing principles. These principles include: a) continuous (vs discrete) processing over time; b) interactivity (i.e. bi-directional connections) between processing layers; and c) the restriction of excitatory influences to between-module connections (information flow) and inhibitory influences to within-module connections (competition). Simulation work within this new, more highly integrated framework has addressed performance in a wide variety of tasks, including ones involving response competition, classical conditioning, covert spatial attention, and eye movements (Cohen *et al.* 1992; Cohen *et al.* 1994b; Armony *et al.* 1995; Forman & Cohen 1995). Most importantly, refinement of our earlier models has allowed us to address new, more detailed empirical data from tasks such as the AX-CPT.

For example, an important limitation of our original model of the CPT (Cohen & Servan-Schreiber 1992) was that it treated time in a discrete fashion (activation updates occurred only at whole-trial intervals). Therefore, while it could simulate accuracy data, it could not simulate the delay manipulations in our experiments, nor could it address the dynamics of performance (e.g. RT data). Our revision of the model overcomes these limitations, allowing us to simulate performance in continuous time (see Braver *et al.* 1995a for details). Thus, with the new model we can simulate reaction time as well as accuracy. To take full advantage of this feature of the new model, we have modified our version of the AX-CPT, so that responses are generated on every trial (one button for target, another for non-targets), thus providing RT data for correct as well as incorrect trials in every condition. We also added another trial condition to the task ('BY') that provides an important control measure by which to compare performance of the model against empirical data. The architectural addition of recurrent connectivity in the model allows us to directly examine the effects of delay on performance. Recurrent connections among units within the context layer allow it to actively maintain representations in the absence of external input. This makes it possible to interpose a delay between the cue and the probe (see figure 14.3), and then examine performance under conditions of different delay durations. We have tested the model with delays corresponding to both the short and long delays used in our empirical studies, and compared the model's performance with that of human subjects. As shown in figure 14.4, the model (solid line) fits a complex pattern of data concerning normal performance in this task (solid circles).

We have also examined the effects of degrading processing in the context layer of the model, by reducing the gain parameter of units in this layer (see Appendix 1). This manipulation produced a dramatic change in the profile of accuracy and RT data generated by the model across task conditions (dashed line in figure 4). These, in turn, make a number of new, and non-intuitive predictions concerning the accuracy and RT of schizophrenic vs. control subjects (Braver *et al.* 1995*b*). Among these is the prediction that, while schizophrenic RT's will be slower in most conditions, they will be comparable for correct responses in the AY condition (see figure 14.4). This prediction is especially interesting given the almost universal finding of slower RT's for schizophrenics in laboratory tasks. The model makes this prediction because under normal conditions, there is a relative slowing of correct (i.e. nontarget) responses in AY trials. This a result of the fact that the context set up by the occurrence of the 'A' cue is maintained over the delay and serves to prime the target response, which is actually the incorrect response to make in the AY condition. This produces interference with the correct response, slowing RT. Under conditions of reduced gain, however, the context information is less reliably maintained. This produces less priming of the target response, less interference with the correct response, and thus less slowing of RT. We have recently collected data from six schizophrenic subjects in this version of the task (open circles in figure 14.4), which provide preliminary corroboration of these predictions.

We have also used this model to examine the effects that different degrees of PFC disturbance may have on task performance. Panel (*a*) of figure 14.5 shows empirical data from our original study, with the performance of unmedicated subjects shown separately for first episode and multi-episode patients. Panel (*b*) shows the patterns predicted by the model for normal performance and for two levels of impairment of the context layer. If we assume that disturbances of PFC function are progressive with course of illness, then the pattern of empirical

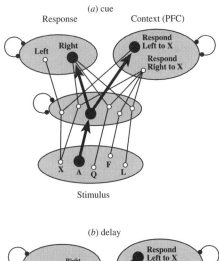

(a) cue

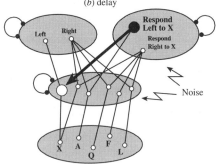

(b) delay

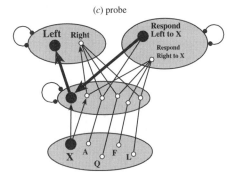

(c) probe

Fig. 14.3 Revised model of the AX-CPT task. Graphic conventions are the same as figure 14.1. Recurrent self-excitatory connections for units in the context module are not shown (see Braver *et al.* 1995a). Panels show sequence of network states during a target sequence (A-X) trial. Panel (*a*) shows the state of the network during presentation of the cue, Panel (*b*) its state during the delay between the cue and the probe, and Panel (*c*) its state during presentation of the probe. Note that the input unit for the letter X has connections to both of the response units, and thus requires additional input from the context layer in order to elicit the correct response.

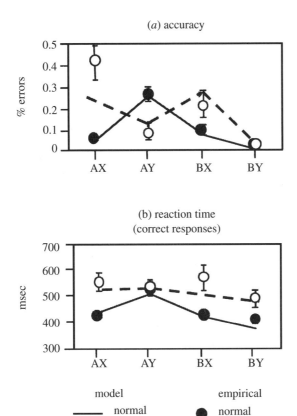

Fig. 14.4 Simulated and empirical performance in the AX-CPT task (long delay condition). Lines designate simulation results (solid: intact network; dashed: reduced gain in
context layer), circles designate empirical results (solid: normal subjects; open: pilot
data from schizophrenic subjects).

results closely matches the predictions of the model. In the model, a moderate
reduction of gain produces a pattern of results similar to that observed for first
episode patients: performance is impaired at the long but not short delay,
suggesting the presence of a 'memory' deficit (see appendix 2). A more severe
disturbance in the model (i.e. a greater reduction of gain) produces further
degradation of performance, similar to that observed for the multi-episode
patients: performance is now impaired at the short as well as the long delay,
suggesting the emergence of an additional 'inhibitory' deficit. Clinically, these
disturbances in 'memory' and 'inhibition' might have been viewed as separate
deficits, arising at different stages of illness. However, the model illustrates that,
in fact, both can be explained in terms of a single, progressive disturbance, that
varies only in severity. Of course, the results of these preliminary studies are by
no means definitive (given that the empirical findings are confounded by a

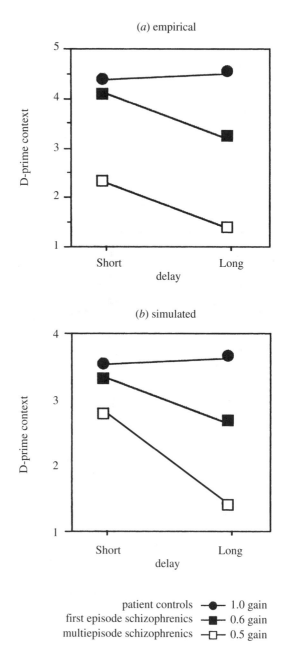

Fig. 14.5 Effects of severity of disturbance on performance in the AX-CPT task. Panel (*a*) compares performance of normal subjects to schizophrenic patients suffering from their first psychotic episode and those at a later stage of illness. Panel (*b*) shows performance of the model under different degrees of gain reduction.

number of factors, including the potential chronic effects of neuroleptic administration that may endure even with temporary discontinuation). Nevertheless,
they serve to highlight the potential value of computational models, both in
providing mechanistic and explicit accounts of empirical phenomena that may
elude less formal accounts, and in making subtle, and sometimes even counterintuitive predictions regarding new phenomena.

14.3 Current challenges and new directions

We believe that we have made significant headway in using computational
models to develop an explicit account of the mechanisms underlying the role
of PFC in cognitive control, using these to account for cognitive disturbances in
schizophrenia, and acquiring empirical support for the predictions made by
our account. At the same time, the mechanisms we have implemented are still
highly simplified, and lack several critical components necessary for a more
general account of cognitive control. First, although we assume that a characteristic of PFC function is its ability to actively maintain context representations, our models have used relatively limited mechanisms for active
maintenance, and have focused on tasks that do not include intervening stimuli
that could interfere with maintained representations. Our models do not incorporate mechanisms for managing such interference, a function typically
ascribed to PFC. Second, we have not specified how task-relevant information
is identified, gains access to PFC, and is updated at appropriate junctures
in processing. Finally, we have argued that context information can be used
to support task-relevant processing in a variety of ways—by representing
relatively abstract information (e.g. the relevant stimulus dimension in
the Stroop task), or more detailed, specific information (e.g. a particular previous stimulus in the AX-CPT). This requires that the representational scheme
within PFC be flexible enough to support a wide range of information. We
have not yet specified what this scheme is, nor the principles that might
characterize it.

To address these issues, we have begun to construct a new, more detailed
theory, that builds on our previous work using neurobiologically plausible
mechanisms to understand the role of PFC in cognitive control. The basic
structure of this theory is as follows: In order for a system to be able to
maintain information in the face of intervening, and potentially interfering
stimuli, a mechanism is required to stabilize these representations. We propose
that dopaminergic neuro-modulation of PFC implements a gating function,
that governs which representations gain access to PFC and when this occurs,
thus protecting them from interference. We assume that this gating mechanism
is driven by top-down projections from cortical areas and is able to learn when
to update PFC based on general principles of reward-based learning, thus
circumventing a potential regress in the locus of control. Furthermore, we
argue that the need to maintain representations in PFC has direct implications

for the nature of these representations. Specifically, we hypothesize that this leads to attractor-based representations that are both categorical and combinatorial, and that this provides a flexible scheme by which PFC can effectively bias processing in other parts of the system. Finally, we assume that, in order to perform controlled processing in novel domains, the system must be able to rapidly learn new associations, that can be used to guide behaviour. We hypothesize that this adaptability arises through interactions between PFC and the episodic storage capabilities of the hippocampal memory system.

Simulation studies are currently under way to establish the computational plausibility of this theory, and its ability to account for human performance in tasks that rely on cognitive control, that are more complex than those we have studied to date. In the remainder of this chapter, we briefly review the components of this theory that address the mechanisms of active maintenance within PFC, and the nature of the representations involved. Our theory concerning the interactions between PFC and hippocampus is presented elsewhere (Cohen & O'Reilly 1996), and thus is omitted from this discussion.

(a) Mechanisms of active maintenance within PFC

A large body of converging evidence suggests that PFC plays a crucial role in maintaining task-relevant information in an active state. It is well established that populations of neurons in monkey PFC exhibit sustained, stimulus-specific activity during delays between a stimulus and a contingent response (Barone & Joseph 1989; Fuster & Alexander 1971; Goldman-Rakic 1987; Kubota & Niki 1971). Neuropsychological studies of frontally-damaged patients also provide strong support for the idea that PFC plays a role in active maintenance (Damasio 1985; Petrides & Milner 1982; Stuss et al. 1994), and a growing number of neuroimaging studies have strengthened this view (Cohen et al. 1994a; Grasby et al. 1993; Jonides et al. 1993; Petrides et al. 1993). However, the specific mechanisms by which neural activity in PFC is sustained has not been clearly elucidated.

(i) Attractor systems

A number of different computational approaches have been reported to deal with tasks requiring short-term storage in neurobiologically plausible terms. One of the most common is the use of recurrent connections between neuron-like processing units (Hopfield 1982). With sufficiently strong recurrent connections, networks of these units will develop 'attractors', defined as stable states in which a particular pattern of activity is maintained. Thus, attractors can be used to actively store information. Indeed, a number of computational models have demonstrated that both physiological and behavioural data regarding PFC function can be captured in simple tasks using an attractor-based scheme (Braver et al. 1995a; Dehaene & Changeux 1989; Zipser et al. 1993). However, in simple attractor systems, the state is strongly determined by its inputs. Thus, presentation of a new input will interfere with the state of the system and drive it into a new attractor state. Although attractor networks can be configured to display resistance to disruption from input (i.e. hysteresis), this impairs their ability to be updated in a precise and flexible manner. One way in which attractor networks can overcome these difficulties is through the addition of a gating mechanism. Such systems only respond to inputs, and change their attractor state, when the 'gate' is opened. Below, we examine the possibility that the DA system provides a gating signal in PFC which acts to maintain context representations in an active, stable, and flexible manner.

(ii) *Modulatory effects of DA*

A number of lines of evidence suggest that DA acts in a modulatory fashion in PFC, which is consistent with a role for DA in gating access to active memory. DA agonists have been found to improve memory performance in humans (Luciana *et al.* 1992), while in primates DA antagonists interfere with performance in delayed-response tasks (Sawaguchi & Goldman-Rakic 1991) and directly affect PFC neuronal activity (Williams & Goldman-Rakic 1995). Electron microscopy studies of the local connectivity patterns of DA in PFC have revealed that DA typically makes triadic contacts with prefrontal pyramidal cells and excitatory afferents, and also with inhibitory interneurons (Lewis *et al.* 1992; Williams & Goldman-Rakic 1993). The triadic synaptic complexes formed in PFC suggest that DA can modulate both afferent input and local inhibition. Electrophysiological data support this view, indicating that DA potentiates both afferent excitatory and local inhibitory signals (Chiodo & Berger 1986; Penit-Soria *et al.* 1987).

(iii) *DA as a gating signal*

In our previous work, we have simulated the modulatory effects of DA as a change in the gain (slope) of the activation function of processing units in PFC (Cohen & Servan-Schreiber 1992; Cohen & Servan-Schreiber 1993; Servan-Schreiber *et al.* 1990), thus influencing the active maintenance of information. In this work, we assumed that DA effects were prolonged (tonic), consistent with the widely-held assumption that neuromodulatory systems (such as DA, noradrenaline (NA), 5-hydroxytryptamine (5-HT)) are slow-acting, diffuse, and non-specific in informational content. However, recent findings suggest a revision of this view. Schultz and colleagues (Schultz 1986, 1992) observed in behaving primates that during learning of a spatial delayed response task, stimuli that failed to activate ventral tegmental area DA neurons on initial presentation, came to elicit transient activity when the animal learned that they were significant for the task. Specifically, Schultz's group observed transient, stimulus-locked activity in response to stimuli that were themselves unpredictable, but predicted later meaningful events. This is precisely the timing required for this information to be gated into and maintained in active memory. These findings, together with the modulatory effects of DA on PFC afferents, suggest that DA may serve as a gating signal for attractor networks housed within PFC.

(iv) DA as a learning signal

At the same time, DA is widely thought to be involved in reward learning (Wise & Rompre 1989). Indeed, in Schultz's experiments, DA activity was found for cues that were predictive of a reward. Montague *et al.* (1996) have built on these findings, and recently reported a computational model that treats DA as a widely distributed error signal, driving the learning of temporal predictors of reinforcement. Intriguingly, the parameter they used to simulate the learning effects of DA is formally equivalent to the gain parameter used in our model to simulate its modulatory effects on active maintenance in PFC (Thimm *et al.* 1996). Furthermore, it is well established that DA neurons in VTA receive strong cortical projections, particularly from PFC (Oades & Halliday 1987). These observations have lead us to the following refinements of our original theory (Cohen & Servan-Schreiber 1992): a) DA implements gating and learning functions, both of which rely on the same mechanism; b) the gating function is used to regulate the access of information to active memory within PFC, and protect it from interference; c) the learning function produces training signals in the cortex; d) both of these functions can be elicited by descending cortical signals; e) the coincidence of the gating and learning signals produces cortical associations between the information being gated, and a triggering of the gating signal in the future. The power of this theory, if confirmed, is that it will describe a system that has both the capacity to control its behaviour (by gating and stabilizing representations within PFC) and, critically, the ability to learn how and when to do so on its own, thus avoiding the perennial problem of a homunculus in most theories of executive control.

In recent simulation studies, we have implemented a gating mechanism, and shown that it can successfully account for the phenomena addressed by our earlier models involving active maintenance. However, the assumption that DA has phasic, in addition to tonic effects in PFC changes the dynamics of processing in our simulations, and makes a number of new predictions regarding both normal and schizophrenic performance in delay tasks. It also allows us to simulate performance in tasks not possible with our previous models (e.g. ones involving intervening distractors). Our work has currently turned to the empirical validation of these simulation studies, and an integration of the gating mechanism with one for reward learning.

(b) Nature of representations within PFC

In addition to maintaining representations in active memory, our theory requires that PFC be able to use these to control behaviour, by biasing processing in other parts of the system. This was illustrated in the Stroop model, where activation of a unit representing the colour dimension biased processing in favour of colour naming over word reading. Here, the relevant representation was a stimulus dimension (colour vs word form). However, as we have noted, this might be any bit of information that specifies the dimensions of information relevant to the task. Important questions remain about how this information is actually represented, and how representations can emerge that provide the flexibility characteristic of human behaviour, without requiring unlimited capacity. It would be unreasonable to expect, for example, that a separate, dedicated unit (or set of units) exists to bias processing for every task that people are able to perform. In this section, we propose a representational scheme that we believe can address these issues. We consider two functional requirements that constrain the nature of representations within PFC: a) the need to be self-maintaining; and b) the ability to flexibly bias processing in the rest of the neocortex. Our hypothesis is that these dual constraints shape the nature of PFC representations in a synergistic fashion: The constraint imposed by the need to be self-maintaining leads to representations that can be used in a combinatorial, and therefore highly flexible way.

(i) *Independent*

The strong recurrent excitation required for self-maintenance imposes the constraint that if two representations are to be reliably distinguishable, they must also be independent of one another. This can be illustrated by the simple case shown in figure 14.6, where three processing units are used to store three different representations. Panel (*a*) shows how this can be done using distributed representations of features (e.g. keyboard, monitor and speaker) that efficiently encode the shared structure among the items (terminal, synthesizer, and television). This supports spreading-activation like computations (pattern completion, content-addressable memory, etc.) that are considered to be characteristic of posterior neocortex (e.g. McClelland *et al.* 1995; Plaut *et al.* 1996). However, problems arise when recurrent connections are made strong enough to maintain activity in the absence of external input. This can be seen in the example, by noting that no value of excitatory weights between these features would allow one pair of units to remain active without activating the third. This can be solved by making each feature independent of the others, with its own recurrent self-excitation (Panel (*b*)). However, this eliminates the representation of the items (e.g. terminal) as a related (connected) set of features (keyboard and monitor). Items can still be stored by activating the appropriate combination of features, but without the benefits of spreading activation among them. Thus, this scheme sacrifices the representation of the internal structure of each item, and its relationship to others. An alternative is to dedicate a separate unit to each item (e.g. a new unit for terminal), since semantic structure is already lost. This would add units to the system, but might only occur for frequently encountered or important items. Either way, the critical point is that there is a trade-off between the capacity for self-maintenance and the ability to represent structured (semantic) relationships among features and/or items.

(ii) *Flexible*

Representations in PFC must be flexible enough to account for the variety of tasks of which humans are capable. We propose that this flexibility is provided by the independence of self-maintaining representations. Precisely because they

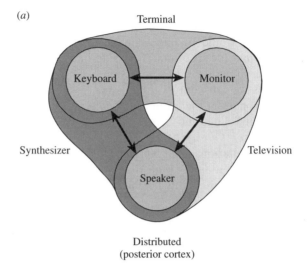

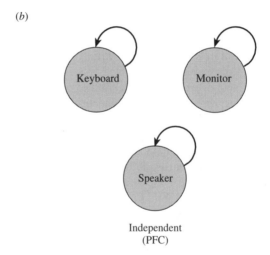

Fig. 14.6 An example of distributed versus independent representations. Panel (*a*) shows the associative connections between features used in the distributed representation of three different concepts. Panel (*b*) shows these units as independent features, which can be used to support self maintenance and combinatorial representations, but at the expense of capturing the associative relationships between the concepts being represented.

are independent of one another, there are no constraints on which representations can be active at the same time, and so they can be used in arbitrary combinations. The ability to rapidly adapt behaviour to novel situations (e.g. problem solving) requires just this capacity for the arbitrary recombination of existing knowledge, and the idea that this capacity resides within PFC is consistent with the neuropsychological literature suggesting that damage to PFC impairs this flexibility, and problem solving abilities (Shallice & Burgess 1991*b*). However, while combinatoriality is a necessary requirement for flexibility, it is not sufficient. The representations themselves must correspond in appropriate ways to information stored in the rest of system, so that their activation can bias processing in behaviourally useful ways.

(iii) *Categorical*

We assume that the content of PFC representations is constrained by the functional characteristics we have just described —self-maintaining and independent—in interaction with posterior neocortex, under conditions of Hebbian learning. The independence of PFC representations frees them to become associated with arbitrary dimensions of information in the neocortex. We suggest that these effects will generate representations within PFC that are categorical in character. That is, PFC representations will become associated with the central tendency of similar representations within the neocortex. We use the term 'categorical' here guardedly, as we do not want to suggest that all representations within PFC correspond directly to 'basic level', or even verbalizable categories. For example, we imagine that PFC representations will exist for very general categories of information, such as stimulus dimensions (e.g. colour, shape, size, etc.) or natural and/or functional kinds (e.g. animals, tools), but also much more specific ones (e.g. a particular colour, word, or person which, though more specific, also correspond to invariants in the world) and non-obvious or abstract ones (i.e. ones that do not correspond directly to recognizable concepts). Finally, we assume that a primary determinant of these representations is their behavioural relevance—that is, their ability to successfully bias the interpretation of stimuli and the selection of responses to produce task-appropriate behaviour. Thus, dimensions that are frequent, or particularly relevant to behaviour are most likely to be represented.

(iv) *Properties of PFC vs posterior neocortex*

The preceding discussion highlights features of representations and processing within PFC that distinguish it from other parts of association neocortex. We assume that posterior neocortex uses distributed representations, and attractor states that are not constrained to be self-maintaining. Thus, we view PFC and posterior neocortex as having complementary properties. Each is specialized along particular dimensions of representation and processing, that involve tradeoffs in functionality (e.g. self-maintaining and flexible vs representation of structured knowledge). We propose that the benefit of such a scheme is fully realized only when these systems interact with one another. Semantically rich, distributed representations in posterior neocortex are not only required to encode the statistical structure of the environment, and support the processing pathways responsible for task performance, but also serve as the base for developing the appropriate set of representations in PFC. These, in turn, provide representations that enable the flexible biasing of representations in posterior neocortex, and maintenance over intervals required to guide task performance in a temporally extended manner.

14.4 Summary and conclusions

The prefrontal cortex is the region of the brain most significantly expanded in humans compared to other species, and appears to be at the heart of those faculties that we consider to be uniquely human, such as execution of the complex behaviours involved in planning and problem solving. Consistent with these observations, schizophrenia, which is thought to involve frontal dysfunction, is an illness that is unique to humans. At best, the effort to understand the function of PFC, and its role in schizophrenia promises to be a complex endeavor, and will require the most powerful conceptual tools we have available. We believe that computational modelling represents one such tool. We began this article by reviewing initial progress in the use of computational models to understand the role of PFC in cognitive control, and its impairment in schizophrenia. We illustrated how such models can provide new insights into the mechanisms underlying cognitive control, can make new predictions about the behavioural performance of both normal and schizophrenic subjects, and provided examples of empirical support for such predictions. We then identified some of the limitations of our current approach, and outlined a set of new principles that we believe can be used to define a more complete theory of PFC function and cognitive control. According to this theory, PFC governs processing in a top-down manner, while at the same time remaining responsive to bottom-up input from other parts of the system. We believe that this interplay of bottom-up and top-down processing, that we hypothesize is mediated by the DA system, can give rise to a system of 'regulated interactivity' that accounts for the full flexibility of control exhibited in human behaviour. These are bold claims. However, as our previous work has shown, by pursuing such ideas within a computational framework, we are able to make them explicit in simulation models. This not only provides a check on their conceptual validity, but also allows us to explore, in detail, their implications for behaviour. Success in this effort would not only provide insights into the mechanisms underlying some of our highest and uniquely human faculties, but might also allow to us to contend better with their failings, which appear to lie at the heart of our deepest vulnerabilities.

Acknowledgements

We thank David Servan-Schreiber, Marius Usher, Jay McClelland, and David Plaut, for the many hours of productive discussion that we have shared with them, and for their comments and insights which helped substantially to shape the ideas presented in this chapter. We also thank Deanna Barch, Cameron Carter, Grace Nah and Vijoy Abraham, without whom the empirical studies described may never have been completed.

This work was supported by a NIMH Physician Scientist Award (MH00673), a NIMH FIRST Award (MH47073), and a research grant from the Scottish Rite Schizophrenia Research Program, N.M.J., U.S.A. to the first author, as well by a NIMH Program Project (MH47566) and a NIMH Center (MH45156) in which the first author is a participant.

Appendix 1

The gain parameter regulates the responsivity of units to their input, so that a reduction of gain degrades the fidelity of representations in this layer. In our previous work, we have used this parameter to approximate the influence that brain catecholamines have on network processing characteristics and behaviour (Servan-Schreiber et al. 1990). The relationship of dopamine to gain, and its influence on PFC function is discussed in greater detail in the last section of this paper. In the current model, gain was reduced exactly the same amount as in our previous work (from 1.0 to 0.6), to simulate the effects of reduced dopamine in PFC that we and others have hypothesized to occur in schizophrenia (Cohen & Servan-Schreiber 1992, 1993; Geraud et al. 1987; Karoum et al. 1987; Levin 1984; Weinberger et al. 1988).

Appendix 2

The reader will note that, even at the long delay, BX errors still involve a failure of inhibition, in addition to a memory failure. Thus, impairment of first-episode patients in this condition could reflect the dual burden of a requirement for memory + inhibition, rather than a specific sensitivity to the memory load. To address this concern, we have also examined performance in the AY condition. This provides a measure of memory function unconfounded by inhibitory demands: AY trials will induce a tendency to respond only to the extent that the subject has an intact representation of context, which primes a target response; in the absence of such information, there should be no such tendency to respond. This is confirmed in our simulations, which exhibit a reduction of such errors at the long vs short delay, even with a moderate disturbance in the processing of context, and an accentuation of this effect at both delays when the disturbance to the context layer is worsened. These effects have the added virtue of predicting improvements of performance as the severity of disturbance is increased. Our empirical data conform to these predictions: first episode subjects showed a significant number of AY errors at the short delay (16%), comparable to the rate observed in control populations, indicating intact processing of context. At the long delay, however, they showed a reduction of this effect (6% errors), indicating a memory deficit unconfounded by inhibitory demands. The multi-episode subjects showed a general accentuation of this effect (7% and 1% AY errors at the long and short delays, respectively).

References

Abramczyk, R. R., Jordan, D. E. & Hegel, M. 1983, 'Reverse' Stroop effect in the performance of schizophrenics. *Perceptual and Motor Skills* **56**, 99–106.
Anderson, J. R. 1983 *The architecture of cognition.* Cambridge, MA: Harvard University Press.
Armony, J. L., Servan-Schreiber, D., Cohen, J. D. & LeDoux, J. E. 1995 An anatomically constrained neural network model of fear conditioning. *Behavioural Neuroscience* **109** (2), 1–12.
Asarnow, R. F. & MacCrimmon, X. 1978 Residual performance deficit in clinically remitted schizophrenics: a marker of schizophrenia? *J. Abnormal Psychology* **87**, 597–608.
Baddeley, A. D. 1986 *Working memory.* New York: Oxford University Press.
Barone, P. & Joseph, J. P. 1989 Prefrontal cortex and spatial sequencing in macaque monkey. *Experimental Brain Res.* **78**, 447–64.
Bianchi, L. 1922 *The mechanism of the brain and the function of the frontal lobes.* Edinburgh: Livingstone.
Braver, T. S., Cohen, J. D. & Servan-Schreiber, D. 1995*a* A computational model of prefrontal cortex function. In *Advances in neural information processing systems* (ed. D. S. Touretzky, G. Tesauro & T. K. Leen), vol. 7, pp. 141–48. Cambridge, MA: MIT Press.
Braver, T. S., Cohen, J. D. & Servan-Schreiber, D. 1995*b* Neural network simulations of schizophrenic performance in a variant of the CPT-AX: a predicted double dissociation. *Schizophrenia Res.* **15**(1–2), 110.
Carter, C. S., Robertson, L. C., Nordahl, T. E., O'Shora Celaya, L. J. & Chaderjian, M. C. 1993 Abnormal processing of irrelevant information in schizophrenia: the role of illness subtype. *Psychiatry Res.* **4**, 178–26.
Chapman, L. J. & Chapman, J. P. 1978 The measurement of differential deficit. Journal of *Psychiatric Res.* **14**, 303–11.
Chapman, L. J., Chapman, J. P. & Miller, G. A. 1964 A theory of verbal behaviour in schizophrenia. In *Progress in experimental personality research* (ed. B. A. Maher), vol. 4, pp. 135–67. New York: Academic Press.
Chiodo, L. & Berger, T. 1986 Interactions between dopamine and amino-acid induced excitation and inhibition in the striatum. *Brain Res.* **375**, 198–203.
Cohen, J. D. & Carter, C. S. 1996 Schizophrenic performance in the Stroop task: empirical findings and a theoretical model of differences between faciliation and interference effects. (In preparation.)
Cohen, J. D. & O'Reilly, R. C. 1996 A preliminary theory of the interactions between prefrontal cortex and hippocampus that contribute to planning and prospective memory. In *Prospective memory: theory and applications* (ed. M. Brandimonte, G Einstein & M. McDaniel). Hillsdale, NJ: Erlbaum.
Cohen, J. D. & Servan-Schreiber, D. 1992 Context, cortex and dopamine: a connectionist approach to behaviour and biology in schizophrenia. *Psychological Review* **99** 45–77.

Cohen, J. D. & Servan-Schreiber, D. 1993 A theory of dopamine function and cognitive deficits in schizophrenia. *Schizophrenia Bull.* **19**(1), 85–104.

Cohen, J. D., Dunbar, K. & McClelland, J. L. 1990 On the control of automatic processes: a parallel distributed processing account of the Stroop effect. *Psychological Rev.* **97**(3), 332–61.

Cohen, J. D., Servan-Schreiber, D. & McClelland, J. L. 1992 A parallel distributed processing approach to automaticity. *Am. J. Psychology* **105**, 239–69.

Cohen, J. D., Forman, S. D., Braver, T. S., Casey, B. J., Servan-Schreiber, D. & Noll, D. C. 1994*a* Activation of prefrontal cortex in a nonspatial working memory task with functional MRI. *Human Brain Mapping* **1**, 293–304.

Cohen, J. D., Romero, R. D., Farah, M. J. & Servan-Schreiber, D. 1994*b* Mechanisms of spatial attention: the relation of macrostructure to microstructure in parietal neglect. *J. Cognitive Neuroscience* **6**(4), 377–87.

Cohen, J. D., Barch, D. M., Carter, C. S. & Servan-Schreiber, D. 1996 Schizophrenic deficits in the processing of context: converging evidence from three theoretically motivated cognitive tasks. (Submitted.)

Cornblatt, B. A. & Keilpk, J. G. 1994 Impaired attention, genetics, and the pathophysiology of schizophrenia. *Schizophrenia Bull.* **20**(1), 31–62.

Damasio, A. R. 1985 The frontal lobes. In *Clinical neuropsychology* (ed. K. M. Heilman & E. Valenstein), pp. 339–75. New York: Oxford University Press.

Dehaene, S. & Changeux, J. P. 1989 A simple model of prefrontal cortex function in delayed-response tasks. *J. Cognitive Neurosci.* **1**, 244–61.

Forman, S. D. & Cohen, J. D. 1995 Modelling saccadic eye movements in schizophrenia: insights into memory mechanisms. *Schizophrenia Res.* **15**(1–2), 175.

Fuster, J. M. & Alexander, G. E. 1971 Neuron activity related to short-term memory. *Science* **173**, 652–54.

Gathercole, S. E. 1994 Neuropsychology and working memory: a review. *Neuropsychology* **8**(4), 494–505.

Geraud, G., Arne-Bes, M. C., Guell, A. & Bes, A. 1987 Reversibility of hemodynamic hypofrontality in schizophrenia. *J. Cerebral Blood Flow Metabolism* **7**, 9–12.

Goldman-Rakic, P. S. 1987 Circuitry of primate prefrontal cortex and regulation of behaviour by representational memory. In *Handbook of physiology—the nervous system* (ed. F. Plum & V. Mountcastle), vol. 5, pp. 373–417. Bethesda, MD: American Physiological Society.

Goldman-Rakic, P. S. 1991 Prefrontal cortical dysfunction in schizophrenia: the relevance of working memory. *Psychopathology and the Brain* 1–23.

Grasby, P. M., Frith, C. D., Friston, K. J., Bench, C., Frackowiak, R. S. J. & Dolan, R. J. 1993 Functional mapping of brain areas implicated in auditory-verbal memory function. *Brain* **116**, 1–20.

Hopfield, J. J. 1982 Neural networks and physical systems with emergent collective computational abilities. *Proc. Natn. Acad. Sci.* **79**, 2554–58.

Jonides, J., Smith, E. E., Koeppe, R. A., Awh, E., Minoshima, S. & Mintun, M. A. 1993 Spatial working memory in humans as revealed by PET. *Nature* **363**, 623–25.

Karoum, F., Karson, C. N., Bigelow, L. B., Lawson, W. B. & Wyatt, R. J. 1987 Preliminary evidence of reduced combined output of dopamine and its metabolites in chronic schizophrenia. *Arch. General Psychiatry* **44** (July), 604–07.

Kimberg, D. Y. & Farah, M. J. 1993 A unified account of cognitive impairments following frontal lobe damage: the role of working memory in complex, organized behaviour. *J. Experimental Psychology: General* **122**(4), 411–28.

Kopfstein, J. H. & Neal, J. M. 1972 A multivariate study of attention dysfunction in schizophrenia. *J. Abnormal Psychology* **3**, 294–98.

Kolb, B. & Whishaw, I. Q. 1983 Performance of schizophrenia patients on tests sensitive to left or right frontal, temporal. *J. Nervous Mental Disease* **171**(7), 435–43.

Kornetsky, C. & Orzack, M. H. 1978 Physiological and behavioural correlates of attention dysfunction in schizophrenic patients. *J. Psychiatric Res.* **14**, 69–79.

Kraeplin, E. 1950 *Dementia praecox and paraphrenia* (transl. J. Zinkin). New York: International Universities Press, Inc.

Kubota, K. & Niki, H. 1971 Prefrontal cortical unit activity and delayed alternation performance in monkeys. *J. Neurophysiology* **34**, 337–47.

Levin, S. 1984 Frontal lobe dysfunctions in schizophrenia. II. Impairments of psychological and brain functions. *J. Psychological Res.* **18**, 57–82.

Lewis, D. A., Hayes, T. L., Lund, J. S. & Oeth, K. M. 1992 Dopamine and the neural circuitry of primate prefrontal cortex: implications for schizophrenia research. *Neuropsychopharmacology* **6**(2), 127–34.

Luciana, M., Depue, R. A., Arbisi, P. & Leon, A. 1992 Facilitation of working memory in humans by a D_2 dopamine receptor agonist. *J. Cognitive Neurosci.* **4**(1), 58–68.

Luria, A. R. 1969 Frontal lobe syndromes. In *Handbook of clinical neurology* (ed. P. J. Vinken & G. W. Bruyn), vol. 2, pp. 725–57. New York: Elsevier.

Manschreck, T., Maher, B. A., Milavetz, J. J., Ames, D., Weisstein, C. C. & Schneyer, M. L. 1988 Semantic priming in thought disordered schizophrenic patients. *Schizophrenic Res.* 61–66.

McClelland, J. L., McNaughton, B. L. & O'Reilly, R. C. 1995 Why there are complementary learnings systems in the hippocampus and neocortex: insights from the successes and failures of connectionist models of learning and memory. *Psychological Rev.* **102**, 419–57.

Montague, P. R., Dayan, P. & Sejnowski, T. J. 1996 A framework for mesencephalic dopamine systems based on predictive Hebbian learning. *J. Neurosci.* **16**, 1936–47.

Nuechterlein, K. H. 1991 Vigilance in schizophrenia and related disorders. *In Handbook of schizophrenia* (ed. S. R. Steinhauer, J. H. Gruzelier & J. Zubin), vol. 5. *Neuropsychology, psychophysiology, and information processing*, pp. 397–433. Amsterdam: Elsevier.

Oades, R. D. & Halliday, G. M. 1987 Ventral tegmental (A10) system: neurobiology. 1. Anatomy and connectivity. *Brain Res. Rev.* **12**, 117–65.

Parasuraman, R. 1979 Memory load and event rate control sensitivity decrements in sustained attention. *Science* **205**, 924–27.

Park, S. & Holzman, P. S. 1992 Schizophrenics show spatial working memory deficits. *Arch. General Psychiatry*, **49**, 975–82.

Penit-Soria, J., Audinat, E. & Crepel, F. 1987 Excitation of rat prefrontal cortical neurons by dopamine: an *in vitro* electrophysiological study. *Brain Res.* **425**, 263–74.

Petrides, E. & Milner, B. 1982 Deficits on subject-ordered tasks after frontal-and temporal-lobe lesions in man. *Neuropsychologia* **20**, 249–62.

Petrides, M. E., Alivisatos, B., Evans, A. C. & Meyer, E. 1993 Dissociation of human mid-dorsolateral from posterior dorsolateral frontal cortex in memory processing. *Proc. Natn. Acad. Sci.* **90**, 873–77.

Plaut, D. C., McClelland, J. L., Seidenberg, M. S. & Patterson, K. 1996 Understanding normal and impaired word reading: computational principles in quasi-regular domains. *Psychological Rev.* **103**, 56–115.

Roberts Jr, R. J., Hager, L. D. & Heron, C. 1994 Prefrontal cognitive processes: working memory and inhibition in the antisaccade task. *J. Experimental Psychology: General* **123**(4), 374–93.

Rosvold, H. E., Mirsky, A. F., Sarason, I., Bransome, E. D. & Beck, L. H. 1956 A continuous performance test of brain damage. *J. Consulting Psychology* **20**(5), 343–50.

Rumelhart, D. E. & McClelland, J. L. 1986 *Parallel distributed processing: explorations in the microstructure of cognition*, vols 1 and 2. Cambridge, MA: MIT Press.

Sawaguchi, T. & Goldman-Rakic, P. S. 1991 D1 dopamine receptors in prefrontal cortex: involvement in working memory. *Science* **251**, 947–50.

Schultz, W. 1986 Responses of midbrain dopamine neurons to behavioural trigger stimuli in the monkey. *J. Neurophysiology* **56**, 1439–62.

Schultz, W. 1992 Activity of dopamine neurons in the behaving primate. *Seminars in Neurosciences* **4**, 129–38.

Servan-Schreiber, D., Cohen, J. D. & Steingard, S. 1996, Schizophrenic deficits in the processing of context: A test of a theoretical model. *Arch. General Psychiatry* **53**, *110–112.*

Servan-Schreiber, D., Printz, H. & Cohen, J. D. 1990 A network model of catecholamine effects: gain, signal-to-noise ratio, and behaviour. *Science* **249**, 892–95.

Shallice, T. 1982 Specific impairments of planning. *Phil. Trans. R. Soc. Lond.* **B298**, 199–209.

Shallice, T. & Burgess, P. 1991*a* Higher-order cognitive impairments and frontal lobe lesions in man. In *Frontal lobe function and dysfunction* (ed. H. S. Levin, H. M. Eisenberg & A. L. Benton). New York: Oxford University.

Shallice, T. & Burgess, P. W. 1991*b* Deficits in strategy application following frontal lobe damage in man. *Brain* **114**, 727–41.

Storms, L. H. & Broen, W. E. 1969 A theory of schizophrenic behavioural disorganization. *Arch. General Psychiatry* **20** (Feb), 129–44.

Stuss, D. T., Eskes, G. A. & Foster, J. K. 1994 Experimental neuropsychological studies of frontal lobe function. In *Handbook of neuropsychology* (ed. F. Boller & J. Grafman), vol. 9. Amsterdam: Elsevier.

Thimm, G., Moerland, P. & Fusler, E. 1996 The interchangeability of learning rate and gain in back-propagation networks. *Neural Computation* **8**, 451–69.

Wapner, S. & Krus, D. M. 1960 Effects of lysergic acid diethylamide, and differences between normals and schizophrenics, on the Stroop colour-word test. *J. Neuropsychiatry* 76–81.

Weinberger, D., Berman, K. & Illowsky, B. 1988 Physiological dysfunction of the dorsolateral prefrontal cortex. III. A new cohort and evidence for a monoaminergic mechanism. *Arch. General Psychiatry* **45**, 609–15.

Weinberger, D. R., Berman, K. F. & Zec, R. F. 1986 Physiological dysfunction of dorsolateral prefrontal cortex in schizophrenia. I. Regional cerebral blood flow evidence. *Arch. General Psychiatry* **43**, 114–25.

Williams, G. V. & Goldman-Rakic, P. S. 1995 Modulation of memory fields by dopamine D1 receptors in prefrontal cortex. *Nature* **376**, 572–75.

Williams, M. S. & Goldman-Rakic, P. S. 1993 Characterization of the dopaminergic innervation of the primate frontal cortex using a dopamine-specific antibody. *Cerebral Cortex* **3**, 199–222.

Wise, R. A. & Rompre, P.-P. 1989 Brain dopamine and reward. *Ann. Rev. Psychology* **40**, 191–225.

Wynne, L. C., Cromwell, R. L. & Matthysse, S. 1978 *The nature of schizophrenia: new approaches to research and treatment.* New York: John Wiley and Sons, Inc.

Wysocki, J. J. & Sweet, J. I. 1985 Identification of brain damaged, schizophrenic, and normal medical patients using a brief neuropsychological screening battery. *Int. J. Clinical Neuropsychology* **7**(1), 40–44.

Zipser, D., Kehue, B., Littlewort, G. & Fuster, J. 1993 A spiking network model of short-term active memory. *J. Neurosci.* **13**, 3406–20.

Zubin, J. 1975 Problem of attention in schizophrenia. *In Experimental approaches to psychopathology* (ed. M. I. Kietzman, S. Sutton & J. Zubin), pp. 139–66. New York: Academic Press.

15

Discussions and conclusions

A. C. Roberts, T. W. Robbins and L. Weiskrantz

The Meeting was proposed as a discussion of the cognitive and *executive* processes of the prefrontal cortex. The decision to denote cognitive and executive separately was deliberate, as it cannot be assumed that all of the cognitive functions of the prefrontal cortex are 'executive' in nature. Of course, this begs the question of what exactly is meant by the term 'executive'. There was a good deal of consensus in the Meeting about the general meaning of this term, but everyone recognized the difficulties of defining this loose set of cognitive functions in unitary terms. Thus, for most of the investigators, the term executive functioning connotes the optimal scheduling of operation of different components of complex tasks that depend on more dedicated or modular mechanisms (generally mediated by posterior cortical structures). This collection of operations would include the types of processes summarized in Chapter 3 by Shallice & Burgess (under the umbrella of 'supervisory' functions), including, for example, appropriate inhibitory mechanisms (e.g. for selective attention and switching between two or more tasks, see Baddeley & Della Sala, Chapter 2) and also the monitoring of processes such as retrieval from long-term memory and also of performance of intended actions (see Frith, Chapter 13). The controversy about the term 'executive function' comes not so much from disagreements about candidate cognitive mechanisms, but more from their inter-relationships. To what degree, for example, can they be considered unitary in nature? This issue was considered by several of the participants, and there was general convergence of evidence that different tests of executive function did not necessarily inter-correlate to a high degree (Duncan *et al.* 1995; see also Chapters 2, 3 and 9). This implies that the term 'executive function' cannot be a unitary construct and, currently, the implications of this form an area of considerable theoretical interest in cognitive psychology (see, for example, the recent volume edited by Rabbitt (1997)). On the other hand, the notion of dissociable executive functions that may be organized in a hierarchical or heterarchical manner (see Chapter 2) may be entirely compatible with emergent concepts about the anatomical and functional organization of the prefrontal cortex (see, for example, Barbas & Pandya 1989).

On logical grounds, however, it makes little sense to equate executive functioning to the prefrontal cortex alone. Caution was urged in the often interchangeable usage of the terms 'frontal' and 'executive' functioning by Baddeley & Della Sala, who showed that not all 'frontal' patients display behavioural disturbances characteristic of the dysexecutive syndrome and, likewise, there are some patients that display the dysexecutive syndrome in the absence of obvious frontal lobe damage. This point is a reworking of the familar principle in neuropsychology that there can be no 'pure' tasks for the purpose of localizing brain functions. However, it is also apparent from Chapter 5 by Pandya & Yeterian that the anatomical connections of the prefrontal cortex have many ramifications in different sets of neural networks where malfunction outside of the prefrontal cortex itself would thus be likely to impair prefrontal functions.

The finding that not all frontal patients display dysexecutive behaviour does of course imply that the prefrontal cortex itself is not unitary in function, suggesting instead heterogeneity of cognitive and executive processing within the prefrontal cortex. The fact that it has proven so difficult to provide unequivocal evidence to support this viewpoint was suggested to represent shortcomings in the approaches that have so far been used. In the past, the classic neuropsychological approach, whether it be in humans or experimental monkeys, has been to attempt to map the location of a lesion onto a particular deficit. This has met with only limited success in identifying functionally distinct subregions within the prefrontal cortex, perhaps as a consequence of far greater emphasis on differentiating prefrontal regions according to specific tasks rather than specific cognitive processes. However, even when the emphasis has been towards localizing processes rather than tasks, progress has still been hampered by a failure to define adequately the component processes being investigated. This is exemplified by attempts to characterize the prefrontal cortex in terms of working memory and inhibitory control processes.

Working memory and the prefrontal cortex: how good is the fit?

Working memory, as defined by Baddeley & Hitch (1974) is composed of at least two subsidiary slave systems, the phonological loop which deals with speech-based information and the sketchpad that deals with visuospatial information. The central executive component was proposed to be responsible for the attentional control of working memory and hence in the attentional control of the two slave systems. Since the original formulation of this theory, working memory deficits have been ascribed to the impaired performance of humans and non-human primates with frontal lobe damage on a range of tests without clear specifications as to which component of working memory may have been disrupted. It can be seen how this may lead to discrepancies between results with regard to localization of function when the same term may be used to describe different functional deficits. For example, an issue raised at the meeting concerned the distinction between short-term and working memory deficits. Short-term memory, within the context of the Baddeley & Hitch working memory model, is considered to represent the processing that takes place in the subsidiary slave systems with deficits in short-term memory being associated primarily with posterior cortical damage, such as patient KF (Warrington & Shallice 1969) rather than with frontal cortical damage. In contrast, the description of the role of the prefrontal cortex in 'on-line' processing as described by Goldman-Rakic (1987) has obvious parallels with short-term memory. However, consideration of the spatial delayed response task, which has been used to study 'on-line' processing within the prefrontal cortex suggests that it requires additional processes over and above the short-term memorial requirement including that of inhibitory control which prevents the monkey responding to the previously rewarded spatial location on the subsequent trial (Diamond 1990). Indeed, it is the need for additional processes such as inhibition that may determine the involvement of the prefrontal cortex and potentially the central executive in task performance. Whether the prefrontal cortex is required solely for passive short-term memory in the absence of additional control processes such as in tests of spatial and digit span is unclear although subtle deficits in attaining the maximum span have been identified in frontal patients (Owen & Robbins, unpublished data). In contrast, monkeys with dorsolateral prefrontal lesions have been reported to perform well at the first location of the A not B task, errors appearing only when location of the reward changes (Diamond 1990) suggesting that in this case simple short-term spatial memory processes remain intact after such a lesion.

Thus, at present, whether the subsidiary slave systems of the working memory model of Baddeley & Hitch fall partially within or outside of the prefrontal cortex remains unclear. What has been postulated though is that there are at least two different levels of contribution made by the prefrontal cortex to mnemonic processing (Petrides, Chapter 8), both levels probably being component processes of the central executive. While ventrolateral prefrontal cortex may be involved in first-order executive processes such as 'active selection and comparison and judgement of stimuli held in short-term memory', the mid-dorsolateral frontal cortex becomes involved when several pieces of information need to be monitored and manipulated in working memory, processes presumably essential for strategic planning. However, whether holding information in short-term memory is a necessary prerequisite for prefrontal involvement in task performance is less than clear, with recent evidence suggesting that it may not be. This theme will be taken up in more detail in the section on the functional organization of the prefrontal cortex where it will be considered in relation to hierarchical organization of processing.

Inhibitory control: an intrinsic property of all prefrontal circuitry?

It became clear as the meeting progressed that there was a certain consensus with regard to the organization of inhibitory control processes within the prefrontal cortex. The original hypothesis that inhibitory control was a function residing exclusively within the ventral prefrontal cortex [(Mishkin 1964; Fuster 1989)] was laid to rest. Instead, converging evidence from neuropsychological, electrophysiological, and computational studies has led to the notion that the ability to suppress inappropriate prepotent response tendencies is an intrinsic property of the prefrontal cortex as a whole. A paper by Dias *et al.* (1996*a*) and discussed in Chapter 9 by Robbins demonstrated that distinct processes of response inhibition are recruited to control extra-dimensional shifting and associative reversal learning, represented in separable processing domains within lateral and orbital prefrontal cortex. Ablation (Diamond & Goldman-Rakic 1989) and electrophysiological recording studies (Funahashi *et al.* 1993) have demonstrated that inhibitory control mechanisms operate together with 'on-line' processing within the region of the sulcus principalis to control performance on the spatial delayed response task. Finally, Cohen, Braver, & O'Reilly (in Chapter 14) incorporate active memory and behavioural inhibition functions into the context layer of their computational model of prefrontal functioning, proposing that these functions may reflect the operation of the context layer in different behavioural conditions. Their model predicts that memory and inhibition effects are differentially sensitive to disturbances of the context layer with memory deficits emerging earlier than inhibitory deficits following partial degradation of context information. Interestingly, such a prediction would account for the findings from a series of studies by Roberts and colleagues which demonstrate that removal of the dopaminergic input to the prefrontal cortex in monkeys, using the neurotoxin 6-hydroxydopamine, only disrupts performance on prefrontal tasks requiring active memory, such as spatial delayed response, but not those requiring inhibitory control, such as attentional set-shifting, associative reversal, and response sequencing (Roberts *et al.* 1994; Collins *et al.* (in the press)).

What was not resolved at the meeting was the role that inhibitory processing plays within the orbitofrontal cortex with respect to the control of social behaviour. There is overwhelming evidence that the orbitofrontal cortex is involved in processing motivational and emotional stimuli. Damage to this region of cortex produces disturbances in emotional and social behaviour (Butter *et al.* 1970; Myers *et al.* 1973) as well as in learning and reversing stimulus–reinforcement associations (Iversen & Mishkin 1970; Jones & Mishkin 1972). Taking into account the facts that this region of cortex contains secondary taste cortex and higher-order olfactory cortex, receives information about the sight of objects from temporal cortex, and contains neurons that are able to detect non-reward and which change their responding rapidly following discrimination reversal, Rolls (Chapter 6) proposed that one function of this region was rapid stimulus–reinforcement association learning and the correction of these associations when reinforcement contingencies in the environment change. These reinforcing signals can then influence behaviour by way, for example, of the basal ganglia. Rolls suggests that this ability to rapidly readjust the reinforcement value of visual signals is crucial to emotional and social behaviour with euphoria, irresponsibility, lack of affect, and impulsivity all related to a dysfunction in this ability. Damasio, in contrast, emphasizes the importance of this region in detecting somatic markers (bodily responses) that occur at the time of reinforcement evaluation and which influence the decision-making process as to which behavioural response to make. In this account, random and impulsive behaviour is the outcome of the absence of such a marker.

Clearly, these two accounts differ with respect to the emphasis placed upon the role of inhibitory control processes. In the former account the ability to process stimuli in a rapidly changing social environment is considered to be central to the ability of humans and non-human primates to survive in a social environment and thus the rapid inhibitory processing that can occur in orbito-frontal cortex underlies the importance of this region in social behaviour. In contrast, in the latter account, greater emphasis is placed upon the difficulty of decision-making in social situations in which seldom is there an obvious solution. It is the proposed role of somatic markers in biasing decision-making and the importance of the orbitofrontal cortex in providing the neural underpinnings of this process that makes the orbitofrontal cortex in this account important for social behaviour, with inhibitory control an integral component of such decision-making machinery. Certainly this latter account is in keeping with the hypothesis that inhibitory control processes are a general property of all prefrontal cortex and that what differentiates individual regions are the kinds of information that are processed and the functions or operations that are performed. However, it was noted in the discussion that in the 'gambling task', which has been used recently to test many of the predictions of the somatic marker hypothesis, the core requirement is for subjects to reverse their responding and to choose the low-paid decks in preference to the high-paid decks. Consequently, the impaired performance of patients with orbito-frontal damage may be due primarily to their difficulty in inhibiting their prepotent response tendency to choose the high-paid decks, rather than an impairment simply in forming associations. In reply, Damasio admitted that this could be a possibility but thought that the most intriguing aspect of the results was that the patients' failure could not be compensated by their realization that their strategy had led them to losses. In addition, Damasio provided evidence that the same patients who failed the gambling task could acquire classical conditioning normally, implying that certain simple types of associative learning were intact. This could be taken as support for the somatic marker hypothesis, in that the solution to a simple classical conditioning paradigm is unambiguous and therefore would be predicted not to require complex decision-making processes to bias responding towards a particular outcome. However, the hypothesis of Rolls emphasizing the importance of inhibitory control processes within the orbitofrontal cortex would also not predict an impairment of simple classical conditioning.

Of potential relevance to this debate is the finding by Iversen & Mishkin (1970) that the marked impairment in visual discrimination reversal learning following lesions of the orbitofrontal cortex may be the result of two independent disorders. While monkeys with lesions of the lateral orbital region perseverated, i.e. they continued to respond to the previously rewarded stimulus for many more trials than controls, monkeys with lesions of the medial orbital region were no slower than controls to inhibit their responding to the previously rewarded stimulus. Instead, the medial orbital lesioned monkeys took many more trials than controls to learn to respond to the previously unrewarded stimulus. Based upon this study alone, it is not possible to define precisely the nature of the cognitive deficits underlying these two types of impairment. However, more recent studies have shown that lesions of the medial orbital region do disrupt the ability of monkeys to learn stimulus–reward associations (Baylis & Gaffan 1991), an impairment that would certainly explain the original deficit of monkeys with medial orbital lesions on reversal learning. Hence, these findings suggest that impairments in learning about the affective properties of stimuli, which may underlie some of the emotional impairments associated with damage to orbitofrontal cortex, can, in certain situations, be divorced from deficits in inhibitory control.

Functional organization of the prefrontal cortex: factors determining its heterogeneous character

While the general consensus of the meeting was that the prefrontal cortex was functionally heterogeneous, one of the main areas of disagreement was in defining those factors that were responsible for that heterogeneity. As outlined in the section on 'working memory' Goldman-Rakic strongly supported the hypothesis that 'on-line' and inhibitory control processes were emergent functions of neuronal circuitry throughout much of the prefrontal cortex and that the regions differed primarily with respect to informational domain, spatial processing taking place in dorsolateral prefrontal cortex and feature processing taking place in ventrolateral prefrontal cortex. A logical extension of this hypothesis would be that ventromedial prefrontal cortex is involved in the processing of reinforcing or 'affective' stimuli. In contrast, Petrides proposed that regions were differentiated primarily according to the functional operations that they performed. Thus, ventrolateral prefrontal cortex was involved in first-order executive processes such as active selection and comparison of stimuli held in short-term memory while dorsolateral prefrontal cortex was involved in higher-order executive components of working memory including monitoring and manipulation of several pieces of information. Although evidence has been provided to support both viewpoints (see Chapters 7 and 8 by Goldman-Rakic and Petrides respectively) a recent critical review of functional neuroimaging studies, including both PET and fMRI, suggests that contrary to popular opinion, the available data do not support the domain-specific account (Owen 1997). Instead it is argued that neuroimaging data support the hypothesis that specific regions within dorsolateral and ventrolateral prefrontal cortex make identical functional contributions to both spatial and non-spatial working memory, differing only with respect to the nature of the processing that they perform. This view is supported by the recent findings of Rao et al.

(1997) that the firing of cells located throughout dorsolateral and ventrolateral regions can convey both spatial and object information.

More general support for the differential localization within the prefrontal cortex of a number of different functional operations comes from human neuropsychological studies that have used factor analytical techniques. Such studies demonstrate low correlations across frontal tasks which involve the same type of material, thereby ruling out the possibility that any differences were due to the different material used rather than to the different operations being performed. This is highlighted in Chapter 3 by Shallice & Burgess and Chapter 9 by Robbins, who hypothesize that multiple functional operations would be a necessary requirement of a supervisory attentional system or central executive. 'On-line' processing and inhibitory control can be recognized as sub-components of some of these operations which may explain why these particular processes are quite widely distributed throughout the prefrontal cortex, while the operations themselves may turn out to be more localized. For example, using the Haylings Sentence Completion Test A and B, it was shown that while the process of strategy production and realization and the process of error monitoring and correction were both impaired by frontal lesions, they were shown to be separable (see Chapter 3 by Shallice & Burgess). Moreover, differences in the kinds of operations engaged during encoding and retrieval of episodic memories have been proposed to underlie the differential activity in the left and right prefrontal cortices that have been reported in functional neuroimaging studies investigating encoding and retrieval mechanisms respectively (Tulving et al. 1994; Fletcher et al. 1997). If so, these results provide additional support for the view that distinct cognitive operations are anatomically separable within the prefrontal cortex, in this case additionally providing evidence of lateralization. Finally, strategic components of executive functioning have been separated from 'on-line' processing. Comparison of performance on a verbal, visual, and spatial version of a working memory task revealed that only on the spatial task was performance correlated with the ability of subjects to generate an effective strategy and only on this task was performance impaired following frontal lesions and shown to be the direct result of failing to use such a strategy (Owen et al. 1996 and discussed in Chapter 9 by Robbins). There was no obvious explanation for the difference in terms of the exact sites of the patients' lesions in the prefrontal cortex.

A rather different approach to the study of the component processes of executive function was adopted by Baddeley & Della Sala at this Discussion Meeting. They suggested that the failure in the past to determine the nature of the organization within the prefrontal cortex was due to the assumption that prefrontal cortex was synonomous with executive functioning. Therefore, they have taken the alternative approach of studying dysexecutive syndromes, i.e. behavioural disturbances associated with poor control in monitoring one's own performance in daily life including disinhibition or apathy, regardless of the locus of brain pathology, hypothesizing that executive processing may be a product of a number of different brain regions. Using the Baddeley & Hitch model of working memory as a starting point they have suggested that a necessary component of the central executive is the coordination of activity in the two slave systems. Consequently, they have studied dual task performance in a variety of different patient groups and shown that in those with a putative dysexecutive syndrome, performance was markedly impaired. Indeed, the dual task paradigm was shown to differentiate between two groups of frontal patients with and without the dysexecutive syndrome, adding further support for the hypothesis that different functional operations are distributed within different regions of the prefrontal cortex—although no direct evidence for the anatomical localization of dual task performance is provided. However, parallels are drawn between these findings and those of Shallice & Burgess of a subgroup of frontal patients with behavioural disturbance who perform normally on the majority of standard frontal tests but are impaired on the 'six elements test' which requires subjects to perform six tests in parallel. Since it is not clear yet whether this capacity to perform parallel tasks is made up of component processes or a single process, care must be taken not to return to differentiating regions by task rather than process.

A somewhat different approach to dual task performance and its usefulness in studying prefrontal function was adopted by Passingham. Rather than evolving from a theoretical model of working memory as a necessary operation for a central executive to perform, it arose from the hypothesis that the decrement in performance when performing two tasks in parallel may be due to competition for resources centrally within the prefrontal cortex. Since functional neuroimaging studies had provided evidence to suggest that the prefrontal cortex was engaged during performance of novel, but not pre-learned, automatic tasks (for review see Chapter 10 by Passingham) it was predicted that decrements in dual task performance would be greatest when two novel tasks, rather than a novel and an automatic task, were paired in a dual task paradigm, a prediction that was borne out by subsequent behavioural studies. What is not clear, however, is how Passingham's and Baddeley & Della Sala's approaches relate to one another. For example, it is not made explicit how the factors of novelty and automaticity are dealt with within the working memory model of Baddeley & Hitch, although it is assumed that this is encompassed within the supervisory attentional model of Shallice & Burgess which was previously adopted as a plausible set of mechanisms governing the operation of the central executive. If so, then it is probably the case that the prefrontal cortex is involved in dual task performance regardless of whether the two tasks are novel or automatic, but that, as Passingham states, marked decrements in performance are only seen if there is competition for resources within the prefrontal cortex.

That dual task performance does activate the prefrontal cortex even when neither of the component tasks activate prefrontal cortex has been demonstrated by D'Esposito *et al.* (1995). This same study also showed that prefrontal activation occurred even though neither component task required the holding of information 'on-line' over a delay period. Therefore, not only do these results support the hypothesis that the prefrontal cortex is involved in the allocation and coordination of attentional resources but they also suggest that the requirement for 'on-line' processing may not be necessary for prefrontal involvement in task performance. Certainly, deficits in performance of discrimination reversal and go–no go tasks have never been accommodated easily into a working memory account of prefrontal function. Moroever, recent (1997) findings by Dias *et al*. (1997) demonstrate that over a range of visual discriminations, all of which could be solved using on-line processing, performance was impaired by prefrontal lesions only on those discriminations that involved the inhibition of a previously acquired response or rule. Finally, Rushworth *et al*. (1997) have demonstrated that lesions of ventral prefrontal cortex impair dramatically the ability to relearn simultaneous colour matching while subsequent matching with delays is unimpaired. Although not inconsistent with the two-level hypothesis of Petrides, the authors suggest that their results extend the hypothesis by suggesting that the ventrolateral prefrontal cortex is important in the active selection, comparison, and judgement of stimuli even in those situations in which 'on-line' processing of information is not required.

At first sight this extended hypothesis of Rushworth *et al*. (1997) would appear to fit the available lesion data in monkeys. However, upon further reflection it is apparent that it does not account for the most well-described result within the non-human primate literature on prefrontal function, namely the impairment upon spatial delayed response following lesions of the banks and depths of the sulcus principalis. According to the two-stage hypothesis of Petrides, classical delayed response paradigms, including spatial delayed response, do not require higher-order executive processes and are not impaired by lesions of the mid-dorsolateral prefrontal cortex which do not include the sulcus principalis (see Chapter 8 for a detailed review of monkey lesion data). Instead, such paradigms are proposed to involve lower-order executive processes and, since this is the function given to ventrolateral prefrontal cortex which lies below the sulcus principalis, this implies that the region of the sulcus principalis which impairs spatial delayed response performance is probably functionally related to the ventrolateral region. Limited support for such an interpretation comes from the developmental studies of Barbas & Pandya (1989) which suggest that the ventral and dorsal banks of the sulcus principalis originate from two separate components or moieties of neocortical development, the insular and cingular regions respectively. Based upon this hypothesis it would not be surprising if the ventral part of the sulcus principalis was associated functionally with ventrolateral rather than dorsolateral regions. Since lesion studies have always removed the entire sulcus principalis there are no experimental data at present that can address the issue of possible functional differences between dorsal and ventral banks of the sulcus principalis.

However, any functional similarity of the sulcus principalis with the ventrolateral prefrontal cortex is lost when taking into account the extended two-stage hypothesis proposed by Rushworth *et al*. (1997) in which the ventrolateral region is proposed to play a more general role in stimulus selection and attention beyond those situations in which stimuli must be held in memory. Indeed, they emphasize the fact that, unlike ventrolateral prefrontal cortex, the sulcus principalis only appears to be involved in tasks which have both spatial and delay components. In this respect the findings of Rushworth *et al.* are not consistent with the two-stage theory of Petrides in which the sulcus principalis and the spatial delayed response task are linked with lower-order executive processing. The most parsimonious explanation would be that the regions of ventrolateral prefrontal cortex involved in lower-order executive mnemonic processes, as described by Petrides, are distinct from those regions involved in the more general function of stimulus selection and attention, as described by Rushworth *et al.* This would appear plausible since the ventrolateral prefrontal cortex, which includes not only the inferior convexity of the dorsal surface but also regions on the ventral surface lateral to the lateral orbital sulcus, has been subdivided into at least two (Petrides & Pandya 1994) and in some cases four (Carmichael & Price 1994) subregions. However, the original lesion of ventrolateral prefrontal cortex in the Rushworth *et al.* study included tissue on the dorsal surface (area 47/12l) only and that lesion did not impair performance on delayed matching to colour in either the simultaneous or delay conditions. Only when the lesion was enlarged to include the tissue on the ventral surface (area 47/12l and 47/12o) was any impairment observed. Thus, at present, discrepancies between these two different theories cannot be fully resolved.

Heterogeneity of prefrontal cognitive function: relevance to psychopathology

The specification of component 'executive' processes and their localization to particular regions of the prefrontal cortex or distributed networks involving this structure is potentially relevant to many forms of psychopathology, including depression and schizophrenia (see Masterman & Cummings 1997, for a recent review). This meeting concentrated on the possibly special relationship between prefrontal dysfunction and schizophrenia because this has been a converging focus of several different types of investigation of the prefrontal cortex: cognitive neuropsychology; animal models of some of the cognitive deficits highlighted in schizophrenia (e.g. the delayed saccade task); functional neuroimaging, psychopharmacology, and computational modelling. However, it should be made clear that several psychiatric and developmental disorders have been associated with prefrontal dysfunction. In particular, while not discussed at this meeting, there has recently been much interest in possible frontal deficits in depression (see Goodwin 1997), although it is significant that this disorder also seems particularly associated with changes of functioning of the cingulate cortex and basal ganglia (see, for example, Elliott *et al.* 1997*a*). Moreover, it is often the case that a study of mechanisms underlying particular symptoms can be applied across psychiatric diagnostic categories (e.g. Dolan *et al.* 1993). The characterization of cognitive deficits in conditions such as schizophrenia is important for two distinct reasons. First, although schizophrenia is associated with a range of profound impairments, including those in certain forms of perception and memory, it is becoming increasingly evident that the 'executive' deficits possibly related to prefrontal cortical dysfunctioning are especially important for determining the full rehabilitation of schizophrenics into the community (see, for example, Levin *et al.* 1989). Second, according to the emergent discipline of 'cognitive neuropsychiatry', the nature of the symptoms themselves can best be elucidated by a careful analysis of their cognitive basis.

Utility of the functional neuroimaging approach for studying psychopathology

Although recent evidence of structural imaging has indicated surprisingly large losses of tissue in the sub-genual region of the frontal cortex in bipolar and unipolar depressed patients (Drevets *et al.* 1997), functional imaging or 'cognitive activation' studies seem to offer the most promise for establishing neural correlates of common psychiatric conditions. The functional neuroimaging approach illustrated in Chapter 12 by Weinberger & Berman, and also by Frith in Chapter 13, has had a particularly stimulating effect on hypothesis generation and testing in this field. It led to the initial formulation of the influential 'hypofrontality' hypothesis, which suggested that schizophrenic patients have a functional lesion of the frontal lobe that accounts for at least a sub-set of their cognitive deficits, as exemplified especially by their poor performance on the Wisconsin Card Sort Test (WCST), and correlated with the severity of 'negative' symptoms. Weinberger & Berman critically reviewed the subsequently somewhat chequered history of the 'hypofrontality' hypothesis for schizophrenia, identifying two factors that may account for some of the disagreements: (1) measurements made in the resting versus the 'cognitive activation' state, the latter generally being more positive; (2) the possibility of artefacts arising from differences in baseline performance in the two tasks. Thus, as argued forcibly by Frith and colleagues, if the task is performed worse by Group A than B, it might be considered unsurprising that there is also a reduction in regional cerebral blood flow (rCBF), arising from the lesser degree of engagement in the task by this group. This essentially reiterates the methodological recommendations of earlier research into core cognitive deficits in schizophrenia (Oltmans & Neale 1975) that it is necessary to 'equate' performance in Groups A and B, before making any interpretation of the differences or patterns of blood flow. However, as acknowledged by Frith, making the task easier for the patients in absolute terms carries with it another set of interpretative problems. An alternative view might be that a matching manoeuvre to equate task performance runs the risk of rejecting an excellent discriminator of dysfunction in the psychiatric group; regional cerebral blood flow is reduced not because the patient is not attending to the task or is not motivated by it, but simply because they cannot perform the key cognitive operations required by the task. This issue may be best approached from a number of approaches to help resolve it by a convergence of evidence.

A good deal of the chapter by Weinberger & Berman considers the various implications and conclusions that may be drawn from data of this type. The issues are of considerable theoretical interest for normal, as well as abnormal, cognition. For example, Weinberger & Berman review their results that indicate that patients with Huntington's disease, who similarly are impaired on the WCST, actually exhibit 'hyperfrontality' in a cognitive activation paradigm with this task. Therefore, hypofrontality is not an invariable consequence of impaired task performance. This can, of course, be explained by postulating that WCST performance depends on a widespread network of cortical and subcortical (probably in this case including fronto-striatal circuitry) activity of which the prefrontal component is but one part. (Incidentally, this anatomical point perhaps makes it clear, in general, why the so-called 'dysexecutive' syndrome does not always appear to arise from damage simply to the prefrontal cortex itself.) More problematic, however, for the view that this activity in the prefrontal cortex is somehow central to task performance is the observation made by Weinberger & Berman that pharmacological blockade of gonadal steroid hormones by lupron in normal women significantly attenuated prefrontal activation (averaged across the group) during WCST performance without affecting task performance. Possible explanations of this fascinating result are that other non-frontal mechanisms are recruited to sustain performance, or that rCBF is not providing a sufficiently sensitive index of prefrontal functioning. The subjects were overtrained on the task before drug treatment, which would be compatible with the former hypothesis.

The attempt to test the nature of the relationship between task performance and regional cerebral blood flow by Weinberger & Berman opened up some additional avenues of theoretical interest. In particular, it appeared that patients may activate different regions of the prefrontal cortex than normal, specifically more anteriorly, than is usually seen in controls. Intriguingly, those normal subjects that showed relatively more activation in this region were the ones that also tended to perform worse on the task, suggesting that the normal inhibition of activity in this prefrontal region (and presumably, in some sense its functioning) is conducive to efficient task performance.

This latter example raises two related matters, namely the nature and interpretation of 'deactivation' in functional imaging studies, and the interactions in patterns of regional cerebral blood flow that occur between different brain regions, including regions in the prefrontal cortex. The possibility of 'deactivation' arising as an artefact of data analysis was considered. The typical practice of comparing brain activity during a condition of interest to a 'baseline' condition has two possible consequences. The first can occur if a shift in global activity occurs in one condition, but not the other, and if the shift is not uniform across the brain but a product of large regional changes. Thus, when the regional data are 'normalized' to the global mean, a region of the brain that actually exhibited increases in rCBF, but less so than other areas, will appear to be 'deactivated' when normalized data are compared to the baseline condition. The best way of resolving this is by consideration of the absolute rCBF data. The second possible consequence concerns possible increases that occur in a 'baseline' condition, as a result of the nature of the processes engaged by this control task, resulting in apparent 'deactivation' when subtracted from the condition of primary interest. This highlights the problems of using simple 'subtractive' designs in cognitive activation studies, as the necessary assumption of the existence of additive, orthogonal cognitive components for complex tasks can rarely be made with confidence.

Ultimately, the interpretation of 'deactivations' must be based on theoretical considerations, as well as the experimental design. A good example is the relative increase in activation of regions specialized for colour processing in the prestriate cortex and decrease in motion areas caused by the simple instruction to attend to the colours of a visual display rather than its motion (Corbetta et al. 1991). It is plausible that the activations and deactivations seen within prefrontal cortex could also be interpreted as reflecting attention to or competition between different cognitive processes. These occur, for example, in the Tower of London planning task described by Robbins (Baker et al. 1996), where increases in dorsolateral and fronto-polar activity are paralleled by reductions in medial prefrontal cortical rCBF. McGuire et al. (1996) have recently shown that activity in medial prefrontal areas is associated with 'stimulus independent thoughts', i.e. thoughts that come to mind unbidden and unrelated to the task in which we are engaged. Such thoughts are known to decrease in frequency when subjects engage in 'executive' tasks such as the Tower of London, and conversely to increase during control tasks. Whether the reciprocal changes within the prefrontal cortex reflect direct interactions between different areas or the result of influences of intermediary structures such as the anterior cingulate cortex is unknown, and will likely probably remain obscure until methods of imaging with better temporal, as well as spatial, resolution, such as fMRI, become established. In general, we remain ignorant about the functional routes of communication within the prefrontal cortex in complex settings. However, there are advances in understanding through functional studies (e.g. of the 'two-stage' hypothesis of processing within the prefrontal cortex (Petrides) and combined neuroanatomical and electrophysiological investigations of the gustatory and olfactory functions of orbitofrontal cortex (see Chapter 6 by Rolls). Moreover, neuroanatomists are making strides in defining neural systems that operate within the prefrontal cortex, but have apparently quite specific routes for intercommunication (see Pandya & Yeterian, Chapter 5, and also the dorsal and ventral 'trends' of Barbas & Pandya (1989)).

The other main form of neural interaction to be considered is between frontal and posterior cortical systems. Several of the contributions (e.g. Goldman-Rakic, Robbins) emphasized that there were important interactions between posterior cortical structures, such as the temporal and parietal lobes and the prefrontal cortex, so that, for example, complex tasks can be affected in different ways by damage to the anterior and posterior cortical regions. Using the asymmetrical crossed lesion approach, Gaffan & Parker (1997) have also recently shown important synergism between the temporal and frontal lobes in monkeys in conditional discrimination tasks.

In the context of the new 'cognitive neuropsychiatry', Frith outlined how hallucinations could potentially arise because of deficits in a set of processes by which schizophrenic patients experience an auditory–verbal percept in the absence of sensation, mistakenly perceive self-generated activity as coming from an external source, such as an 'agent' intending to influence the patient. The hypothesis is that these aberrations arise, at least in part, from failures of integration of temporal and prefrontal cortical activity. For example, auditory hallucinations appear to arise from a failure to recognize one's own inner speech as one's own, perhaps because of a failure of an executive monitoring process controlled by the frontal lobe (not dissimilar to the higher-order corollary discharge mechanism envisaged by Teuber (1964)). Frith reviews much of the data that indicate that inner speech activates Broca's area in normal controls and that imagining another person's voice recruits additional areas such as the left superior temporal gyrus (McGuire et al. 1996).

The perception of agency is an important part of Frith's theory, especially as it bears on the hypothesis that schizophrenics may be impaired in 'Theory of Mind' type processes, that is the ability to predict and even control what other people do, through analysing their beliefs and knowledge. The notion is that deluded patients falsely attribute intentions to other people or even to objects, such erroneous beliefs being driven by 'overactive' Theory of Mind processes. The application of this theory to schizophrenia arises from a strong tradition of work that has developed in autism, in which autistic individuals often fail elementary requirements of having a theory of mind, such as the capacity to understand the significance of false beliefs in others (see Frith et al. 1991). According to recent functional activation studies the perception of mental states of others, as inferred from stories, depends on the left medial prefrontal cortex, specifically area 8 (Fletcher et al. 1995). Frith points out that this part of the brain is activated in many other conditions which converge on the hypothesis that the region is concerned with the detection of agents and in coping with them, as well as in hallucinations. It was also pointed out that similar tasks used by Goel et al. (1995) produced activations in a zone quite close to the area of peak activity in the Fletcher et al. study, but that the activation extended to regions of the left temporal lobe (areas 21, 38, and 39). This was relevant to the key issue of the possible modularity of 'Theory of Mind' processes, the cognitive nature of which, however, remains unspecified at present.

If 'Theory of Mind' processes are impaired in schizophrenia, this would predict that patients with this disorder would have difficulty in solving such tasks, just as many autistic individuals do. Recently, Frith & Corcoran (1996) have reported that patients with negative features perform worse on 'Theory of Mind' tasks than would have been expected on the basis of their current IQs. There was also evidence that patients with delusions about the intentions of others were impaired, perhaps as would be expected from the earlier discussion. Finally, patients in remission had no problems with these tasks, suggesting that the Theory of Mind deficits were operating as state, rather than trait, variables.

The picture was less clear in patients with frontal excisions; indeed it was queried in discussion whether patients with frontal excisions had any greater incidence, not only of Theory of Mind' abnormalities, but also of schizophrenic psychopathology. Several investigators are currently examining the capacity of patients with frontal lesions to do Theory of Mind tasks. Rather unusually, predictions can be made from the functional neuroimaging evidence surveyed that excisions centred on area 8 would be particularly effective. The same critical scrutiny will have to be made, however, of the degree to which any such deficits are secondary to more general impairments in executive functioning, a debate that continues to be lively in the case of autism (see Russell 1997). For example, area 8 has been linked with the learning of conditional discrimination tasks in non-human primates (of the form, if A, then B) (Petrides 1991), and it is the case that many of the Theory of Mind tasks embody similar forms of reasoning.

The question of the apparent lack of schizophrenic symptoms in patients with frontal lesions can be countered in several ways. The first main point is that frontal lesions may lead to a greater incidence of psychotic symptoms if they occur earlier in life, e.g. in adolescence (Weinberger 1987). In a recent analysis of the psychopathology associated with metachromatic leucodystrophy which is associated with frontal damage, Hyde *et al.* (1992) reported that the disease presents as a schizophrenia-like illness in many cases when it is expressed early. The second counter-argument would be that schizophrenia may not reflect reduced frontal functioning, but rather a pathological over-functioning in some cases (compare the 'overactive' Theory of Mind hypothesis, above). The neurochemical pathology is not consistent with massive structural lesions, but with more subtle deficits, for example in glutamate receptor markers (Deakin *et al.* 1997) and in the mesocortical dopamine projection which has a neuromodulatory influence that may lead to deficits that are qualitatively distinct from those produced by lesions of the prefrontal cortex itself (Roberts *et al.* 1994, and discussed in Chapter 9). The heterogeneity of schizophrenia may indicate that the executive deficits that can be so prominent in this condition are a province of frontal changes, as well as the negative symptomatology, whereas its other features result from neural changes elsewhere. The apparent discrepancies that arise from studying effects of excisions and neuroimaging are, however, by no means limited to schizophrenic symptoms; presumably these discrepancies are telling us something more about how the system normally operates.

The computational approach to understanding psychopathology

The contribution by Cohen *et al.* helped to bring together disparate themes of the Discussion Meeting. This represents a distinct cognitive approach to that presented by Frith to schizophrenia, while also making contact with some of the main topics discussed during the course of the meeting such as working memory and behavioural inhibition. They have developed a connectionist approach towards a theory for understanding prefrontal cortical functioning, and its postulated dysfunctioning in schizophrenia. There is a variety of computational approaches being used to simulate prefrontal and executive processes (e.g. Cooper *et al.* 1995; Dehaene & Changeux 1995) and it is unclear at present which will be the most appropriate and productive. Most of them attempt to model particular functions that might be expected to be within the domain of prefrontal/executive functioning; for example, the WCST (Dehaene & Changeux 1995), oculomotor associations and sequences (Dominey *et al.* 1995), or complex actions such as making a cup of coffee (Cooper *et al.* 1995). The utility of the approach is that it provides a check on the internal consistency of a theory such as Shallice & Norman's SAS model that incorporates contention scheduling, and helps to generate novel predictions that can be tested empirically.

The approach by Cohen *et al.* focuses on the Stroop task, which clearly has some executive components (suppression of attention), and the performance of which has been shown to be associated with the anterior cingulate, and possibly with that of prefrontal cortex (see Vendrell *et al.* 1995). They also employ a lexical disambiguation test to assess language processing and the 'continuous performance task', a test of sustained attention that also incorporates measures of processing of the context, as well as working memory for that context. It is interesting that this task has been linked with cingulate as well as medial prefrontal cortical functioning (e.g. Stuss *et al.* 1995). Based on the literature, Cohen *et al.* argue that many of the cognitive deficits in schizophrenia can be understood in terms of impairments of attention and behavioural inhibition. As mentioned above, their simulation studies bear directly on the issue of the relationship between working memory and behavioural inhibition by indicating their relative susceptibility to disturbances of the 'context layer' of their model. This leads to a prediction that memory disturbances should occur before behavioural inhibitory deficits during the course of schizophrenia. The authors mention some preliminary empirical evidence in unmedicated patients with first episode schizophrenia which appears to support the predictions that the deficits are specific to schizophrenia and appear in the predicted sequence. Such investigations will prove invaluable in the future for addressing theories about the nature and basis of the intellectual deficits in schizophrenia, especially if the possible confounding influences of medication with neuroleptic (dopamine receptor blocking) drugs are taken into account.

Neurotransmitter modulation of prefrontal function in the context of psychopathology

The Cohen *et al.* paper also served as a focal point for assessing the importance of neuromodulation of prefrontal function, for example by the ascending dopaminergic and noradrenergic neurotransmitter systems. Their previous theoretical perspectives failed to differentiate separable roles for the dopaminergic and noradrenergic systems, and formerly proposed that dopamine influences the active maintenance of information. However, in this most recent formulation they have focused on the hypothesis that mesocortical dopamine provides a gating signal for attractor networks housed within the prefrontal cortex.

Understanding the role of the neuromodulation provided by subcortical neurotransmitter systems was not a major theme, as it was complemented by a dedicated meeting on this topic at about the same time (published as a special issue of *Journal of Psychopharmacology* **11**(2) 1997). However, there is no doubt that this is a potential growth area and it is worth summarizing some of the main issues that extended across both meetings. The first is what the significance of such neuromodulation may be, especially bearing in mind that the frontal cortex itself is able reciprocally to influence it because of its descending projections to the relevant cell groups of origin in the subcortical brain (see Goldman-Rakic 1987). Evidence has accumulated that these chemically defined neurotransmitter systems, especially including the mesocortical dopamine system, are tonically responsive to stressors (see review by Arnsten 1997), as well as to phasic 'reward signals' (Schultz 1992). There is also accumulating evidence that their actions within the prefrontal cortex can be quite complex, including, in the case of dopamine, the potentiation of both afferent excitatory input and local inhibitory signals. Recently, it has been shown that low doses of the D1 dopamine receptor antagonist SCH-23390 may enhance neuronal firing in the prefrontal cortex in monkeys, apparently enhancing the 'signal-to-noise ratio' whereas higher doses may have the reverse effect (Williams & Goldman-Rakic 1995). The net effect of increased activity of mesocortical dopamine may even appear to be reciprocally related to changes in dopamine functioning in the subcortical striatum (see Roberts *et al.* 1994).

These considerations are relevant especially to the effects of dopaminergic activity on cognitive functions of the prefrontal cortex. It is plausible that at least some of the 'somatic markers' postulated by Damasio to affect decision-making mechanisms within the prefrontal cortex are actually mediated by activity within these systems. However, Damasio cautions that this activity is more likely to be of importance developmentally when learning about the central representation of visceral events. Thus, a straightforward pharmacological approach to manipulating autonomic activity, for example, with beta blockers in normal adult subjects, may be insufficient to affect performance in Damasio's 'gambling task'. This remains a fertile area for future research.

Cohen *et al.* cite two or three major pieces of evidence to support the notion that dopamine acts to facilitate cognitive functions characteristic of the prefrontal cortex, such as delayed response performance. In her contribution, Diamond (Chapter 11) made the case, partly based on rodent models of spatial working memory function, that the cognitive deficits of PKU children are dependent in part on depletions of prefrontal dopamine. Arnsten (1997) recently reviewed the evidence for facilitation of cognitive performance by catecholaminergic agents, especially in aged monkeys. However, it is clear that enhancing catcholaminergic function may not always boost cognitive performance. Recent evidence is accumulating that increased catecholaminergic turnover within the prefrontal cortex may be associated with impaired performance on 'frontal' tasks such as delayed alternation and delayed response, in rats and monkeys respectively (Murphy *et al.* 1996). This would seem to suggest that in certain circumstances, reduced prefrontal cortical dopamine transmission might lead to enhanced functioning. Indeed, Robbins referred to data (Roberts *et al.* 1994) that performance on a primate analogue of the WCST was *improved* by substantial prefrontal cortical dopamine depletion in monkeys, even though lesions of the prefrontal cortex *per se* had the expected effect (Dias *et al.* 1996b). What was of even greater interest, however, was the finding that this sparing, and even apparent, enhancement of the attentional set-shifting performance was accompanied by impairments in spatial delayed response performance. Therefore, it is apparent that a simple inverted U-shaped function for describing the relationship between levels of mesocortical dopamine activity and 'cognitive performance' is insufficient; instead, this relationship depends on the precise nature of the task. This suggests that there are 'costs' as well as 'benefits' for cognitive functioning affected by fluctuations in prefrontal catecholaminergic function, perhaps related adaptively to modes of cognitive function that are appropriate under varying degrees of 'stress' or 'arousal'. This formulation makes it clear that another major function of the prefrontal cortex may be to organize the behavioural response to varying motivational demands. The formulation may also be of considerable therapeutic significance, as it seems likely that the effects of drugs, for example, in the treatment of dementia (Coull *et al.* 1996; Goodwin *et al.* 1997) and in attention deficit disorder (Elliott *et al.* 1997b) may variably affect different aspects of 'executive functioning'. This possibility is consistent with one of the main theoretical suggestions to arise from this meeting; that executive processes may not be unitary and may be organized somewhat independently in different regions of the prefrontal cortex.

Conclusions

One of the aims of this Discussion Meeting was to determine to what extent it was possible to use cross-species comparisons to advance theoretical knowledge about the prefrontal cortex in man and how far evidence from a number of disciplines could converge to provide a coherent evolutionary perspective about the functions of the prefrontal cortex. For example, the delayed response task in primates and the Wisconsin Card Sort Test in humans have both been used to make inferences about prefrontal functioning which appear radically to contrast with one another despite imaginative attempts to unify in the context of striking neurobiological advances (e.g. Goldman-Rakic 1987). From the outcome of this meeting it can seen that the development of ingenious new variants of basic paradigms is providing measures capable of dissecting different components of tasks suitable for the testing of both monkey and human subjects. For humans, such tasks can be employed in the neuroimaging as well as the clinical context, and are beginning to be defined sufficiently precisely for the purposes of computational modelling. These exciting developments are facilitating the multi-disciplinary neurobiological endeavour that is now necessary to make further progress in this field.

Acknowledgements

Supported by the Wellcome Trust.

References

Arnsten, A. F. T. 1997 Catecholaminergic regulation of the prefrontal cortex. *J. Psychopharmacology* **11**, 151–162.
Baddeley & Hitch 1974 Working memory. In *The psychology of learning and motivation* (ed. I. S. A. Bower), pp. 47–90. New York: Academic Press.
Baker, S. C., Rogers, R. D., Owen, A. M., Frith, C. D., Dolan, R., Frackowiak, R. S. J. & Robbins, T. W. 1996 Neural systems engaged by planning: a PET study of the Tower of London task. *Neuropsychologia* **34**, 515–526.
Barbas & Pandya 1989 Architecture and intrinsic connections of the prefrontal cortex in the rhesos monkey. *J. Comp. Neurol.* **286**, 353–75.
Baylis, L. L. & Gaffan, D. 1991 Amygdalectomy and ventromedial prefrontal ablation produce similar deficits on food choice and in simple object discrimination learning for an unseen reward. *Exp. Brain Res.* **86**, 617–622.
Butter, C. M., Snyder, D. R. & McDonald, J. A. 1970 Effects of orbital frontal lesions on aversive and aggressive behaviors in rhesus monkeys. *J. Comp. Physiol. Psychol.* **72**, 132–144.
Carmichael, S. T. & Price, J. L. 1994 Architectonic subdivision of the orbital and medial prefrontal cortex in macaque monkey. *J. Comp. Neurol.* **346**, 403–434.
Collins, P., Roberts, A. C., Dias, R., Everitt, B. J. & Robbins, T. W. 1997 Perseveration and strategy in a novel spatial self-ordered sequencing task for non-human primates: effects of excitotoxic lesions and dopamine depletions of the prefrontal cortex. *J. Cog. Neurosci.* (In the press.)
Cooper, R., Shallice, T. & Farringdon, J. 1995 Symbolic and continuous processes in the automatic selection of actions. In *Hybrid problems, hybrid solutions* (ed. J. Hallam). Amsterdam: IOS Press.

Corbetta, M., Miezin, F. M., Dormeyer, S., Schulman, G. L. & Petersen, S. E. 1991 Attentional modulation of neural processing of shape, colour and velocity in humans. *Science* **248**, 1556–1559.

Coull, J. T., Sahakian, B. J. & Hodges, J. R. 1996 The alpha-2 antagonist idazoxan remediates certain attentional and executive forms of dysfunction in dementia of the frontal type. *Psychopharmacology* **123**, 239–249.

Deakin, J. F. W., Simpson, M. D. C., Slater, P. & Hellewell, J. S. E. 1997 Familial and developmental abnormalities of frontal lobe function and neurochemistry in schizophrenia. *J. Psychopharmacology* **11**, 133–142.

Dehaene, S. & Changeux, J.-P. 1995 Neuronal models of prefrontal cortical functions. *Ann. N. Acad. Sci.* **769**, 305–319.

D'Esposito, M. D., Detre, J. A., Alsop, D. C., Shin, R. K., Atlas, S. & Grossman, M. 1995 The neural basis of the executive system of working memory. *Nature* **378**, 279–281.

Diamond, A. 1990 The development and neural bases of memory functions as indexed by the AB and delayed response tasks in human infants and infant monkeys. *Ann. N. Y. Acad. Sci.* **608**, 266–309

Diamond, A. & Goldman-Rakic, P. S. 1989 Comparison of human infants and rhesus monkeys on Piaget's AB task: evidence for dependence on dorsolateral prefrontal cortex *Expl. Br. Res.* **74**, 24–40.

Dias, R., Robbins, T. W. & Roberts, A. C. 1996*a* Dissociation in prefrontal cortex of affective and attentional shifts. *Nature, Lond.* **380**, 69–72.

Dias R., Robbins, T. W. & Roberts, A. C. 1996*b* Primate analogue of the Wisconsin Card Sort Test: effects of excitotoxic lesions of the prefrontal cortex in the marmoset. *Behav. Neurosci.* **110**, 870–884.

Dias, R., Robbins, T. W. & Roberts, A. C. 1997 Dissociable forms of inhibitory control within prefrontal cortex with an analogue of the Wisconsin Card Sort Test: restriction to novel situations and independence from 'on-line' processing. *J. Neurosci.* **17**, 9285–97.

Dolan, R. J., Bench, C. J., Liddle, P. F., Friston, K., Frith, C. D., Grasby, P. M. & Frackowiak, R. S. J. 1993 Dorsolateral prefrontal cortex dysfunction in the major psychoses: symptom or disease specificity? *J. Neurol. Neurosurg. Psychiat.* **56**, 1290–1294.

Dominey, P. F., Ventre-Dominey, J., Brousolle, E. & Jeannerod, M. 1995 Analogical transfer in sequence learning. Human and neural-network models of fronto-striatal function. *Ann. N.Y. Acad. Sci.* **769**, 369–373.

Drevets W. C., Price, J. L., Simpson, J. R. Jr., Todd, R. D., Reich, T., Vannier, M. & Raichle, M. 1997 Subgenual prefrontal cortex abnormalities in mood disorders. *Nature* **386**, 824–827.

Duncan, J., Burgess, P. & Emslie, H. 1995 Fluid intelligence after frontal lobe lesions. *Neuropsychologia* **27**, 1329–1344.

Elliott, R., Baker, S. C., Rogers, R. D., O'Leary, D. A., Paykel, E. S., Frith, C. D., Dolan, R. & Sahakian, B. J. 1997*a* Prefrontal dysfunction in depressed patients performing a complex planning task: a study using positron emission tomography. *Psychol. Med.* **27**, 931–942.

Elliott, R., Sahakian, B. J., Matthews, K., Bannerjea, A., Rimmer, J. & Robbins, T. W. 1997*b* Effects of methylphenidate on spatial working memory and planning in healthy young adults. *Psychopharmacology* **131**, 196–206.

Fletcher, P., Happe, F., Frith, U., Baker, S. C., Dolan, R. J., Frackowiak, R. S. J. & Frith, C. D. 1995 Other minds in the brain: a functional imaging study of 'theory of' mind' in story comprehension. *Cognition* **57**, 109–128.

Fletcher, P. C., Frith, C. D. & Rugg, M. D. 1997 The functional neuroanatomy of episodic memory. *TINS* **20**, 213–218.

Frith, C. D. & Corcoran, R. 1996 Exploring the 'theory of mind' in people with schizophrenia. *Psychol. Med.* **26**, 521–530.

Frith, U., Morton, J., & Leslie, A. M. 1991 The cognitive basis of a biological disorder: autism. *TINS* **14**, 433–438,

Funahashi, S., Chafee, M. V. & Goldman-Rakic, P. S. 1993 Prefrontal neuronal activity in rhesus monkeys performing a delayed anti-saccade task. *Nature* **365**, 753–756.

Fuster, J. M. 1989 *The prefrontal cortex.* New York: Raven Press.

Gaffan, D. & Parker, A. 1997 Memory after frontal–temporal disconnection in monkeys: conditional and nonconditional tasks, unilateral and bilateral frontal lesions. *J. Neurosci.* (in press)

Goel V., Grafman, J., Sadato, N. & Hallett, M. 1995 Modelling other minds. *Neuroreport* **6**, 1741–1746.

Goldman-Rakic, P. S. 1987 Circuitry of primate prefrontal cortex and regulation of behavior by representational memory. In *Handbook of physiology. The nervous system* (ed. F. Plum), pp. 373–417. Bethesda, MD: American Physiological Society.

Goodwin, G. M. 1997 Neuropsychological and neuroimaging evidence for the involvement of the frontal lobes in dementia. *J. Psychopharmacology* **11**, 115–122.

Goodwin, G. M., Conway, S. C., Peyro-Saint-Paul, H., Glabus, M. F., O'Carroll, R. E. & Ebmeier, K. P. 1997 Executive function and uptake of ^{99m} Tc-exametazime shown by single photon emission tomography after oral idazoxan in probable, Alzheimer-type dementia. *Psychopharmacology* **131**, 371–378.

Hyde, T. M., Ziegler, J. C. & Weinberger, D. R. 1992 Psychiatric disturbances in metachromatic leukodystrophy. Insights into the neurobiology of psychoisis. *Arch. Neurol.* **49**, 401–406.

Iversen, S. D. & Mishkin, M. 1970 Perseverative interference in monkeys following selective lesions of the inferior prefrontal convexity. *Exp. Brain Res.* **11**, 376–386.

Jones, B. & Mishkin, M. 1972 Limbic lesions and the problem of stimulus–reinforcement associations. *Exp. Neurol.* **36**, 362–377.

Levin, S., Yurgelin-Todd, D. & Craft, S. 1989 Contribution of clinical neuropsychology to the study of schizophrenia. *J. Abn. Psychol.* **98**, 341–356.

Masterman, D. L. & Cummings, J. L. 1997 Frontal-subcortical circuits: the anatomic basis of executive, social and motivated behaviors. *J. Psychopharmacology* **11**, 107–114.

McGuire, P. K., Paulesu, E., Rackowiak, R. S. J. & Frith, C. D. 1996 Brain activity during stimulus independent thought. *Neuroreport* **7**, 2095–2099.

Mishkin, M. 1964 Perseveration of central sets after frontal lesions in monkeys. In *The frontal granular cortex* (ed. J. M. Warren & K. Akert), pp. 219–241, New York: McGraw-Hill.

Murphy B. L., Arnsten, A. F. T., Goldman-Rakic, P. S. & Roth, R. H. 1996 Increased dopamine turnover in the prefrontal cortex impairs spatial working memory in rats and monkeys: pharmacological reversal of stress induced impairment. *J. Neurosci.* **16**, 7768–7775.

Myers, R. E., Swett, C. S. & Miller, M. 1973 Loss of social group affinity following prefrontal lesions in free-ranging macaques. *Brain Res.* **64**, 257–269.

Oltmans, T. F. & Neale, J. M. 1975 Schizophrenic performance when distractors are present: attentional deficits or differential task difficulty? *J. Abn. Psychol.* **84**, 205–209.

Owen, A. M. 1997 The functional organisation of working memory processes within human lateral frontal cortex: the contribution of functional neuroimaging. *Eur. J. Neurosci.* **9**, 1329–1339.

Owen, A. M., Morris, R. G., Sahakian, B. J., Polkey, C. E. & Robbins, T. W. 1996 Double dissociations of memory and executive functions following frontal lobe excisions, temporal lobe excisions or amygdalo-hippocampectomy in man. *Brain* **119**, 1597–1615.

Petrides, M. 1991 Learning impairments following excision of the primate frontal cortex. In *Frontal lobe function and dysfunction* (ed. H. S. Levin, H. M. Eisenberg & A. L. Benton), pp. 256–272. New York: Oxford University Press.

Petrides, M. & Pandya, D. N. 1994 Comparative architectonic analysis of the human and the macaque frontal cortex. In *Handbook of neuropsychology*, vol. 9 (ed. F. Boller & J. Grafman), pp. 17–58. Amsterdam: Elsevier Science B.V.

Rabbitt, P. M. A. (ed.) 1997 *Methodology of frontal and executive function*. London: Psychology Press. (In the press.)

Rao, S. C., Rainer, G. & Miller, E. K. 1997 Integration of what and where in the primate prefrontal cortex. *Science* **276**, 821–824.

Roberts, A. C., De Salvia, M. A., Wilkinson, L. S., Collins, P., Muir, J. L., Everitt, B. J., & Robbins, T. W. 1994 6-Hydroxydopamine lesions of the prefrontal cortex in monkeys enhance performance on an analogue of the Wisconsin Card Sorting test: possible interactions with subcortical dopamine. *J. Neurosci.* **14**, 2531–2544.

Rushworth, M. F. S., Nixon, P. D., Eacott, M. J. & Passingham, R. E. 1997 Ventral prefrontal cortex is not essential for working memory. *J. Neurosci.* **17**, 4829–4838.

Russell, J. (ed.) 1997 *Autism as an executive disorder*. Oxford: Oxford University Press.

Schultz, W. 1992 Activity of dopamine neurons in the behaving primate. *Semin. Neurosci.* **4**, 129–138.

Stuss D. T., Shallice, T., Alexander, M. P. & Picton, T. W. 1995 A multidisciplinary approach to anterior attentional functions. *Ann. N.Y. Acad. Sci.* **769**, 191–211.

Teuber, H. L. 1964 The riddle of frontal lobe function in man. In *The frontal granular cortex and behavior* (ed. J. M. Warren & K. Akert), pp. 410–444, New York: McGraw-Hill.

Tulving, E., Kapur, S., Craik, F. I. M., Moscovitch, M. & Houle, S. 1994 Hemisphere encoding/retrieval asymmetry in episodic memory: positron emission tomography findings. *Proc. Natl. Acad. Sci.* **91**, 2016–2020.

Vendrell, P., Junque, J., Pujol, M., Jurado, A., Molet, J. & Grafman, J. 1995 The role of the prefrontal regions in the Stroop task. *Neuropsychologia* **33**, 341–352.

Warrington, E. K. & Shallice, T. 1969 The selective impairment of auditory verbal short-term memory. *Brain* **92**, 885–896.

Weinberger, D. 1987 Implications of normal brain development for the pathogenesis of schizophrenia. *Arch. Gen. Psychiat.* **44**, 660–669.

Williams, G. V. & Goldman-Rakic, P. S. 1995 Modulation of memory fields by dopamine D1 receptors in prefrontal cortex. *Nature* **376**, 572–575.

Index

Page numbers which appear in **bold** indicate a more significant portion of the text